# FIRST EXPOSURE TO
# PEDIATRICS

# Notice

Medicine is an ever-changing science. As new research and clinical experience broaden our knowledge, changes in treatment and drug therapy are required. The authors and the publisher of this work have checked with sources believed to be reliable in their efforts to provide information that is complete and generally in accord with the standards accepted at the time of publication. However, in view of the possibility of human error or changes in medical sciences, neither the authors nor the publisher nor any other party who has been involved in the preparation or publication of this work warrants that the information contained herein is in every respect accurate or complete, and they disclaim all responsibility for any errors or omissions or for the results obtained from use of the information contained in this work. Readers are encouraged to confirm the information contained herein with other sources. For example and in particular, readers are advised to check the product information sheet included in the package of each drug they plan to administer to be certain that the information contained in this work is accurate and that changes have not been made in the recommended dose or in the contraindications for administration. This recommendation is of particular importance in connection with new or infrequently used drugs.

# FIRST EXPOSURE TO

# PEDIATRICS

## Joseph Gigante, MD

Associate Professor
Department of Pediatrics
Vanderbilt University School of Medicine
Vice Chairman of Education
Department of Pediatrics
Vanderbilt Children's Hospital
Nashville, Tennessee

**McGRAW-HILL**
**MEDICAL PUBLISHING DIVISION**

New York / Chicago / San Francisco / Lisbon / London / Madrid / Mexico City
Milan / New Delhi / San Juan / Seoul / Singapore / Sydney / Toronto

**First Exposure to Pediatrics**

Copyright © 2006 by The McGraw-Hill Companies, Inc. All rights reserved. Printed in the United States of America. Except as permitted under the United States Copyright Act of 1976, no part of this publication may be reproduced or distributed in any form or by any means, or stored in a data base or retrieval system, without the prior written permission of the publisher.

1 2 3 4 5 6 7 8 9 0  DOC/DOC  0 9 8 7 6

ISBN 0-07-144170-0

This book was set in Palatino by Pine Tree Composition, Inc.
The editors were Jason Malley, Karen Edmonson, Selina Connor,
    and Lester Sheinis.
The production supervisor was Catherine H. Saggese.
The cover designer was Janice Bielawa.
The text designer was Marsha Cohen/Parallelogram.
The indexer was Alexandra Nickerson.


This book is printed on acid-free paper.


**Library of Congress Cataloging-in-Publication Data**

First Exposure to Pediatrics/[edited by] Joseph Gigante
   p. ; cm.
ISBN 0-07-144170-0 (alk. paper)
  1. Pediatrics.  I. Gigante, Joseph, 1963-
[DNLM:  1. Pediatrics.  WS 100 P3704 2006]
RJ45.P39666 2006
618.92–dc22                                                     2005056147


INTERNATIONAL EDITION ISBN 0-07-110522-0
Copyright © 2006. Exclusive rights by The McGraw-Hill Companies, Inc., for manufacture and export. This book cannot be reexported from the country to which it is consigned by McGraw-Hill. The International Edition is not available in North America.

To my family, especially my parents,
Giovanni and Caterina,
my daughters, Isabelle and Cecilia,
and my wife, Felice Apolinsky.
Thank you for all of your patience, love, and support.


In memory of
Dr. Richard Sarkin and Dr. Steve Miller,
two wonderful educators, colleagues, and friends.
You continue to inspire us to be better teachers and better people.


In loving memory of
Jane McEvoy and Mary McEvoy.
I love and miss you both.

# CONTENTS

# CONTRIBUTORS

**Michael A. Barone, MD, MPH**
Director, Medical Student Education
Assistant Dean for Student Affairs
Department of Pediatrics
Johns Hopkins University School of Medicine
Baltimore, Maryland
Chapters 21, 22, 38

**M. Robin English, MD**
Associate Professor of Pediatrics
Department of Pediatrics
Louisiana State University Health Sciences Center
New Orleans, Louisiana
Chapters 9, 20, 23, 25, 36

**Joseph Gigante, MD**
Associate Professor, Department of Pediatrics
Vanderbilt University School of Medicine
Vice Chairman of Education, Department of Pediatrics
Vanderbilt Children's Hospital
Nashville, Tennessee
Chapters 1, 2, 3, 27, 30, 31, 35

**Lynn M. Manfred, MD, EdD**
Assistant Professor of Medicine and Pediatrics
University of Massachusetts Medical School
Worcester, Massachusetts
Chapters 13, 14, 24, 26, 39

**Gregory Plemmons, MD**
Assistant Professor of Pediatrics
Division of General Pediatrics
Vanderbilt Children's Hospital
Nashville, Tennessee
Chapters 7, 10, 32, 37

**Sandra M. Sanguino, MD, MPH**
Assistant Professor of Pediatrics
Northwestern University
Feinberg School of Medicine
Chicago, Illinois
Chapters 4, 5, 6, 8, 12

**Stephanie Starr, MD**
Assistant Professor
Mayo Clinic College of Medicine
Rochester, Minnesota
Chapters 15, 16, 17, 18, 19

**Aida Yared, MD**
Assistant Professor of Pediatrics
Division of General Pediatrics
Vanderbilt Children's Hospital
Department of Pediatrics
Nashville, Tennessee
Chapters 11, 28, 29, 33, 34

# PREFACE

*First Exposure to Pediatrics* was written with medical students in mind, although any student who wishes to learn more about pediatrics will benefit from reading this book. The book is intended to provide an orientation to pediatrics and the basics of what a student is expected to get out of the pediatrics clerkship. The content of the book is based on the Council on Medical Student Education in Pediatrics (COMSEP) curriculum that is used in most of the pediatrics clerkships in the United States and Canada. It contains the amount of clinically relevant material that can be reasonably learned during a 4- to 6-week clerkship. Many clerkship books that are currently on the market are too fact-intense. In this era of instant access to information, good data gatherers can easily find the answer to a question but do not always get the concept that prompted the search for that question. My intent was to write a book that is built on the comprehension of concepts rather than the memorization of facts.

Each chapter begins with a list of learning objectives. The first section of the book is an introduction to pediatrics, which includes the pediatric history and physical examination. The next section is devoted to topics in general pediatrics, such as health supervision, behavior, growth, and development, which are unique to pediatrics. The chief complaints section includes common acute illnesses commonly seen in both the inpatient and outpatient setting. Each chief complaint includes a "Don't Miss Diagnoses" table. The final section of selected topics includes specific diseases in the major pediatric subspecialties that are likely to be seen during the clerkship. The pathophysiology, history, physical examination, laboratory and radiographic evaluation, diagnosis, and management for each disease are presented.

*Joseph Gigante*

# ACKNOWLEDGMENTS

I first want to thank my fellow authors, Michael A. Barone, M. Robin English, Lynn M. Manfred, Gregory Plemmons, Sandra M. Sanguino, Stephanie Starr, and Aida Yared. This book would not have been possible without their dedication and hard work. I also want to recognize my fellow clerkship directors in the Council on Medical Student Education in Pediatrics (COMSEP). This group of individuals is dedicated to teaching medical students and is committed to innovations in education. Through their efforts, I am inspired to become a better educator. The content of this book is based on the COMSEP curriculum. I would like to acknowledge Dr. William Altemeier III for teaching me to always "do the right thing" and Dr. Jerry Hickson for his past and continuing support and mentorship.

A number of individuals at McGraw-Hill have been instrumental in making this book a reality. Fred Rose first contacted me about writing this book and Andrea Seils helped to develop the book's content. Jason Malley, Karen Edmonson, Selina Connor, and Lester Sheinis kept me on track and oversaw the completion of this effort. Finally, my special thanks to Lane Newsom, whose secretarial support was invaluable to me.

# INTRODUCTORY
# INFORMATION

# CHAPTER 1

# INTRODUCTION TO PEDIATRICS

*Joseph Gigante*

## LEARNING OBJECTIVES

1. Describe the ways in which pediatrics is different from other medical specialties.
2. Describe the ways in which child development affects the interaction between physician and patient.
3. Discuss the importance of communication skills in interactions with pediatric patients.
4. Perform a concise, goal-directed verbal patient presentation.

## INTENT

This book was written with the intent of providing a firm foundation for medical students who are pursuing a rotation in pediatrics but not necessarily planning to specialize in pediatrics. It is concise enough to be read in its entirety in 4 weeks in conjunction with working on inpatient wards and outpatient sites and attending lectures. Thus, only selected topics in pediatrics are covered. A section covering general pediatrics, including topics such as growth, development, and immunizations, is presented. The information is presented in a clinical format to facilitate the evaluation of children in both the inpatient and the outpatient settings. Although some basic science information is presented, the focus of the discussion is a problem-oriented approach to the evaluation and management of patients with specific complaints and disease entities that cannot be misdiagnosed without harming the patient or are encountered commonly in pediatrics.

3

Particular attention should be paid to excluding the "'Don't Miss' Diagnoses" outlined in each discussion of common chief complaints. The remainder of the book discusses specific disease entities in enough detail to be clinically relevant while covering information that frequently is used as testable material.

Learning objectives are included at the beginning of each chapter to direct the reader to the most important information contained in the text. The overall objectives of this entire book are fourfold:

1. To contrast the practice of pediatrics with that of other medical specialties in the hospital and outpatient settings
2. To describe some of the aspects of general pediatrics that are unique to the specialty
3. To describe the basic evaluation and management of chief complaints and common acute illnesses in pediatrics
4. To outline the pathophysiology, diagnosis, and management of common diseases in selected pediatric subspecialties

The specific chapter objectives are designed to facilitate these overall objectives as they pertain to each topic.

This book is designed to provide only an overview of the specialty. Numerous comprehensive texts are available for more in-depth study of pediatric topics. Pediatric residency programs commonly use one or more of the following general pediatric texts as their main sources of reading material: *Rudolphs' Pediatrics*, *Nelson's Textbook of Pediatrics*, *Oski's Pediatrics*, and *Primary Pediatric Care*, edited by R. A. Hoekelman. In addition to these texts, several other textbooks are available for specialized study in pediatrics. One popular text is *Atlas of Pediatric Physical Diagnosis*, edited by Zitelli. That book contains many photographs and illustrations that aid the reader in diagnosing pediatric disorders through the use of visual findings. *The Color Textbook of Pediatric Dermatology*, edited by Weston, contains many photographs of rashes and may be helpful because rashes commonly occur in children. *The Red Book, 2003 Report of the Committee on Infectious Diseases* (it actually has a red cover), is a valuable resource with regard to pediatric infectious diseases. The book is updated every 3 years and is available online at www.aapredbook.org. Finally, *The Harriet Lane Handbook*, edited by Robertson and Shilkofski, is the one reference book most pediatric house staff members carry with them at all times. This list represents only a fraction of the available books dealing with pediatric topics. The ones listed here are some of the most commonly utilized.

Most pediatric clerkships range in length from 4 to 8 weeks. The clerkships usually are divided into an inpatient experience and an outpatient experience, with about an equal amount of time devoted to each. It is impossible to learn all of pediatrics in such a short period. During the time you are on the rotation, you should try to generate a knowledge base predicated on the pediatric clinical entities that are the "bread and butter" of pediatric practice. The Ambulatory Pediatrics Association and the Committee on Medical Student Education in Pediatrics (COMSEP) developed *The General Pediatric Clerkship Curriculum* (www.comsep.org) in 1995 to provide clerkship directors with a framework on which to build a program for medical student education in pediatrics. Most clerkships around the country use part, if not all, of that curriculum. This book has been structured on the basis of the COMSEP curriculum. CLIPP (Computer Assisted Learning in Pediatrics Project) cases offer an educational program that comprehensively covers the learning objectives of the COMSEP curriculum, using interactive Web-based patient simulations. CLIPP cases are available on the Internet at www.clippcases.org to any COMSEP member school.

## CHARACTERISTICS OF PEDIATRICS

Those in pediatrics devote themselves to the care and development of children and adolescents, with the goals of prevention and treatment of disease. Family, community, environment, and society affect children during illness and in health. Growth and development are areas that are followed closely and emphasized in children. Pediatricians often play a vital role in helping children with a variety of issues, some of which are not strictly medical, such as school and behavioral problems and issues involving social adjustment. Pediatricians focus on areas of health promotion and prevention more than do physicians who care for adults. During a general health maintenance (well-child) visit, discussing topics such as car seats and bike helmets with parents will help prevent injury in children. The administration of immunizations prevents many of the diseases that caused significant morbidity and mortality not long ago.

Some students are intimidated by neonates and infants. Others feel that they cannot relate well to adolescent patients. Being aware of the various developmental milestones and behaviors of children of different ages will help you in your clinical encounters. Reading about these milestones and behaviors before you see a patient will help make the encounter go more smoothly. There is an old cliché in pediatrics: "Children are not little adults." This is true not only with regard to their development and behavior but also with regard to their anatomy and physiology. Drug absorption, metabolism, and elimination vary with the patient's age and weight. Weight and surface area are used to calculate medication doses, as opposed to the single standard dose administered to adult patients.

You will develop your communication skills during the pediatrics clerkship. One of the unique aspects of pediatrics is that you often are dealing not only with the patient but with the patient's parents and family as well.

An infant obviously cannot provide a history, and so you will rely on parents and other family members to provide information. Thus, not only do you have to develop rapport with your patient, you have to develop rapport with the family as well. The success of the clinical care you deliver will depend on the relationship you develop with your patient and that patient's family. Dealing with an uncooperative patient during a physical examination is another situation you will encounter. You may have to play games with infants, learn to distract verbal children by engaging them in conversations about topics of interest to them, or have them help you with the physical examination. Sometimes, regardless of the technique you use, you may not be able to perform the physical examination. This scenario is not uncommon even for a seasoned pediatrician. There are times when you have to leave the room and come back later to try again. Children who were crying and fussy just moments ago may be more cooperative in the physical examination after they have been calmed by their parents.

## BEING SUCCESSFUL IN THE PEDIATRICS CLERKSHIP

A team of physicians, nurses, and ancillary staff will take care of patients on the inpatient service. Be respectful of all the members of the team. One can learn a lot from nurses, social workers, physical therapists, pharmacists, and other members of the team. Students often play a key role in patient care. Take responsibility for your patients and know their histories, physical examination findings, and laboratory and radiographic results, along with the outcome of subspecialty consultations. The house staff appreciates being kept up to date on any new data regarding its patients. Talk to your patients and families but do not share bad news with them without your resident or attending physician present. Residents are often very busy and may not have time to give you specific duties. Be self-motivated to work up patients and help residents with their daily activities and tasks. You are not expected to do "scut work," but residents appreciate a "team player." Volunteer to look up articles and bring information to the team. They will appreciate the knowledge you share with them, and you will be playing a key role in providing evidence-based medicine for the care of your patients.

New patient presentations on the inpatient service will be much more thorough than are the daily updates given on morning rounds. When presenting patients, do so in an organized fashion. Begin with the chief complaint and its duration and identifying information such as age and sex. Next, discuss the history of the present illness, giving a summary of the pertinent events that preceded the admission. Review the patient history, including information that rules out major differential diagnoses or suggests the diagnosis. Then present the physical examination, being sure to note the child's general appearance, pertinent positive findings, and negative findings that help eliminate major differential diagnoses. Although the whole history should be present in your written admission history and physical, all the information should not be presented on rounds. Remember that the team members have short attention spans and that a few of the listeners may be postcall; thus, a brief, concise presentation that offers the highlights of the problem and is arranged in a manner that leads to a diagnosis or differential diagnosis will be appreciated by all who listen to your presentation.

On the outpatient service you will see both well children coming in for general health maintenance visits and sick children coming in for an acute problem. General pediatric practices are busy, and so time and efficiency are important. Before you do a well-child examination, familiarize yourself with the components of the specific visit (e.g., the 2-week checkup) so that you can be organized and prepared to collect all the information pertinent to that visit. Ask your preceptor how much time is allotted for a well-child visit. As a general rule, for sick visits, a patient evaluation, including the history and physical examination, should not exceed approximately 10 min. This requires the evaluation to be concise and goal-directed; this is why it is helpful to have a differential diagnosis in mind when entering the room. Pertinent positive and negative historical and examination characteristics must be the focus of the evaluation. Performing a complete family history and review of systems is often not necessary.

When you are presenting a sick patient to the precepting physician, the same rules about being concise and including pertinent positive and negative information about the history and physical examination (including abnormal vital signs) apply. Conclude the presentation by stating what the most likely diagnoses are and what evaluation and treatment are required at this time to differentiate those entities. This demonstrates to the preceptor that you have collected and organized the information at your disposal. Your presentation of a well-child visit will be more thorough, including issues such as growth, development, nutrition, behavior, immunizations, and anticipatory guidance.

# THE PEDIATRIC HISTORY

*Joseph Gigante*

1.  Describe the differences between a pediatric history and an adult history.
2.  Be able to obtain a nutritional history that is age-specific.
3.  Be able to obtain past, family, and social histories in an appropriate manner from the child or the primary caregiver.

Most students will have had some experience obtaining a history and performing a physical examination before beginning a pediatrics clerkship either through a physical diagnosis course in the preclinical years or during a previous clerkship. The format of the pediatrics history and physical examination (H&P) is similar to that of an adult H&P. Certain aspects of the history are emphasized more in children than they are in adults. These aspects include the prenatal, birth, and neonatal histories; nutrition; immunizations; and development. Another major difference in the pediatric history is that the patient may not be the individual from whom you obtain the history. Depending on the age of the patient, the primary caregiver (usually a parent) may be the historian. The reason for the visit should be ascertained. Most children come to a physician's office for a health maintenance visit (checkup) or a sick visit.

## GENERAL PRINCIPLES

Smile as you enter the room and introduce yourself. Shake hands with the primary caregivers and with the child if he or she is old enough. It is important to try to help the patient and family feel comfortable; most often this is accomplished by trying to establish rapport with those in the examination room.

## IDENTIFYING INFORMATION

Chart the date of the H&P; the patient's name, date of birth, and gender; and the informant, including the relationship of the informant to the patient and the informant's reliability.

## CHIEF COMPLAINT

Ask the patient or informant to use his or her own words if possible. Be aware that the concern that brought the patient in may or may not be related to the patient's underlying problem. For example, an adolescent female may have a chief complaint of a "rash" but really wants a pregnancy test.

## HISTORY OF PRESENT ILLNESS

More information concerning the chief complaint should be elicited here. Questions should be asked about symptoms, time course, and interventions. What are the symptoms? How long have they been present? Who else is sick (family members, day-care contacts, etc.)? Has this patient ever had a similar illness? What treatments have been tried for this problem? A pertinent review of systems (ROS) and a past medical history should be included here.

## PAST MEDICAL HISTORY

The following should be included in the past medical history of pediatric patients:

### PRENATAL

The information that should be obtained includes maternal age at delivery, gravida/para status (number of pregnancies, number of deliveries), abortions (spontaneous or elective), onset of prenatal care, weight gain, maternal past medical history (e.g., diabetes, hypertension), pregnancy complications (e.g., bleeding, preterm labor, infections, medications, gestational diabetes), results of maternal laboratory work (e.g., rubella immunity status, rapid plasma reagin, purified protein derivative, human immunodeficiency virus, group B streptococcus, hepatitis B), blood type, maternal medications, alcohol, and tobacco and illicit drug use.

## BIRTH HISTORY

This information should include duration of pregnancy, duration of labor and whether it was spontaneous or induced, duration of rupture of membranes before delivery, maternal treatment with medications or anesthesia, vertex or breech presentation, vaginal or cesarean section delivery, meconium staining of amniotic fluid, and complications.

## NEONATAL

This information should include birthweight, estimated gestational age, Apgar score, resuscitation in delivery room, problems in the nursery (e.g., respiratory distress, hypoglycemia, jaundice, feeding difficulty), length of stay in the hospital after birth, and reasons for prolongation of stay.

## PREVIOUS HOSPITALIZATIONS

This should include age, length of stay, reason, and hospital name.

## PREVIOUS SURGERY

This should include transfusions as well as age, reason for procedure, and complications.

## CHILDHOOD ILLNESSES OR EXPOSURES

This should include age, complications, frequency, treatment, recent exposures, date, nature of exposure, travel, and animal exposure.

## TRAUMA

This should include injuries, ingestions, and burns, along with age, circumstances surrounding event, treatment, and complications.

## ALLERGIES

This should include medications, names of medications, timing of reaction, signs and symptoms, and who made the diagnosis of allergy. Information on other allergies, including signs and symptoms and management should be elicited.

## MEDICATIONS

This should include current or recent prescription medications, over-the-counter medications, dosage, frequency, indications and reactions, and timing of most recent dose.

## NUTRITION

The nutrition history will vary with the age of the patient.

*Infants*: Elicit whether the infant is breast-feeding or formula feeding. With breast-feeding infants, ask about the frequency and duration of feedings, the presence of maternal letdown, whether the infant is latching on well, and whether the mother hears the infant swallowing during feeding. With a formula-fed infant, ask about formula type, duration, quantity, and frequency of feedings. In both situations, ask if there are any problems with feeding.

*Older infants and toddlers*: Ask when baby foods and cereal were introduced, volume of milk intake, when the transition from formula or breast milk to cow's milk occurred, problems with feeding (e.g., "picky eater"), and peculiar eating habits (e.g., pica).

*Older children*: Does the child have a good appetite or is the child a "picky eater," special diets, milk intake, "junk foods," concerns about weight.

## IMMUNIZATIONS

List immunizations and any adverse reactions. Don't rely on parents' memory; *ask to see the shot record.*

## GROWTH

List weight, height, and head circumference and evaluate the rate of growth compared with prior values; onset of puberty and menarche; list any concerns.

## DEVELOPMENT AND BEHAVIOR

Ask about the child's developmental progress. Developmental milestones such as gross motor and fine motor milestones, social interactions, and speech and language development can be assessed by using a developmental screening tool such as the Denver Developmental Screening Test II. Ask about the results of age-appropriate hearing and vision tests. In older children, ask about school performance. Assess the child's general disposition and behavior (see Chap. 7).

## FAMILY HISTORY

Ask about parents, siblings, grandparents, and extended family. Focus on inherited diseases, diseases that "run in the family," miscarrages, infant or childhood deaths, congenital anomalies, developmental delay, mental retardation, seizures, early cardiovascular diseases, sickle cell disease, consanguinity, and family members with problems similar to the patient's current complaint. Draw a family tree that includes the last two generations.

## SOCIAL HISTORY

This is one of the most important components of the pediatric history. Observe interactions between the family and the child. Seek information about the home environment, which will affect the way the child and family cope with illness. Find out what resources are available for support for the child and family. Find out if there are underlying concerns that have not been brought out (e.g., a neighbor died from a brain tumor and the mother fears that this child's headache is a sign of a tumor). Typical questions may include the following: Who lives at home (including extended family members and family friends)? Who is the primary caregiver or disciplinarian? What are the levels of education of the parents and their occupations? Does the child attend school or day care or have a baby-sitter? Who helps the mother? Does anyone in the household smoke? How much television does the child watch? Is he or she involved in any extracurricular activities? In the outpatient setting, important questions may include the following: Do you have a way to pay for this prescription? Do you have transportation to return if your child gets worse?

## REVIEW OF SYSTEMS

The review of systems is similar in general to that of adult patients with a few important differences. You may include organ systems that are pertinent to the chief complaint in the history of the present illness.

*General*: Include fever, weight loss, and overall appearance as in adults but also include patient's activity level, playfulness, appetite, sleep habits, days of school missed.

*Head*: Trauma, headaches.

*Eyes*: Visual acuity, use of eyeglasses, tendency to cross, edema, erythema, discharge.

*Ears*: Hearing, history of otitis media or otitis externa, discharge, myringotomy tube placement.

*Nose*: Nasal drainage or congestion, frequent colds or sneezing, nosebleeds, foreign bodies, snoring.

*Mouth and throat*: Frequency of sore throats and infections, teething, dental problems/cavities, mouth lesions or ulcers.

*Neck*: Tenderness or pain, swollen lymph nodes or masses, stiffness.

*Respiratory*: Cough, wheezing, apnea, stridor, shortness of breath, chest pain, exercise intolerance.

*Cardiovascular*: History of murmur, exercise or feeding intolerance, cyanosis, syncope, diaphoresis, feeling of heart racing.

*Gastrointestinal*: Frequency of bowel movements, diarrhea, constipation or encopresis, nausea (young children often do not complain of nausea), vomiting (include whether it is bilious or bloody), appetite. In infants, suck and swallow, colic, abdominal pain, jaundice.

*Genitourinary*: Urine output (number of wet diapers), history of previous urinary tract infections, dysuria, frequency, urgency, enuresis, change in urinary pattern such as enuresis in a previously toilet-trained child, hematuria, vaginal or penile discharge, menarche, menstrual history.

*Musculoskeletal*: Joint or muscle pain, swelling, edema, erythema, warmth, cramps, strength, deformities.

*Neurologic/psychiatric*: Seizures, headaches, dizziness, loss of consciousness, gait, weakness, mental status changes, hyperactivity, development, school achievement, mood, personality.

*Skin*: Rashes, dry skin, itching, hair loss, color, easy bruising, bleeding.

## BIBLIOGRAPHY

Algranati, PS. *The Pediatric Patient: An Approach to History and Physical Examination.* Baltimore: Williams & Wilkins, 1992.

Barness LA. The pediatric history and physical examination. In McMillan JA, ed., *Oski's Pediatrics*, 3d ed., Philadelphia: Lippincott, 1999: 39–52

# CHAPTER 3

# PEDIATRIC PHYSICAL EXAMINATION

## Joseph Gigante

● LEARNING OBJECTIVES

1. Recognize when a child is critically ill and/or toxic.
2. Recognize the importance of observation in examining a child.
3. List the aspects of the physical examination that are unique to pediatrics.
4. Be able to perform a pediatric physical examination and interpret both normal and abnormal findings.

After you complete a physical examination of a child and present the patient to a preceptor, one of the first questions that is asked, especially in an acute care or inpatient setting, is: "Is the child sick?" Knowing whether a child is critically ill and in need of immediate support is often the most critical information one must have when examining a child. An experienced clinician often can make this determination within a few seconds. What comes as a surprise to many students is the fact that one often can determine if a child is sick solely by using one's observation skills, before one even lays hands on the patient and performs a physical examination. By assessing a child's color, respiratory status, resting position, and level of activity, one can determine quickly whether the child is sick (Table 3-1):

*Color*: Color is probably the most important indicator of a child's cardiorespiratory function. It is therefore important to determine whether the child is cyanotic. In making this determination, it is important to distinguish between peripheral cyanosis and central cyanosis. Peripheral

Table 3-1 **Assessing a Sick/Toxic Child versus a Not Sick Child**

|  | *Sick/Toxic* | *Not Sick* |
| --- | --- | --- |
| Color | Blue | Pink |
| Respiratory status | Respiratory distress | No respiratory distress |
| Position | Extended | Flexed |
| Activity | Not interested in environment | Interested in environment |

cyanosis is due to decreased blood flow to the distal extremities; this can be seen in children when there is vasoconstriction caused by exposure to cold water or air. Central cyanosis, which refers to a bluish discoloration of the mouth and mucous membranes, implies decreased arterial oxygen saturation. Central cyanosis is present in sick children who have cardiac disease, respiratory disease, or sepsis. In Caucasian children a "good color" is a reddish-pink hue all over, except for newborn infants, who may have cyanosis of the hands and feet after birth (acrocyanosis). Mucous membranes are more reliable indicators of cyanosis in dark-skinned children.

*Respiratory status*: An examiner can determine if a child is in respiratory distress before auscultating the chest. Children in respiratory distress have tachypnea and increased work of breathing. Signs of increased work of breathing include grunting, flaring, and retractions. *Grunting* is a sound infants and toddlers may produce on expiration as a means of increasing end-expiratory pressure and expelling air. Nasal *flaring* (enlargement of the nares) is seen in infants during the respiratory cycle and is a way of increasing airflow, since infants are obligate nasal breathers. *Retractions* may be present when accessory muscles are used to maximize respirations. They are observed as indrawing of the skin between the ribs (intercostals), above the sternum (suprasternal), or below the costal margin (subcostal). Chest retractions are seen most commonly in children less than 2 years of age because their chest walls are more compliant.

*Resting position*: The normal position for infants at rest is to have flexion of the extremities. An infant or young child who has decreased tone will have extension of the extremities. A variety of different diseases can cause hypotonia and extension.

*Level of activity*: Healthy infants and children typically are interactive with the environment: smiling, making eye contact, playing, and running around the examination room. A sick child will not be interested in the environment. Such a child may lie on the examination table, not interact with the examiner or family members, and be lethargic (difficult to arouse).

## GENERAL CONSIDERATIONS

Before and after each physical examination you perform, be sure to wash your hands. Not only will this prevent the spread of disease from patient to patient but you also will keep yourself healthy (it is not uncommon for students to get sick with fever, vomiting, and diarrhea shortly after they begin a pediatrics clerkship).

As was mentioned previously, start by observing the patient. Not only will this give you an opportunity to determine whether the child is sick, it may give the child a chance to become comfortable with you. Another way to minimize fear in the child is to introduce instruments and let the child check them. Explain everything you will be doing to both the child and the parent and be sure to use age-appropriate nonthreatening terms. The child should be undressed for the examination, but this can be done gradually. Once children reach 8 years of age or so, they can be examined in the standard adult fashion. The order of the examination can be individualized on the basis of the age of the child. For instance, in infants and young children, the head and neck examination is often disturbing to the patient, and so you may want to defer this part of the examination until the end. In general, it is a good idea to leave invasive (examination of the genitalia) or painful parts for the end. Infants and young children feel more comfortable and secure in their parents' arms, and so it may be wise to conduct most of the physical examination with the child in the parents' arms. Engaging an older child in conversation about favorite toys and activities or school may alleviate some of the anxiety the patient might have and make it easier to perform the examination. Be sure to treat older children and adolescents as individuals and respect their requests for modesty. This may mean that you ask a parent to leave the room or have a chaperone present during the examination, especially if you are performing a breast or genital examination.

## VITAL SIGNS

Vital signs in pediatrics include temperature, heart rate, respiratory rate, blood pressure, weight, height/length, and head circumference. Temperature is often more labile in children than it is in adults. A normal temperature in a child is 37°C (98.6°F). Be aware that age-appropriate normal values are available for heart rate, respiratory rate, and blood pressure. When measuring blood pressure, be sure that the cuff covers half to two-thirds of the child's arm. A cuff that is too narrow often results in a falsely elevated blood pressure reading.

Weight, height/length (length is measured until 2 to 3 years of age), and head circumference should be obtained and plotted on an age- and gender-appropriate growth chart.

## GENERAL APPEARANCE

It is extremely important to make a comment about the child's general appearance. Noting the child's general level of activity (smiling and playful versus tired and lethargic) is indicated here. Other topics that can be commented on include nutritional status (well nourished versus malnourished), hydration status (well hydrated versus dry), and any gross abnormalities that are present.

## HEAD

Size and symmetry should be noted. Macrocephaly (large head size) may be due to hydrocephalus or an intracranial mass. Microcephaly (small head size) may be due to a congenital infection. Molding occurs when the cranial bones of a newborn overlap at the suture lines. This usually disappears within 2 days. Head asymmetry may be present in infants with craniosynostosis (premature fusion of the sutures). Fontanelles ("soft spots") occur in areas where the major sutures intersect. The anterior fontanelle measures 4 to 6 cm at birth and usually closes some time between 4 and 26 months of age (90 percent close between 7 and 19 months of age). The anterior fontanelle may be depressed in infants who are dehydrated and bulging in infants with increased intracranial pressure caused by meningitis or hydrocephalus. The posterior fontanelle measures 1 to 2 cm at birth, although it is closed in many neonates. It usually closes by 2 months of age. Caput succedaneum is a soft tissue swelling with edema and bruising of the scalp that occurs when a portion of the scalp is drawn into the cervical os at the time of delivery. A cephalohematoma typically appears either immediately after birth or within the first 24 h of life and is due to subperiosteal bleeding involving the outer table of one of the cranial bones. The swelling therefore does not cross the suture line.

## EYES

Nystagmus in one direction or many directions is common immediately after birth. This should resolve completely within a few days. Small subconjunctival, scleral, and retinal hemorrhages are common in newborns. Nasolacrimal duct obstruction is the most common cause of eye discharge (usually excessive tearing) in newborns and usually resolves spontaneously at 9 to 12 months of age. Strabismus (misalignment of the eyes) may be reported by the parents in the first 6 months of life. Persistence beyond this time is abnormal and warrants a referral to an ophthalmologist. To detect esotropia (eye turning in) or exotropia (eye turning out), look for a change in the corneal reflection pattern of lateral gaze. The reflections on each cornea should be symmetrically placed. Some infants have pseudostrabismus: the appearance of strabismus as a result of epicanthal folds and a flat nasal bridge.

The red reflex is tested by setting the opthalmoscope at "0" diopters and viewing the pupil at a distance of approximately 12 in. A reddish-orange color should be seen through the pupil. A white pupillary reflex (leukocoria) may be present in children with cataracts, retinoblastoma, or retinal detachment. Papilledema is seen only rarely even with markedly increased intracranial pressure because the fontanelles and open sutures absorb the increased pressure, sparing the optic discs. Until age 3 the sutures separate sufficiently to prevent papilledema. The "setting sun" sign is a sign of increased intracranial pressure but may be seen transiently in some infants. At 2 to 4 weeks of age, fixation on objects occurs; at 5 to 6 weeks, coordinated eye movements in following an object are seen; at 3 months, the eyes converge and the baby begins to reach for objects. At age 1 year, normal visual acuity is in the 20/200 range. Normal visual acuity at age 3 is approximately 20/40; at age 4 to 5, 20/30; and at age 6 to 7, 20/20. Visual acuity should be tested in a child once the child is able to cooperate with the examination, usually at 3 to 4 years of age. Brushfield's spots (white specks scattered in a linear fashion around the iris), prominent inner epicanthal folds, and an upward outer slant to the eyelids are suggestive of Down syndrome.

## EARS

Note the shape and position of the ears in relation to the eyes. Normally the ear joins the scalp on or above the extension of a line drawn across the inner canthus and outer canthus of the eye. Examination of the ear in the immediate neonatal period only establishes the patency of the ear canal because the tympanic membranes are obscured by accumulated vernix in the external auditory canal. In infancy, the ear canal is directed downward from the outside; therefore, the pinna should be pulled gently downward for the best visualization of the eardrum. To examine the tympanic membranes in older children, the pinna should be pulled upward and backward. Brace the hand used to hold the otoscope against the child's head to help restrain the head and protect the child from injury that might result from sudden head movements. Use pneumatic otoscopy as part of the otoscopic examination. If movement of the tympanic membrane is not seen, this may indicate acute otitis media or otitis media with effusion. Hearing screening is done in the immediate neonatal period in many areas in the United States.

## NOSE

Neonates in whom choanal atresia is suspected should have this condition evaluated by passing a no. 14 French catheter through each nostril into the posterior nasopharynx. Children with infections may have rhinorrhea or mucopurulent material in the nose, whereas those with allergic symptoms may have pale, boggy nasal turbinates with watery rhinorrhea. Nasal polyps may be seen in patients with cystic fibrosis or allergic rhinitis. Nasal flaring may be present in children with respiratory distress.

## MOUTH AND THROAT

The mouth, lips, buccal mucosa, tongue, and palate should be assessed for lesions, clefts, and color. A dusky or bluish color to the mucous membranes indicates cyanosis. The lip and palate should be evaluated for the presence of clefts. Children with bifid uvulas may also have a submucous cleft. Pearl-like keratin retention cysts often are seen on the hard palate (Epstein's pearls) or buccal margins at birth; they disappear within a few weeks or months. Thrush is a lacy white material seen on the surface of oral mucous membranes. Difficulty in removing it distinguishes it from milk, which wipes away easily. Examine the teeth for number and condition. Nursing bottle caries are common in children who take their bottles to bed at night and during naps. In both early and late childhood, the tonsils are relatively larger than they are in infancy and adolescence. The tonsils usually have deep crypts on their surfaces that may have white concretions or food particles. Exudate and erythema may be noted on the tonsils in those with pharyngitis. Cobblestoning of the posterior pharyngeal wall is seen in patients with postnasal drip caused by an infection or chronic allergic rhinitis.

## NECK

Range of motion and mobility of the neck should be assessed by having the patient touch the chin to the chest and move the head from side to side. In any sick child in whom meningitis is suspected, the presence or absence of nuchal rigidity should be documented. Neck masses should be documented. A thyroglossal duct cyst may be seen or felt in the midline immediately superior to the thyroid cartilage. It moves with swallowing. The thyroid gland also may be palpated in the midline of the neck. Lymph nodes are the masses that are palpated most commonly in the neck. Injury to the sternomastoid muscle with bleeding into the muscle belly as it is stretched during birth results in torticollis (wry neck).

## CHEST AND LUNGS

The chest should be assessed for symmetry. A barrel chest may be noted in children with pulmonary disease. Protrusion of the chest and sternum is referred to as pectus carinatum, and a depressed chest and sternum is called pectus excavatum. Tanner staging of adolescent female breast development should be noted. During puberty, adolescent males sometimes develop breast enlargement, which can be unilateral or bilateral.

Before examining the lungs, first inspect the child for signs of respiratory distress (tachypnea, grunting, flaring, or retractions). Fremitus and percussion of the chest wall are not used commonly in the examination of pediatric patients to detect abnormalities (e.g., consolidation or effusions) but may be useful in school-age children and adolescents. Familiarize yourself with pediatric lung anatomy before proceeding with auscultation. It is also helpful to describe abnormal breath sounds in terms of pitch, location, and especially timing (whether they are present in inspiration, expiration, or both).

Breath sounds should be symmetric from lobe to lobe. Decreased breath sounds on one side may suggest an effusion or infiltrate. Rales sometimes are described as the sound of a few hair strands rubbed through the fingers or the sound of crisped rice cereal in freshly poured milk. These sounds are associated with the accumulation of fluid in the airway. Rhonchi often are described as coarser, low-pitched sounds that clear with coughing. Coarse breath sounds are often harsher and louder than rales. Since the distance from the upper airway to the lungs is much shorter in children, any upper airway congestion may be transmitted to the lower airway, making auscultation more difficult in young children. The term *coarse breath sounds* sometimes is used to describe this phenomenon; sometimes the term *transmitted upper airway noise* may be used. In states of extreme bronchoconstriction, the listener may hear little. In some asthmatic patients, wheezing may be absent if there is extreme reduction of air movement. There must be movement of air to produce a sound, whether normal or abnormal. Wheezing may be heard on inspiration, on expiration, or throughout the respiratory cycle. It may be described as polyphonic (simultaneous emission of different tones) or monophonic (a single tone).

## HEART

When examining the chest, first palpate the point of maximal impulse (PMI) and note its location on the chest and its intensity. The PMI may be prominent in children with thin chest walls and those with fever. The rate and the rhythm of the heart sounds should be noted in both the supine and the sitting positions. Listen over the whole precordium, including the aortic area (right second interspace), the pulmonic area (left second intercostal space), the tricuspid valve area (fourth interspace over the sternum), and the apex. Murmurs should be described with regard to intensity (grade 1 to grade 6), phase in cardiac cycle (systolic or diastolic), pitch (high or low), quality (rough or blowing), location on chest, and radiation to the axilla, neck, or back. Any additional sounds, such as rubs, gallops, or clicks, should be noted.

## ABDOMEN

First inspect the abdomen. A distended abdomen may be a sign of an abdominal mass, obstruction, ascites, infection, or celiac disease. Many toddlers have protuberant abdomens. A scaphoid abdomen may be present in children with a diaphragmatic hernia. Diastasis recti (vertical separation of the rectus abdominis muscles) is seen commonly in infants. Umbilical hernias should be noted, and their size measured. An umbilical granuloma is the most common cause of umbilical drainage after the cord falls off. However, a patent urachus or omphalomesenteric duct remnant, though rare, is also in the differential diagnosis of umbilical drainage. Infants with an obstruction such as pyloric stenosis may have visible peristaltic waves.

Auscultation of the abdomen should occur before palpation since palpation may change peristalsis and alter bowel sounds. Warm your stethoscope (and your hands) before performing auscultation. Absent bowel sounds may suggest a paralytic ileus or peritonitis. High-pitched frequent bowel sounds may occur in patients with gastroenteritis or intestinal obstruction. Before you palpate the abdomen, have the patient lie supine on the examination table, with the knees bent. Children are often ticklish during an abdominal examination. Distracting a child with conversation about topics he or she is interested in is sometimes helpful. Having the child place his or her hand on yours also may reduce giggling.

A rigid abdomen may be present in a child with a surgical abdomen. Check for abdominal pain and tenderness. The location of the abdominal tenderness may provide a clue to the cause of the pain. Right upper quadrant pain may be due to hepatitis, hepatomegaly, or cholecystitis. Pain in the right lower quadrant may be caused by appendicitis, an abscess, or intussusception. Pain in the left upper quadrant may be due to splenomegaly, whereas pain in the left lower quadrant is often present in children with constipation. Cystitis often results in tenderness in the midline suprapubic region. The liver may be palpated 1 to 2 cm below the right costal margin and is usually soft. A spleen tip may be palpable in infancy. In newborns, the kidneys can be palpated between your hands, allowing you to assess for masses. All four quadrants of the abdomen should be percussed to assess for dullness and tympany.

*Table 3-2* **Stages of Puberty (Tanner Stages)**

**Female breast**

1. Preadolescent. The breast has an elevated papilla (nipple) and a small flat areola.
2. Breast bud. The papilla and areola elevate as a small mound, and the diameter of the areola increases.
3. The breast bud enlarges further. The areola continues to enlarge. No separation of breast contours is noted.
4. The areola and papilla separate from the contour of the breast to form a secondary mound.
5. Mature. The areolar mound recedes into the general contour of the breast. The papilla continues to project.

**Pubic hair**

| *Male* | *Female* |
| --- | --- |
| 1. Preadolescent. No pubic hair. | 1. Preadolescent. No pubic hair. |
| 2. Sparse distribution of long, slightly pigmented hair at the base of the penis. | 2. Sparse distribution of long, slightly pigmented straight hair appears bilaterally along the medial border of the labia majora. |
| 3. The pubic hair pigmentation increases; it begins to curl and spread laterally in a scanty distribution. | 3. The pubic hair pigmentation increases; it begins to curl and spread sparsely over the mons pubis. |
| 4. The pubic hair continues to curl and become coarse in texture. An adult type of distribution is attained, but with fewer hairs. | 4. The pubic hair continues to curl and become coarse in texture. The number of hairs continues to increase. |
| 5. Mature. The pubic hair attains an adult distribution, spreading to the surface of the medial thigh. Pubic hair grows along the linea alba in 80% of males. | 5. Mature. The pubic hair attains an adult feminine triangular pattern, with spread to the surface of the medial thigh. |

*Male genital development*

1. Preadolescent.
2. The testes enlarge. The scrotum enlarges, developing a reddish hue and altering in skin texture. The penis enlarges slightly.
3. The testes and scrotum continue to grow. The length of the penis increases.
4. The testes and scrotum continue to grow; the scrotal skin darkens. The penis grows in width, and the glans penis develops.
5. Mature. The testes, scrotum, and penis are adult in size and shape.

## GENITALIA

When performing a genitourinary examination, always respect the patient's modesty. It is a good idea to have a chaperone present when you perform the examination, preferably of the same sex as the patient.

In males, begin by noting if the patient is circumcised, the penis size, where the urethra is positioned, and whether any scrotal masses are present. In uncircumcised males, the foreskin is usually not retractable until approximately 3 years of age. Phimosis is the inability to retract the foreskin, whereas paraphimosis is the inability to place the foreskin in its natural position after retraction. This can act as a tourniquet, leading to strangulation of the glans. Microphallus is associated with growth hormone deficiency. Hypospadias is ventral displacement of the urethral meatus. Hydrocele (accumulation of fluid in the tunica vaginalis) may cause a scrotal mass. Hydroceles are not reducible, whereas inguinal hernias can be reduced. Hydroceles should resolve by 12 months of age, but inguinal hernias require surgical repair. Both testicles should be palpated. Some infants have retractile testes. The testes can be milked down into the scrotum from the inguinal canal. The testes should be in the scrotum by 12 months of age. Boys who have undescended testes at age 12 months should be referred to an urologist. Tanner staging of pubic hair and genital development is described in Table 3-2.

In females, examine the external anatomy (labia majora, labia minora, clitoris, hymen). Newborn girls may have a white mucoid discharge or vaginal blood from estrogen withdrawal. Any nonphysiologic vaginal discharge should be noted and cultured. Labial adhesions are not uncommon and can be treated with topical estrogen cream. Clitoromegaly is a sign of virilization. Trauma, bleeding, or bruising should be noted because they may be signs of sexual abuse. Pelvic examinations are performed routinely on sexually active females and in adolescents with vaginal discharge or abdominal pain. The possibility of pregnancy always should be considered in adolescent females even if they deny being sexually active. Tanner staging of breasts and pubic hair is described in Table 3-2.

## RECTAL

In a newborn, check for a patent anus. Any evidence of trauma, fissures, or prolapse should be noted. Fissures may be present in children with constipation. This can also be a sign of sexual abuse. Rectal prolapse may be present in children with cystic fibrosis. A rectal examination should be performed on patients with severe abdominal pain, hematochezia, melena, constipation, or encopresis. While performing the examination, check for sphincteral tone, masses (including stool in the rectal vault), and tenderness (which may be seen in patients with appendicitis). A guaiac examination of the stool should be performed to check for occult blood.

## MUSCULOSKELETAL AND EXTREMITIES

The extremities should be examined for clubbing, cyanosis, and edema. Clubbing may be seen in children with congenital heart disease or pulmonary disease (e.g., cystic fibrosis). Acrocyanosis is seen commonly in newborns. The hips are examined routinely in newborns and infants. The *Ortolani maneuver* (a reduction test) is performed with the infant lying supine. The lower limb is grasped with the fingers extended over the greater trochanter and simultaneously lifted and abducted. A palpable clunk is appreciated as the femoral head pops back into the acetabulum. The *Barlow maneuver* (a dislocation test) is performed by grasping the leg in the same manner as in the Ortolani maneuver but pressing down and adducting. If the femoral head pops out, it is felt and confirmed by the Ortolani maneuver. *Galeazzi's sign* describes the equality of knee height when an infant is supine and the knees are bent. The knee heights should be equal. If the hip is dislocated, the affected femur is shifted posteriorly and the knee heights are unequal, with the knee on the affected side lower than the knee on the unaffected side. Decreased range of motion, asymmetric thigh skin folds, and unequal leg lengths also may be signs of developmental dysplasia of the hip (DDH).

In examinations of the legs, genu varum (bowleggedness) and genu valgum (knock knees) are common findings. They may be physiologic or may require further evaluation. Genu varum is seen in infants until approximately 18 months of age. Genu valgum typically is seen in children 2 years of age and older and often persists into adolescence. Metatarsus adductus (inversion of the forefoot that can be brought to a normal position) is seen commonly in neonates. Clubfoot is a fixed foot inversion deformity that requires surgical repair by an orthopedic surgeon.

The spine should be inspected for tufts of hair, dimples, masses, or cysts, which may be present in patients with spina bifida. The child's posture should be observed, looking for abnormal spine curvatures. Scoliosis is a lateral curvature of the spine that is seen most commonly in school-age children and adolescents. To examine a child for scoliosis, have the patient bend forward at the waist and examine the patient from behind, looking for unilateral elevation of the scapula, rib cage, and hip. Any costovertebral tenderness should be noted. Muscles should be examined for tone, mass, and strength. Joints should be examined for range of motion, tenderness, warmth, erythema, and effusion. The patient's gait should be observed, and any abnormality should be noted.

## SKIN

Skin color should be noted. Pallor may be seen in children with anemia or shock. Acrocyanosis is common in neonates. Jaundice may be seen in normal newborns, but it is always abnormal in the first 24 h of life (pathologic jaundice). Skin pigmentation also should be noted. Mongolian spots are bluish-black lesions typically seen in the lower back and buttocks of infants. Hypopigmented lesions can be caused by fungal infections (tinea versicolor), vitiligo, or tuberous sclerosis. Rashes and birthmarks should be described and documented. The location of traumatic lesions such as bruises and petechiae can provide important clues to whether the lesions are a result of an accidental injury or are due to physical abuse.

## LYMPHATICS

The location, size, mobility, and consistency of lymph nodes should be noted. Any tenderness or warmth should be documented. Anterior cervical and inguinal lympadenopathy is common. Posterior occipital lympadenopathy can be seen in scalp infections (e.g., tinea capitis). Enlarged lymph nodes (< 2 cm, not hard or fixed) are usually secondary to viral infections. Concern about malignancy is raised when the enlarged node is > 2 cm and is hard, fixed, supraclavicular, or associated with persistent fever or weight loss over an extended period.

## NEUROLOGIC

Primitive reflexes are noted in Table 3-3. Much of the neurologic examination involves observation of the child. Any abnormalities of movement, strength, tone, or bulk should be investigated further. Deep tendon reflexes are graded the same way they are for adults and should be tested for with a reflex hammer. Ankle clonus may be normal in newborns. Assessment of a child's developmental milestones is an important part of the neurologic

Table 3-3 **Primitive Reflexes**

| Reflex | Appears | Disappears |
|--------|---------|------------|
| Rooting | Birth | 3–4 months |
| Moro | Birth | 4–6 months |
| Tonic neck | Birth | 4–6 months |
| Babinski | Birth | 1–2 years |

examination, and so some type of developmental screening assessment tool should be performed as part of the neurologic assessment. As a child becomes older, it is easier to perform an examination of the cranial nerves. The cranial nerve examination is the same as the cranial nerve examination for adults. Coordination can be assessed by having the patient perform rapid alternating movements of the hands, finger to nose, and heel-toe gait. General sensation can be assessed by checking for response to light touch. Mental status becomes easier to assess as a child becomes older and more verbal. All children in whom meningitis is suspected should be evaluated for signs of meningeal irritation. These signs include decreased range of motion of the neck (although this is not a reliable sign in children less than 18 months of age), a positive Kernig, or Brudzinski sign. A *Kernig sign* is elicited by having a child lie on the back with flexion at the hip and knee. If meningeal irritation is present, extension of the knee causes pain. A *Brudzinski sign* occurs when the hips and knees spontaneously flex after passive flexion of the neck.

## BIBLIOGRAPHY

Barness LA. *Manual of Pediatric Physical Diagnosis*, 6th ed. St. Louis: Mosby, 1991.

Bickley LS. *Bates' Guide to Physical Examination and History Taking*, 8th ed. Philadelphia: Lippincott, 2003.

# GENERAL

# PEDIATRICS

# HEALTH SUPERVISION

*Sandra M. Sanguino*

## ● LEARNING OBJECTIVES

1. List specific objectives for the prenatal visit.
2. Be able to give age-appropriate examples of anticipatory guidance about nutrition, sleep, safety, and discipline.
3. State some of the specific screening tests that are obtained during a health supervision visit.

## INTRODUCTION

The goal of pediatrics is to promote the health and well-being of children and their families. One way to accomplish this is through a health supervision visit. A health supervision visit is used not only to identify, manage, and prevent problems but also to promote health. Components of the health supervision visit may include history, physical examination, screening tests, immunizations, assessment of growth and development, observation of parent-child interaction, counseling, and anticipatory guidance. Anticipatory guidance is the advice and education that the practitioner provides to the patient and the patient's family. It is tailored to the child's developmental level and to anticipated changes in the child's development before the next scheduled visit.

29

## HEALTH SUPERVISION GUIDELINES

The American Academy of Pediatrics (AAP) has specific guidelines for the frequency of assessments, anticipatory guidance, and screening evaluations to be performed at health supervision visits (Fig. 4-1). Additionally, based on a consensus of expert opinion, the AAP Guidelines for Health Supervision III and the National Center for Education in Maternal and Child Health (*Bright Futures: Guidelines for Health Supervision of Infants, Children, and Adolescents*) have issued guidelines regarding recommended anticipatory guidance content for child health supervision visits. Anticipatory guidance topics that are discussed commonly include behavior and development, sleep, nutrition, safety, and family functioning. It is nearly impossible to cover all the suggested anticipatory guidance topics in a health supervision visit. One way many providers succeed in covering the suggested topics is through the use of preprinted handouts. The specific health-care needs of adolescents are expanded in the Guidelines for Adolescent Preventive Services (GAPS). The American Academy of Pediatrics also has published specific guidelines for the health supervision of patients with chronic medical conditions such as Down syndrome, sickle cell disease, and Turner syndrome.

## HEALTH SUPERVISION VISITS

### INTRODUCTION

The next series of sections discuss briefly the anticipatory guidance and screening tests that may be performed as part of a health supervision visit. This is not intended to be a complete overview of everything that should be addressed at each health supervision visit. Rather, it is an overview of the common anticipatory guidance issues that may be discussed. Child development will be discussed in Chap. 6. Many other topics discussed in this chapter will be explored further elsewhere in this book.

## PRENATAL VISIT

One of the main goals of the prenatal visit is to begin to develop a relationship between the physician and the family. The prenatal visit is a good time to start to develop a therapeutic alliance between the physician and the family that should last throughout the child's life. Specific objectives of the visit include learning about the family's health and social history and discussing the anticipated behavior of the newborn and the care provided in the newborn nursery. The pediatrician should explore the family's plan for feeding the infant and discuss the advantages of breast-feeding. Parents also should be given information about circumcision and given an opportunity to discuss the performance, risks, and benefits of the procedure.

## NEWBORN VISIT

### NUTRITION

Mothers who choose to breast-feed should be aware that for the first several days postpartum the infant will be receiving antibody-rich colostrum. At about 3 to 5 days postpartum, a mother's milk will come in. Breast-fed babies should feed on demand anywhere from 8 to 12 times a day (typically every 2 to 3 h). Most formula-fed newborns take about 2 to 3 oz every 2 to 3 h. A newborn should not be allowed to go for more than 4 or 5 h between feedings. Infants should have six to eight wet diapers per day. One should remind parents that it is normal for infants to lose up to 10 percent of their body weight after birth. An infant should regain his or her birthweight by 2 weeks of age.

### SLEEP

Most newborns sleep 18 to 20 h per day. The recommended sleeping position for infants is on the back.

## INFANCY: AGE 1–6 MONTHS

### NUTRITION

It is essential to assess the quantity of breast milk or formula that the infant is taking. For a breast-fed infant, one should assess how long and how frequently the infant is feeding. Most infants breast-feed every 2 to 4 h, 15 to 20 min at each breast. For an infant who is being formula-fed, one should determine how the formula is being prepared. Additionally, one needs to inquire about the amount and frequency of feeds. At this time infants will be taking 24 to 32 oz of formula per day. Breast milk or formula is the major nutritional source during this period. Vitamin D should be given to all infants who consume less than 16 oz of formula a day by 2 months of age. Beginning at 4 to 6 months of age, one may begin to introduce solid foods. In general, it is recommended that infants first be given iron-fortified cereal, vegetables, and then fruits. The cereal should be mixed in a bowl and given to the infant with a spoon. It should not be placed in the bottle. Each new food should be added every 3 to 5 days.

### SLEEP

It is important to assess the sleeping position of the infant. The AAP recommends that infants be placed on their backs to sleep. This position has been shown to decrease the incidence of sudden infant death syndrome (SIDS).

Each child and family is unique; therefore, these **Recommendations for Preventive Pediatric Health Care** are designed for the care of children who are receiving competent parenting, have no manifestations of any important health problems, and are growing and developing in satisfactory fashion. **Additional visits may become necessary** if circumstances suggest variations from normal.

| AGE[5] | | INFANCY[4] | | | | | | | | |
|---|---|---|---|---|---|---|---|---|---|---|
| | PRENATAL[1] | NEWBORN[2] | 2–4d[3] | By 1mo | 2mo | 4mo | 6mo | 9mo | 12mo |
| **HISTORY** <br> Initial/Interval | • | • | • | • | • | • | • | • | • |
| **MEASUREMENTS** <br> Height and Weight <br> Head Circumference <br> Blood Pressure | | • <br> • | • <br> • | • <br> • | • <br> • | • <br> • | • <br> • | • <br> • | • <br> • |
| **SENSORY SCREENING** <br> Vision <br> Hearing | | S <br> O[7] | S <br> S | S <br> S | S <br> S | S <br> S | S <br> S | S <br> S | S <br> S |
| **DEVELOPMENTAL/ BEHAVIORAL ASSESSMENT**[8] | | • | • | • | • | • | • | • | • |
| **PHYSICAL EXAMINATION**[9] | | • | • | • | • | • | • | • | • |
| **PROCEDURES-GENERAL**[10] <br> Hereditary/Metabolic Screening[11] <br> Immunization[12] <br> Hematocrit or Hemoglobin[13] <br> Urnialysis | | ←——•——→ <br> • | • | • | • | • | • | •——→ | •——→ |
| **PROCEDURES-PATIENTS AT RISK** <br> Lead-Screening[16] <br> Tuberculin Test[17] <br> Cholesterol Screening[18] <br> STD Screening[19] <br> Pelvic Exam[20] | | | | | | | | •——→ | * |
| **ANTICIPATORY GUIDANCE**[21] <br> Injury Prevention[22] <br> Violence Prevention[23] <br> Sleep Positioning Counseling[24] <br> Nutrition Counseling[25] | • <br> • <br> • <br> • <br> • | • <br> • <br> • <br> • <br> • | • <br> • <br> • <br> • <br> • | • <br> • <br> • <br> • <br> • | • <br> • <br> • <br> • <br> • | • <br> • <br> • <br> • <br> • | • <br> • <br> • <br> • <br> • | • <br> • <br> • <br> • | • <br> <br> <br> <br> • |
| **DENTAL REFERRAL**[26] | | | | | | | | | ← |

1. A prenatal visit is recommended for parents who are at high risk, for first-time parents, and for those who request a conference. The prenatal visit should include anticipatory guidance, pertinent medical history, and a discussion of benefits of breastfeeding and planned method of feeding per AAP statement "The Prenatal Vist" 1996).
2. Every infant should have a newborn evaluation after birth. Breastfeeding should be encouraged and instruction and support offered. Every breastfeeding infant should have an evaluation 48–72 hours after discharge from the hospital to include weight, formal breastfeeding evaluation, encouragement, and instruction as recommended in the AAP statement "Breastfeeding and the Use of Human Milk" (1997).
3. For newborns dischared in less than 48 hours after delivery per AAP statement "Hospital Stay for Healthy Term Newborns" (1995).
4. Developmental, psychosocial, and chronic disease issues for children and adolescents may require frequent counseling and treatment visits separate from preventive care visits.
5. If a child comes under care for the first time at any point on the schedule, or if any items are not accomplished at the suggested age, the schedule should be brought up to date at the earliest possible time.
6. If the patient is uncooperative, rescreen within 6 months.
7. All newborns should be screened per the AAP Task Force on Newborn and Infant Hearing Statement, "Newborn and Infant Hearing Loss: Detection and Intervention" (1999).

*Figure 4-1* **Recommendations for Preventive Pediatric Health Care (RE9535)** Committee on Practice and Ambulatory Medicine.

These guidelines represent a comsensus by the Committee on Practice and Ambulatory Medicine in consultation with national committees and sections of the American Academy of Pediatrics. The committee emphasizes the great importance of **continuity of care** in comprehensive health supervision and the need to avoid **fragmentation of care.**

| Early Childhood[4] | | | | | Middle Childhood[4] | | | | Adolescence[4] | | | | | | | | | | |
|---|---|---|---|---|---|---|---|---|---|---|---|---|---|---|---|---|---|---|---|
| 15mo | 18 mo | 24mo | 3y | 4y | 5y | 6y | 8y | 10y | 11y | 12y | 13y | 14y | 15y | 16y | 17y | 18y | 19y | 20y | 21y |
| • | • | • | • | • | • | • | • | • | • | • | • | • | • | • | • | • | • | • | • |
| •  • | •  • | • | • | • | • | • | • | • | • | • | • | • | • | • | • | • | • | • | • |
| | | | • | • | • | • | • | • | • | • | • | • | • | • | • | • | • | • | • |
| S  S | S  S | S  S | $O^6$  S | O  O | O  O | O  O | O  O | O  O | S  S | O  O | S  S | S  S | O  O | S  S | S  S | O  O | S  S | S  S | S  S |
| • | • | • | • | • | • | • | • | • | • | • | • | • | • | • | • | • | • | • | • |
| • | • | • | • | • | • | • | • | • | • | • | • | • | • | • | • | • | • | • | • |
| • | • | • | • | • | •  → | | | • | •  ← | • | •14 | • | • | •  ← | | 15 | • | →  | • |
| | | | | | • | | | | | | | | | | | | | | |
| *  *  *  * | *  * | *  * | *  * | *  * | *  * | *  * | *  * | *  * | *  *  *  * | *  *  *  * | *  *  *  * | *  *  *  * | *  *  *  * | *  *  *  * | *  *  *  * | *  *  *  * | ←20 | *  * | *  * |
| •  •  • | •  • | •  • | •  • | •  • | •  • | •  • | •  • | •  • | •  • | •  • | •  • | •  • | •  • | •  • | •  • | •  • | •  • | •  • | •  • |
| • | • | • | • | • | • | • | • | • | • | • | • | • | • | • | • | • | • | • | • |

8. By history and appropriate physical examination: if suspicious, by specific objective developmental testing. Parenting skills should be fostered at every visit.
9. At each visit, a complete physical examination is essential, with infant totally unclothed, older child undressed and suitably draped
10. These may be modified, depending upon entry point into schedule and individual need.
11. Metabolic screening (eg, thyroid, hemoglobinopathies, PKU, galactosemia) should be done according to state law.
12. Schedule(s) per the Committee on Infectious Diseases, published annually in the January edition of *Pediatrics.* Every visit should be an opportunity to update and complete a child's immunizations.
13. See AAP *Pediatric Nutrition Handbook* (1998) for a discussion of universal and selective screening options. Consider earlier screening for high-risk infants (eg, premature infants and low birth weight infants). See also "Recommendations to Prevent and Control Iron Deficiency in the United States. *MMWR.* 1998;47 (RR-3):1–29.
14. All menstruating adolescents should be screened annually.
15. Conduct dipstick urinalysis for leukocytes annually for sexually active male and female adolescents.
16. For children at risk of lead exposure consult the AAP statement "Screening for Elevated Blood Levels" (1998). Additionally, screening should be done in accordance with state law where applicable.

(continued on page 34)

*Figure 4-1* **Continued**

17. TB testing per recommendations of the Committee on Infectious Diseases, published in the current edition of *Red Book: Report of the Committee on Infectious Diseases*. Testing should be done upon recognition of high-risk factors.
18. Cholesterol screening for high-risk patients per AAP statement "Cholesterol in Childhood" (1998). If family history cannot be ascertained and other risk factors are present, screening should be at the discretion of the physician.
19. All sexually active patients should be screened for sexually transmitted diseases (STDs).
20. All sexually active females should have a pelvic examination. A pelvic examination and routine pap smear should be offered as part of preventive health maintenance between the ages of 18 and 21 years.
21. Age-appropriate discussion and counseling should be an integral part of each visit for care per the AAP *Guidelines for Health Supervision III* (1998).
22. From birth to age 12, refer to the AAP injury prevention program (TIPP*) as described in *A Guide to Safety Counseling in Office Practice* (1994).
23. Violence prevention and management for all patients per AAP Statement "The Role of the Pediatrician in Youth Violence Prevention in Clinical Practice and at the Community Level" (1999).
24. Parents and caregivers should be advised to place healthy infants on their backs when putting them to sleep. Side positioning is a reasonable alternative but carries a slightly highter risk of SIDS. Consult the AAP statement "Positioning and Sudden Infant Death Syndrome (SIDS): Update" (1996).
25. Age-appropriate nutrition counseling should be an integral part of each visit per the AAP *Handbook of Nutrition* (1998).
26. Earlier initial dental examinations may be appropriate for some children. Subsequent examinations as prescribe by dentist.

---

**Key: • = to be performed        * = to be performed for patients at risk**
**S = subjective, by history      O = objective, by a standard testing method**
**◄──•──► = the range during which a service may be provided, with the dot indicating the preferred age.**

---

**NB: Special chemical, immunologic, and endocrine testing is usually carried out upon specific indications. Testing other than newborn (eg, inborn errors of metabolism, sickle disease, etc) is discretionary with the physician.**

**The recommendations in this statement do not indicate an exclusive course of treatment or standard of medical care. Variations, taking into account individual circumstances, may be appropriate. Copyright ©1999 by the American Academy of Pediatrics. No part of this statement may be reproduced in any form or by any means without prior written permission from the American Academy of Pediatrics except for one copy for personal use.**

**American Academy of Pediatrics**

*Figure 4-1* **Continued**

By 4 months of age many infants can sleep through the night without waking for feeds. Most infants at this age will sleep 12 to 18 h per day and take two to three naps per day.

## SAFETY

It is important to make sure that the infant is in a rear-facing car seat. As the infant reaches 6 months of age, the need to safeguard the environment should be discussed. Specifically, the need to store medicine and household cleaning products out of the infant's reach should be discussed. One also should ask if any injuries to the infant have taken place.

## INFANCY: AGE 6–12 MONTHS

### NUTRITION

Infants at this age should be eating a variety of soft foods. An infant may need to try a new food at least 10 times before he or she begins to accept it. Finger food should be introduced, and the infant should be encouraged to self-feed. Until the child is 1 year of age, he or she should still receive formula or breast milk. As a result of the introduction of solids, it is common for formula or breast milk consumption to decrease. At 1 year of age, whole milk can be introduced into the diet. A "sippy" cup can be introduced during this period, and parents should be reminded never to let an infant go to bed with a bottle, as this puts the infant at risk for dental caries.

### SLEEP

Between 6 and 12 months of age, most children sleep approximately 10 to 12 h at night and take two daytime naps, each lasting more than an hour, in the midmorning and the afternoon. The infant should be sleeping through the night at this point. Parents should be encouraged strongly to develop a nighttime routine. Infants should be put to bed drowsy so that they can learn to console themselves and fall asleep on their own.

### SAFETY

Children should still be in a rear-facing car seat until they reach 1 year of age and weigh 20 pounds. Parents should be encouraged to get down on the floor to check for hazards. The use of walkers should be discouraged strongly.

### DISCIPLINE

Discipline should consist of distracting the infant from the situation.

### ORAL HEALTH

Parents should be reminded not to put infants to bed with a bottle. They should begin to clean the baby's teeth with a soft brush or cloth.

## AGE 1–2 YEARS

### NUTRITION

At around 1 year of age it is very common to see a decrease in appetite. This often leads to mealtime struggles. Parents should be encouraged not to turn mealtimes into a battle. The family should be encouraged to have structured mealtimes with the children. Milk should be limited to 16 to 24 oz a day. No more than 4 oz of juice per day is recommended. Children should be encouraged to feed themselves, and the use of the bottle should be discouraged strongly. Because of the danger of choking, foods such as hard candy, popcorn, hot dogs, nuts, and whole grapes should be avoided.

## SLEEP

At this age most children are sleeping 10 to 12 h. Around 15 months of age, one nap usually is eliminated. During this period most children who have been sleeping in a crib can be transitioned to a toddler bed. Toddlers frequently resist going to bed. The use of a transition object such as a blanket or stuffed animal may make falling and staying asleep easier. At this age, it is especially important to have an established bedtime routine that allows the child to calm down.

## DISCIPLINE

This is the period when toddlers begin to exhibit more independence and curiosity. It is important to establish clear limits for the child. Providing a toddler with the opportunity to make choices among acceptable options allows the child to express his or her need for control and independence. Praising children for good behavior is also important. If a child is engaging in potentially harmful or disruptive behavior, an effective method for dealing with the situation may be to place the child in a "time-out." Temper tantrums are seen commonly at this age. The most effective method for extinguishing this behavior is to ignore it.

# EARLY CHILDHOOD: AGE 2–4 YEARS

## NUTRITION

After age 2 children no longer require whole milk. They can be transitioned to 2% or skim milk. It is suggested that children drink 16 to 20 oz of milk per day. Children should have three structured meals and two snacks per day. Parents of toddlers often worry about the amount of food the child is eating and the child's eating habits. It is important to inform parents that a child's rate of growth slows down after the first year of life. Reviewing the growth chart with parents can be very reassuring.

Families should sit down together at mealtimes and avoid distracting activities such as television watching. Mealtimes should last 20 to 30 min. Food not finished during that time should be removed, and except for routine between-meals snacks, parents should avoid giving the child additional food until the next meal. Parents should not have unreasonable expectations about the amount of food a child should eat. A child's portion size is roughly the size of the child's fist. At this age it is also very common for children to be picky eaters. Parents should continue to offer children a wide variety of foods. If a child completely avoids one food group, it may be necessary to give the child a multivitamin.

## SLEEP

At this age children still require 10 to 12 h of sleep at night. Most children will continue to have one daytime nap until age 4. The importance of a bedtime routine should be emphasized. Nighttime fears and nightmares are not uncommon at this age. Potentially frightening activities such as watching disturbing television programs and reading scary books should be avoided, especially before bedtime. A night-light or open door may help minimize such fears.

## TOILET TRAINING

Most children are toilet trained during this period, although some children may be ready to be toilet trained by 18 months of age. Girls usually are trained earlier than boys are. Signs that a child may be ready to toilet train include staying dry after a nap and complaining about wet or soiled diapers. Toddlers should be allowed to observe their parents in the bathroom. Parents may chose to buy their children a potty chair and initially have a child sit on the potty chair with the diaper in place. Parents should be reminded to praise children for their successes and avoid punishment for accidents. Although most children are toilet trained by the end of this period, it is still very common to have nighttime wetting.

## MIDDLE CHILDHOOD: AGE 5–10 YEARS

### NUTRITION

Parents should be encouraged to model healthy eating habits. Children should have three structured meals a day. High-fat, low nutrient foods and beverages such as sodas, chips, and candy should be avoided. The importance of physical activity should be emphasized.

### DISCIPLINE

The expectations and responsibilities of the child should be clear to all and enforced consistently. Punishments should be fair and logical.

### HEALTHY HABITS

The promotion of health habits should be discussed. This includes brushing the teeth twice a day and seeing a dentist every 6 months.

## SCREENING TESTS

Screening tests are an essential component of the health supervision visit. For a schedule of when specific screening test should be performed, see Fig. 4-1.

## NEWBORN SCREENING

Newborn screening involves testing for metabolic and genetic diseases. Since all states differ in the tests that are included in the newborn screen, it is important to know what diseases are tested for in the state in which you reside. Currently all state newborn screening programs include tests for phenylketonuria (PKU) and congenital hypothyroidism. Also, most states test for galactosemia and sickle cell disease. Additional diseases screened for in some state programs include congenital adrenal hyperplasia, homocystinuria, maple syrup urine disease, biotinidase deficiency, tyrosinemia, other metabolic conditions, cystic fibrosis, and toxoplasmosis. It is extremely important that infants with a positive test receive close follow-up.

### BLOOD PRESSURE

The benefits of controlling high blood pressure have been known for many years. High blood pressure may result in long-term damage to the heart, kidneys, or brain. It is recommended that blood pressure screening at health supervision visits begin at age 3. If a child is known to have a renal or cardiovascular abnormality, a blood pressure reading should be obtained at each visit regardless of age. To determine blood pressure adequately, one must have a cooperative subject and appropriate equipment. The width of the cuff should be 40 to 50 percent of the circumference of the child's limb. Cuffs that are too small will overestimate, and those that are too wide will underestimate, the true blood pressure.

### HEARING SCREENING

Hearing loss in newborns is not readily apparent by routine observation. Moderate to profound hearing loss in early infancy is associated with impaired language development. Because of this, universal newborn hearing screening is recommended. The two types of audiologic tests used are the brainstem auditory evoked response (BAER) and the evoked otoacoustic emissions (OAE) tests. Infants who do not pass screening or subsequent retesting should have an appropriate medical and audiologic evaluation to confirm hearing loss by 3 months of age. Hearing screening in young infants and toddlers can be done by subjective measures such as asking the parents if the child responds to noises. Beginning at age 4, objective measures of hearing such as pure-tone audiometry can be utilized in the office setting.

### VISION SCREENING

For children from birth to 3 years of age, the eye evaluation consists of examination of the eye and lids, assessment of the red reflex, and pupil examination. Vision is assessed by noting the child's ability to fixate on and follow an object. In children older than age 3, a more formal assessment of visual acuity can be performed. This can be accomplished by using a variety of tests, such as the Snellen number or letter test, the Allen picture test, or the tumbling E test. The random E test is best used for detecting strabismus.

## TUBERCULOSIS SCREENING

The tuberculin skin test it the only practical method for diagnosing tuberculosis (TB) in asymptomatic individuals. It has been determined that routine TB skin testing in children constitutes an inefficient use of health-care resources, and it no longer is recommended. The AAP recommends skin testing for children who are at increased risk of acquiring TB. These children include individuals who have been in contact with people with confirmed or suspected TB as well as children with clinical or x-ray findings suggestive of TB. In addition, children emigrating from countries where TB is endemic and children who travel to countries where TB is endemic should be tested. Children who are infected with human immunodeficiency virus (HIV) or are incarcerated should have yearly testing. Some experts advocate that children should be tested every 2 to 3 years if they have ongoing exposure to HIV-infected people, homeless people, or institutionalized children and adolescents. A tuberculin skin test (TST) should be performed before the initiation of chronic immunosuppressive therapy. Testing should be done with the Mantoux skin test. The tine test no longer is recommended. A TST can be administered during the same visit that immunizations are given. Since measles vaccine temporarily can suppress tuberculin reactivity, if tuberculin testing is indicated and cannot be performed at the same time as measles immunization, tuberculin testing should be deferred for 4 to 6 weeks. Bacillus Calmette-Guérin (BCG) vaccine is not a contraindication to tuberculosis skin testing.

## LEAD SCREENING

Over 400,000 U.S. children age 1 to 5 years have blood lead levels higher than the Centers for Disease Control and Prevention (CDC) recommended level of 10 μg of lead per deciliter of blood. Lead poisoning can cause learning disabilities, behavioral problems, and, at very high levels, seizures, coma, and even death. Lead poisoning often can be asymptomatic in children. There has been a remarkable decrease in blood lead levels since the 1970s. This decrease can be attributed to primary prevention strategies such as the banning of leaded gasoline and improved screening and identification of children with elevated lead levels. Currently, high blood lead levels are thought to be the result of exposure to old paint, interior settled dust, and exterior dust around older housing.

The CDC recommends universal lead screening for communities with a high percentage of old housing. This is defined as more than 27 percent of houses built before 1950. Additionally, universal screening is recommended for communities with a high percentage of children with elevated blood lead levels (>12 percent of children with levels above 10 μg/dL). Communities where data regarding local blood lead levels are inadequate should undergo universal screening. For children living in other areas, the CDC recommends target screening based on risk assessment. Children from ages 6 months to 6 years should have a measurement of the blood lead level if their parents answer yes to any of the following questions: (1) Does your child live in or regularly visit a house or child-care facility built before 1950? (2) Does your child live in or regularly visit a house or child-care facility built before 1978 that is being or recently has been remodeled? (3) Does your child have a sibling or playmate who has or had lead poisoning? In addition, one may consider children for screening if they may be exposed to lead-containing folk remedies, have emigrated from countries where lead poisoning is prevalent, have been exposed to contaminated lead or soil, and have parents who have been exposed to lead. The blood lead level may be determined from blood obtained via a venipuncture or a fingerstick blood sample. The preferred method of obtaining blood is by venipuncture as fingerstick specimens are easily contaminated. Fingerstick values higher than 10 μg/dL should be confirmed with a venipuncture.

## CHOLESTEROL SCREENING

There is evidence to suggest that atherosclerosis begins in childhood and slowly progresses through adulthood. The AAP recommends screening children over the age of 2 if there is evidence of cardiovascular disease in parents or grandparents under age 55. In this case, a lipoprotein analysis should be obtained. If parents have a total cholesterol over 240 mg/dL, a total cholesterol should be obtained in the child. In addition, physicians should consider obtaining cholesterol levels in children and adolescents in whom a family history is unobtainable. Children who are deemed to have other risk factors for cardiovascular disease, such as smoking and obesity, should be screened at the discretion of their physician.

## BIBLIOGRAPHY

American Academy of Pediatrics. *American Academy of Pediatrics Guidelines for Health Supervision III*, 3d ed. Elk Grove Village, IL: American Academy of Pediatrics, 1997.

American Academy of Pediatrics Committee on Psychosocial Aspects of Child and Family Health. The prenatal visit. *Pediatrics* 107(6):1456–1458, 2001.

American Academy of Pediatrics Joint Commission on Infant Hearing. Year 2000 position statement: Principles and guidelines for early hearing detection and intervention programs. *Pediatrics* 106(4):798–817, 2000.

Green M, ed.. *Bright Futures: Guidelines for Health Supervision of Infants, Children, and Adolescents*, 2d ed. Arlington, VA: National Center for Education in Maternal and Child Health, 2002. http://www.brightfutures.org.

# GROWTH

## Sandra M. Sanguino

## LEARNING OBJECTIVES

1. Explain the importance of monitoring growth in a child.
2. Describe the importance of interpreting growth charts in the longitudinal evaluation of weight, height, head circumference, and body mass index.
3. Recognize growth problems in children, including failure to thrive and obesity.
4. Recognize abnormalities of head growth.

## INTRODUCTION

Monitoring a child's growth is an essential component of a health supervision visit. Growth is one of the key features of childhood, and changes in the normal pattern of a child's growth may be an early manifestation of an underlying pathologic process. Growth is determined by a complex interaction of genetics and environmental influences. Although growth is a continuous process during childhood, there are two periods of rapid growth: infancy and puberty. To assess the adequacy of growth, the provider generally monitors weight, length, head circumference, and the appearance of secondary sexual characteristics.

Growth parameters should be measured and plotted at each health supervision visit. Data should be plotted on age-specific and gender-specific growth charts (see Figs. 5-1 and 5-2). The Centers for Disease Control and Prevention (CDC) growth charts published in 2000 represent the revised version of the 1977 National Center for Health Statistics (NCHS) growth charts. Most of the data used to construct these charts came from the National

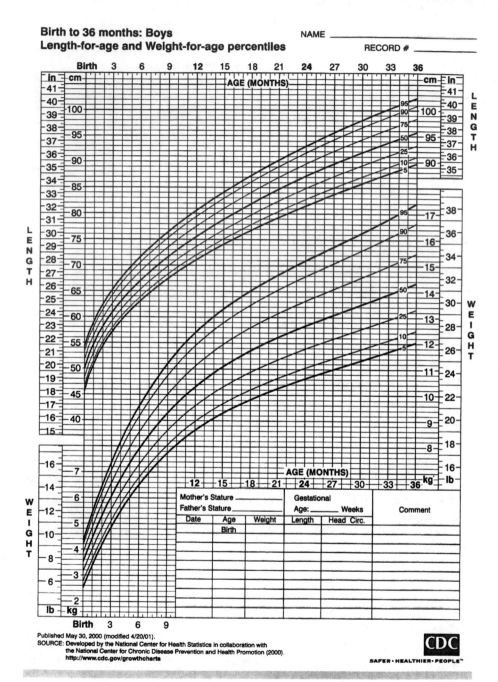

Figure 5-1  *Clinical Growth Chart, Birth to 36 Months: Boys.*

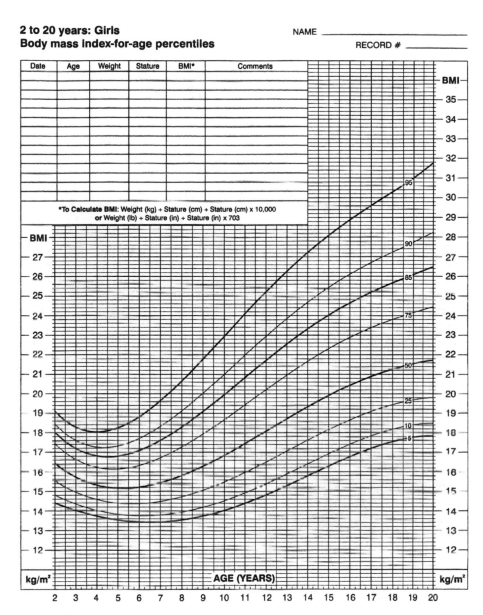

**2 to 20 years: Girls**
**Body mass index-for-age percentiles**

NAME _____

RECORD # _____

Published May 30, 2000 (modified 10/16/00).
SOURCE: Developed by the National Center for Health Statistics in collaboration with
the National Center for Chronic Disease Prevention and Health Promotion (2000).
http://www.cdc.gov/growthcharts

*Figure 5-2 Clinical Growth Chart, 2 to 20 Years: Girls.*

Health and Nutrition Examination Survey (NHANES). The revised charts are based on ethnically diverse national samples. Compared with the original infant charts, which were based on primarily formula-fed infants, the revised growth charts for infants include a mix of both breast-fed and formula-fed infants in the U.S. population. The revised growth charts also include a body mass index for children ages 2 to 20. For children with disorders such as Down syndrome, achondroplasia, and Turner syndrome, special growth charts are available and should be used to plot growth parameters

## MEASUREMENTS

An infant should be unclothed when weighed. A child's weight should be obtained without shoes, and the child should be wearing lightweight clothing or a hospital gown.

From infancy until age 2 to 3 years, length should be obtained in the recumbent position, using an appropriate measuring board. An accurate length can be difficult to obtain in a squirming infant. For older children, length should be obtained without the child's shoes, using a wall-mounted measuring device. If one is obtaining length in the standing position for the 2- to 20-year-old group, a growth chart should be utilized. The head circumference should be measured and plotted on standard growth charts during health supervision visits until age 2. The measurement is obtained by placing a tape measure around the maximum occipitofrontal circumference. After age 3, a special head circumference chart can be utilized to assess children when there is concern about microcephaly or macrocephaly. For infants (birth to 36 months), weight for length also should be plotted. For children ages 2 to 20, the American Academy of Pediatrics (AAP) recommends that body mass index (BMI) be plotted during health supervision visits. The BMI is calculated as follows: body weight in kilograms divided by height in meters squared. This figure is then multiplied by 703. BMI changes with age. A child whose BMI is between the 85th and 95th percentiles is considered to be at risk for overweight. A BMI over the 95th percentile is considered overweight. Pubertal development is assessed by utilizing the sexual maturity rating or Tanner stages. See Chap. 14 for further details.

## NORMAL GROWTH

Infancy is a period of tremendous growth. It is normal for newborn infants to lose up to 10 percent of their birthweight before they begin gaining weight. By 2 weeks of age most infants should have regained their birthweight. Over the first 6 months of life the average infant gains about 20 to

30 g per day, doubling his or her birthweight by about 4 to 5 months of age. During the first 6 months of life infants require approximately 110 to 120 kcal/kg per day in order to grow. In later infancy, the infant's rate of growth slows down to an average of 10 g per day and about 100 kcal/kg per day is required for growth. By 1 year of age a child has tripled his or her birthweight. The rate of weight gain significantly decreases after the first year of life. Toddlers gain about 2 to 3 kg per year. The average school-age child gains 3 to 4 kg per year. The rate of weight gain again increases during adolescence.

Linear growth also follows a relatively consistent pattern. Over the first year of life the average child grows 25 cm per year, increasing birth length by 50 percent at 1 year. Over the next year the expected increase in height is about 12.5 cm. From age 2 until adolescence the average child grows 6.25 cm per year. Birth length doubles by 4 years of age and triples by 13 years of age. Height is genetically determined, and a child's ultimate height can be predicted on the basis of mean paternal height.

$$\text{Boy's predicted stature} = \frac{[(\text{mother's height} + 13 \text{ cm or 5 in.}) + \text{father's height})]}{2}$$

$$\text{Girl's predicted stature} = \frac{[\text{mother's height} + (\text{father's height} - 13 \text{ cm or 5 in.})]}{2}$$

## ASSESSMENT OF GROWTH

In trying to determine whether an infant or child is growing appropriately, the key is to look at the trajectory of the growth curves over time. Serial growth measurements provide the most accurate assessment of whether physical growth is progressing normally for an individual child. A child growing at the 3d percentile may be growing normally, whereas a child growing at the 10th percentile when that child previously was growing at the 90th percentile is worrisome. In general, most children stay within one or two growth channels. An exception to this is seen in the first 2 years of life. Size at birth is a reflection of the intrauterine environment rather than genetic factors. Because of this, one may see a change in growth velocity. There may be a change in growth velocity of more than 25 percent because of a genetic adjustment. Often one will see large neonates begin to shift growth channels at approximately 6 months of age until they find their genetically predetermined growth curves.

## GROWTH PROBLEMS

### *FAILURE TO THRIVE*

#### DEFINITION

The term *failure to thrive* is not a diagnosis or disease but refers to children whose attained weight or rate of weight gain is significantly below that of other children of similar age and the same sex. There is no clear consensus about the definition. Commonly used definitions include growth below the third or fifth percentile or a change in growth that has crossed two major growth percentiles in a short time.

#### ETIOLOGY

The differential diagnosis for failure to thrive is quite extensive, involving almost every organ system (Fig. 5-3). The diagnosis of failure to thrive can be divided in to two categories: organic and nonorganic. Organic failure to thrive is marked by an underlying medical condition; nonorganic failure to thrive generally refers to poor growth caused by factors external to the child. There also may be cases of mixed failure to thrive, which involves a combination of both organic and nonorganic factors. In trying to assess the etiol-

| Gastrointestinal | Gastroesophageal reflux, celiac disease, pyloric stenosis, malrotation, Hirschsprung disease, milk protein intolerance, inflammatory bowel disease, hepatitis |
| --- | --- |
| Cardiac | Congenital heart disease |
| Pulmonary | Bronchopulmonary dysplasia, cystic fibrosis, obstructive sleep apnea |
| Renal | Renal tubular acidosis, chronic renal insufficiency, |
| Endocrine | Hypothyroidism, diabetes mellitus |
| Infectious | Urinary tract infection, human immunodeficiency virus, tuberculosis, parasites |
| Metabolic | Inborn errors of metabolism |
| Neurologic | Hydrocephalus, neurodegenerative disorders, tumor |
| Oncologic | Malignancy |

*Figure 5-3* **Organic Causes of Failure to Thrive.**

ogy of failure to thrive, it is often helpful to think about the causes in the following sequence: (1) inadequate intake, (2) increased losses (i.e., vomiting or diarrhea), and (3) increased metabolic demand.

## EVALUATION

The history, physical, and observation of the parent-child interaction are key in the evaluation of a child with failure to thrive. The history should pay particular attention to the chronology of the development of the growth problem. It is helpful to obtain all previous growth records.

A careful and detailed diet history is essential. Is the infant formula-fed or breast-fed? How often does the infant feed? How is the formula prepared? If the infant is breast-fed, does the mother feel letdown? Does she hear the infant swallowing? For an older child, when were solids introduced? How much juice, soda, and water does the child drink? What are mealtimes like? If the parents cannot give a detailed diet history, it may be helpful to send them home with a nutritional diary to fill out prospectively and bring to the next visit.

One should inquire about the presence of vomiting or spitting up as well as the pattern and frequency of stooling. A family history should be obtained, with particular attention paid to the growth patterns of family members.

The social history should inquire about the relationship among family members as well as the adequacy of resources. During the physical examination, it is essential to obtain growth measurements accurately and plot them on the appropriate growth charts. During the examination, the examiner should pay particular attention to the child's interaction with the parents as well as the examiner.

The use of laboratory studies to determine the etiology of failure to thrive is often not helpful. If the cause of a child's failure to thrive remains unclear after a careful history and physical examination, it may be helpful to obtain a complete blood count, urinalysis and culture, serum electrolytes, blood urea nitrogen and creatinine, and liver enzymes.

## TREATMENT

Regardless of the etiology, the treatment of failure to thrive consists of providing sufficient calories to reverse impaired growth, achieve catch-up growth, and restore normal growth. For a child with organic failure to thrive, the underlying medical condition should be treated. For a patient with nonorganic failure to thrive, the psychosocial factors that are affecting feeding behavior must be evaluated and addressed. In general, nutritional therapy consists of calories 150 to 200 percent above the recommended level for age. In a severely malnourished child, one needs to be careful during the early phase of nutritional therapy because of the risk of refeeding syndrome.

## OBESITY

### EPIDEMIOLOGY

The prevalence of overweight children has increased markedly over the last three decades. In 2001, the surgeon general stated that $117 billion per year was spent managing obesity and obesity-related complications. Data from NHANES for the period 1999–2000 showed that over 10 percent of 2- to 5-year-olds and more than 15 percent of 6- to 9-year-olds in the United States were overweight. The biggest rise in the prevalence of overweight was among African-American and Mexican-American children.

### DEFINITION

Obesity is defined as excess body fat for age. Direct measurement of fat is not feasible in the clinical setting. What is most often used to estimate obesity is BMI. BMI is calculated by body weight in kilograms divided by height in meters squared. This figure is then multiplied by 703. BMI is considered a proxy measure of adiposity.

### COMPLICATIONS

Numerous complications are associated with obesity in childhood. Children who are overweight are at higher risk for disorders of lipid metabolism and cardiovascular disease. Obese children have been demonstrated to have elevated levels of low-density lipoprotein cholesterol and triglycerides and low levels of high-density lipoprotein cholesterol. An increasing number of overweight children have been noted to have impaired glucose tolerance and type 2 diabetes. Many of these children have acanthosis nigricans, a skin disorder characterized by a velvety thickening and hyperpigmentation of the neck, the axilla, and intertriginous areas. This condition has been associated with obesity, hyperinsulinism, and insulin resistance. Menstrual irregularities have been associated with obesity in overweight females. The most common menstrual irregularity is anovulatory cycles with dysfunctional uterine bleeding and amenorrhea. Orthopedic problems and complications also are seen in overweight children. Slipped capital femoral epiphysis (SCFE), a displacement of the femoral neck from the femoral head through the growth plate, is seen more commonly in children who are overweight. Blount disease, which is a bowing of the tibia associated with medial epiphyseal osteochondrosis, also has been associated with obesity. Overweight children are more likely to experience sleep problems and may require treatment for obstructive sleep apnea. One of the most severe consequences of being overweight is the impact on the social and emotional development of the child. Overweight children have been noted to experience a lower quality of life compared with normal-weight children.

## PROGNOSIS AND TREATMENT

Overweight children are more likely to become overweight adults. Twenty percent of individuals who are overweight at age 4 will be overweight as adults. By adolescence this figure rises to 80 percent. Early childhood appears to be a critical period in the development of obesity because of adiposity rebound. Adiposity rebound is the time, generally between 4 and 6 years of age, when a child's adiposity starts to increase after a low point in the earlier years of life. The younger and heavier one is during the adiposity rebound period, the more likely one is to become an overweight adult. One of the advantages of treating overweight children at a younger age is that they seem to respond more readily to interventions than do older children. Successful treatment of childhood obesity requires a multifactorial approach that includes encouraging family behavior modification, increasing physical activity, decreasing sedentary behavior, and improving eating practices. Regular follow-up should be arranged for monitoring intervention effectiveness and providing positive reinforcement for success.

# HEAD GROWTH ABNORMALITIES

## INTRODUCTION

The majority of head growth occurs prenatally and in the first 2 years of life. The normal head is 75 percent of adult head size by 1 year of age. When one is evaluating head growth, the most common abnormalities seen are microcephaly and macrocephaly.

## MICROCEPHALY

### ETIOLOGY

Microcephaly is defined as a head circumference that measures more than two standard deviations below the mean for age and sex. In general, the small size of the head reflects the small size of the brain. The differential diagnosis for microcephaly is quite extensive. The etiologies of microcephaly can be divided into primary and secondary microcephaly.

Primary microcephaly (also referred to as congenital microcephaly) is associated with abnormal development during the first 7 months of gestation. Secondary microcephaly is caused by an insult during the last 2 months of gestation, the perinatal period, or the first year of life. Primary microcephaly results from a variety of genetic and environmental insults that cause abnormal brain growth. There are both autosomal dominant and autosomal recessive forms of familial microcephaly as well. Numerous chromosomal disorders, including trisomies, deletions, and translocations, also may cause primary microcephaly. Dysmorphic syndromes such as Cornelia de

Lange, Hallermann-Streiff, and sickle cell disease also are associated with primary microcephaly. Maternal exposure to drugs and toxins (e.g., fetal alcohol syndrome) also has been associated with primary microcephaly. Other causes of primary microcephaly include early prenatal infection such as human immunodeficiency (HIV) and toxoplasmosis, other infections, rubella, cytomegalovirus, and herpes (TORCH) infections.

Secondary microcephaly is caused by a variety of infectious, traumatic, metabolic, and anoxic insults that occur during the last part of the third trimester, the perinatal period, and early infancy. Causes of secondary microcephaly include but are not limited to meningitis, encephalitis, hypoxic-ischemic encephalopathy, cytomegalovirus, rubella, and toxoplasmosis.

## EVALUATION

The evaluation of a child with microcephaly is determined by the history and physical examination. Serologic studies looking for evidence of intrauterine infections should be considered. If a chromosomal disorder is suspected, a karyotype should be sent. Imaging studies such as a computed tomography (CT) scan to look for intracranial calcifications and magnetic resonance imaging (MRI) to look for structural abnormalities should be considered. Additional studies such as plasma amino acids and urine organic acids may be of value.

## MACROCEPHALY

### ETIOLOGY

Macrocephaly is defined as a head circumference that is more than two standard deviations from the mean for age and gender. Unlike microcephaly, the size of the head in patients with macrocephaly does not reflect the size of the brain. Conditions associated with macrocephaly include hydrocephalus, mass lesions such as a tumor or subdural hematoma, skeletal dysplasias, and an increase in brain substance (megalencephaly). Megalencephaly can be seen in Soto syndrome, neurofibromatosis, achondroplasia, and metabolic storage diseases. Primary macrocephaly also may be seen as a benign familial condition.

### EVALUATION

In evaluating a child with a head that is abnormally large or is growing at an excessive rate, one needs to review carefully the serial head circumference measurements. A detailed developmental history also should be obtained. A thorough neurologic examination for assessment of increased intracranial pressure is also necessary. Measurement of the parents' head circumferences may be useful. If there is evidence of increased intracranial pressure, a CT scan or MRI may be necessary.

## BIBLIOGRAPHY

American Academy of Pediatrics Committee on Nutrition. Prevention of pediatric overweight and obesity. *Pediatrics* 112(2):424–430, 2003.

Ariza AJ, Greenberg RS, Unger R. Childhood overweight: Management approaches in young children. *Pediatr Ann* 33(1):33–38, 2004.

Baucher H. Failure to thrive. In Behrman RE, Kleigman RM, Jensen HB, eds., *Nelson Textbook of Pediatrics*, 17th ed. Philadelphia: Saunders, 2004: 133–134.

Williams CL, Hayman LL, Daniels SR, et al. Cardiovascular health in childhood: A statement for the health professionals from the Committee on Atherosclerosis, Hypertension and Obesity in the Young (AHOY) of the Council on Cardiovascular Disease in the Young, American Heart Association. *Circulation* 106(1): 143–160, 2002.

Williams SD, Wessel HB. Neurology. In Zitelli BJ, Davis HW, eds., *Atlas of Physical Diagnosis*, 4th ed. Philadelphia: Mosby, 2002: 516.

# CHAPTER 6

# DEVELOPMENT

*Sandra M. Sanguino*

● LEARNING OBJECTIVES

● LEARNING OBJECTIVES

1. Describe the importance of developmental assessment.
2. List the domains of development.
3. Outline key developmental milestones at various ages.
4. List developmental screening tools.

## INTRODUCTION

Developmental assessment and surveillance are critical components of a health supervision visit. It is essential that those who care for children have a good understanding of the normal progression of developmental events. This allows a physician to monitor children over time and identify potential delay. Development generally is divided into broad categories or domains. The developmental domains include motor, language, cognition, problem-solving, and psychosocial domains. These domains are not meant to be exclusive; they are closely linked to and influence one another.

## NORMAL DEVELOPMENT

It is beyond the scope of this chapter to give a complete overview of every aspect of child development. This section highlights important developmental milestones at different stages. The assessment of developmental milestones provides a systematic way to assess a child's progress. It is important to realize that there is considerable variability in the attainment of developmental milestones.

## NEWBORN

A neonate's sensory capabilities and ability to interact with the outside world are much more complex than once was realized. An infant's behavior has been recognized to exist in discrete behavioral states. The six states that have been described are quiet sleep, active sleep, drowsy, alert, fussy, and crying. Infants move through the states with some regularity. The behavioral state determines an infant's muscle tone, movements, electroencephalographic pattern, and response to stimuli. In a process called habituation, infants can ignore repeated presentation of lights, noise, or painful stimuli, depending on their behavioral state. For example, in the alert state an infant may show less reaction to repeated loud noises, whereas in the drowsy state the repeated noises may push the infant into crying.

A newborn has a number of primitive reflexes that provide an indication of his or her neurologic integrity. Each reflex has its own age of emergence and disappearance Fig. 6-1). When one is evaluating the primitive reflexes, it is important to note not only the absence or presence of each reflex but also the symmetry of the reflexes. In assessing the motor development of a newborn, one will note that an infant prefers to be in the flexed position with the hands fisted. When placed in the supine position, the infant will turn his or her head from side to side. A neonate can see faces and objects at a focal length of 8 to 12 in. Infants appear to demonstrate differential attention to objects that have high contrast, bright colors, and curved lines. Neonates also are very sensitive to light and often will open their eyes only in dim light.

| Reflex | Age When Appears | Age When Disappears |
|--------|------------------|---------------------|
| Moro | Birth | 2–4 months |
| Palmar grasp | Birth | 2–4 months |
| Plantar grasp | Birth | 9–12 months |
| Rooting | Birth | 4–6 months |
| Tonic neck | Birth | 4–6 months |
| Walking/stepping | Birth | 2 months |

Figure 6-1 **Primitive Reflexes.**

A newborn can hear, and research confirms that a fetus is responsive to sounds in the uterus. By 1 month of age an infant is able to distinguish between the primary caregiver's voice and that of a stranger. Infants also have a well-developed sense of taste and smell. An infant has a greater number of taste buds than an adult does, and the taste buds are distributed more widely. Fetuses in utero have been noted to have changes in sucking frequency when sugar is introduced into the amniotic fluid. An infant can localize odors and may turn away from an unpleasant odor.

## AGE 1–6 MONTHS

This period is characterized by tremendous physical and developmental growth of the infant. Motor development progresses in a cephalocaudal direction. By 2 months of age infants should be able to hold their heads steady while in a sitting position. At 4 months an infant should have no head lag when raised from lying to sitting. Beginning at around 4 to 5 months of age, infants will start rolling, and by 6 months most infants can roll. By 6 months of age many infants can sit without support. The disappearance of the palmar reflex during this period allows infants to hold objects as well as release them. At 2 months of age an infant may hold a rattle briefly. By 4 months of age the infant will be reaching, grasping, and pulling at objects. The grasp is a raking motion that involves the ulnar aspect of the hand at 3 to 4 months of age. At around age 5 months the thumb is added to this motion. By 6 months an infant is transferring objects from hand to hand. Infants also become progressively more vocal. At about 2 months of age an infant will start cooing, and by 6 months of age infants should be babbling consonants. During this stage an infant is becoming increasingly more responsive and interested in the environment. By 2 months of age an infant should have developed a social smile. A 4-month-old will laugh and squeal with delight. One can see some imitative behavior by 4 months of age, such as sticking out the tongue or raising the eyebrows.

## AGE 6–12 MONTHS

This is an extremely exciting stage for infants and their families. The infant is much more responsive and is interested in exploring the environment. As infants begin to explore the environment, they have increasing opportunities to get into trouble. Because of this, a central part of the health supervision visit at this age revolves around a discussion of safety. At 6 months of age most infants are sitting without support. Infants then become progressively more mobile as they begin to creep and crawl at 8 months of age. The infant will pull to a stand and begin cruising at approximately 9 to 10 months of age. By 1 year of age many children may be walking independently, although there is wide variation. Fine motor skills also develop significantly during this time so that by 1 year of age a child should have a precise pincer grasp. An infant's ability to communicate also progresses significantly during this time. Beginning at 6 months of age, an infant will start babbling chains of consonants, and by age 9 months the infant will be stating "dada" and "mama." By 10 months of age the average infant should be able to follow a one-step command without a gesture. By age 1 year most children are able to say "mama" and "dada" as well as one to three other words.

Cognitively, this period is marked by the emergence of object permanence. This generally begins at 6 to 9 months of age. This is the concept that people and objects exist even when the infant cannot see them. As object permanence emerges, stranger anxiety also develops. During stranger anxiety the infant has an apparent and overtly negative reaction to a stranger. This continues until about 18 to 24 months of age. As the concept of object permanence emerges, infants become able to play games such as peek-a-boo.

### AGE 12–15 MONTHS

The developmental milestone that most parents focus on at this age is walking. Many infants begin to walk around 1 year of age, with a range of 9 to 17 months. At first, infants walk with a wide-based gait. They bend their knees and walk with their arms flexed at the elbows, and the torso rotates with each step. Gradually, with practice, the center of gravity shifts back and the torso stays more stable. Children begin to run approximately 6 months after they have been walking well. As a child begins walking, his or her perspective on the world changes. The child's ability to explore interesting things is now under his or her control. Play continues to be primarily solitary, but they use objects appropriately in pretend play. For example, a 15-month-old may pretend to talk on a toy telephone. They also can use a cup appropriately. During this period receptive language continues to precede expressive language. By 15 months of age the average child can point to one or two body parts and use four to six words appropriately. In addition to the words the child is saying, he or she will jargon (babble with mixed constants, inflection, and cadence). Children at this age continue to have a distrust of strangers.

### AGE 18–24 MONTHS

This period is marked by increasing independence and autonomy. In terms of motor development, one sees improvements in balance and agility. During this time children begin running and climbing stairs. Fine motor skills and visual-motor coordination also advance. An 18-month-old will use a cup and spoon and also try to self-feed. An 18-month-old has a much better understanding of cause and effect and will demonstrate problem-solving skills. Despite the child's striving for increased autonomy and independence, the child at this age often exhibits increased clinginess. This may be a reaction to the child's awareness of the possibility of separation. Parents often report that they cannot go anywhere without having the child attached to them. The use of a transitional object such as a blanket or stuffed animal is often useful at this time.

## AGE 2 YEARS

Age 2 years is marked by the rapid development of language. Language development and the increase in a 2-year-old's cognitive abilities allow the child to interact with his or her environment in new ways. By 2 years of age most children can say approximately 50 words, and by the end of the second year of life they can say up to 200 to 300 words. The use of verbs, adjectives, and even some adverbs emerges. After acquiring a vocabulary of about 50 words, children begin to make simple two-word sentences. Receptive language is always ahead of expressive language so that a child always understands more than he or she can say. This may result in some degree of frustration in the child. With respect to receptive language, a 2-year-old should be able to understand a two-step command. In evaluating a child with language delay, one should be more concerned about a child who has difficulty understanding age-appropriate words that are presented without visual cues than about a child who says little but follows verbal commands at an age-appropriate level.

In general, around age 2 many children exhibit signs that they are ready to be toilet trained. Clues that a child may be ready include the fact that the child has increased periods of daytime dryness and tells the parent after having a bowel movement or urinating. Other signs include showing an interest in the toilet, imitating behavior, and showing an interest in orderliness. Although age 2 is the time when many of these signs are present, it may occur earlier for some children and later for others. It may be detrimental to begin toilet training a child who is not showing signs of readiness, as this may create expectations that the child cannot handle. Generally, boys toilet train later than girls do, and the whole process takes several months.

## PRESCHOOL

The preschool period is marked by an increasing ability to communicate as well as the emergence of imagination and magical thinking. Language development continues to emerge, and by age 5 children can say close to 2000 words. Speech gradually becomes more intelligible to a stranger. A stranger should understand approximately 75 percent of a 3-year-old's speech and 100 percent of a 4-year-old's speech. By age 4 children should be able to sustain a conversation. A 4-year-old will use the past tense in conversation and at age 5 will use the future tense. A preschool age child will begin asking a lot of questions using the "w" words (why? what? when? where?). The child should be able to give his or her full name, gender, and age. He or she can identify colors and maybe a few letters and numbers.

Motor skills that are emerging in a preschool-age child include walking up and down the stairs using alternating feet, skipping on one foot, and dressing himself or herself.

The preschool period is marked by the development of magical thinking and fantasy. As the child's imagination becomes more active, the child often develops imaginary friends and has nightmares or fear of monsters. Play during this period becomes more complex. The ability of children to fantasize allows them to play with other children in new ways. At this age a child's play should be interactive as opposed to in parallel. Starting in the preschool period, play shows marked gender differences. Girls play in smaller groups and often play games in which there is no winner or endpoint. In contrast, boys play more physical games in larger groups in which there is a clear winner and loser.

## EARLY SCHOOL AGE (AGE 5–7)

Age 5 is marked by entry into kindergarten. Cognitive development at this stage was described by Piaget as "preoperational thinking," that is, thinking marked by magical qualities. In addition, children age 5 to 6 have difficulty performing tasks that involve changes in more than one variable at a time. Around age 6 children transition to a stage Piaget called "concrete operations" thinking. They are progressively able to think about more than one variable at a time and also begin to understand the concepts of conservation of length, mass, and volume. In kindergarten, children start grouping and recognizing symbols. By first and second grade children can read a simple sentence and add and subtract. Strength, speed, and coordination rapidly improve. At age 5 children may begin to ride a bike, and by age 6 to 7 some children may begin to participate in sports. Fine motor skills also improve as children learn how to write.

## MIDDLE CHILDHOOD (AGE 7–10)

The major developmental tasks of middle childhood involve achievement in school and social acceptance. School becomes increasingly demanding, and the required tasks become more complex. For example, a child may be asked to access previously gained knowledge, organize it, and express it in writing. Problems in the ability to accomplish such a task may be the first evidence of a learning disability. The quest for social involvement and acceptance is integral in middle childhood. Most children try to find a place for themselves among a group of same-sex friends. Peers become more influential, and friendships are important. Children with positive peer relationships have been noted to give and receive positive attention, adhere to rules, and perform well academically. At this age children often are involved in a variety of artistic and athletic activities.

## DEVELOPMENTAL SCREENING TESTS

According to recent estimates, 12 to 16 percent of children have developmental or behavioral issues. The Individual with Disabilities Educational Act (IDEA) of 1997 mandates early identification of and intervention for children with developmental disabilities. The current emphasis is on children from birth to age 2. Since at this age the family and the pediatrician are in frequent contact, the pediatrician can play a central role in identifying and referring children appropriately. The IDEA requires that pediatricians refer children with a suspected developmental delay in a timely fashion. In addition to clinical observation and history during the health supervision visit, an approach to developmental assessment involves the use of developmental screening tests.

Currently, an ideal screening test does not exist. One commonly used test is the Denver Developmental Screening Test II. This is a 125-item test that that generates pass-fail ratings in four domains of development: personal-social, fine motor adaptive, language, and gross motor. It can be used to evaluate children from birth to age 6. Another commonly used screening tool is the Ages and Stages Questionnaires. These are a series of 11 questionnaires that are completed at home by the parents. These tests are administered to children 4 to 48 months of age. The Parents Evaluation of Developmental Status and the Child Development Inventory are also well-validated parent report instruments. The advantage of these types of instruments is that they require much less time to score and interpret. Regardless of the method used to assess development, once a delay is identified, it is critical that the patient be referred for further evaluation and intervention as soon as possible.

## BIBLIOGRAPHY

American Academy of Pediatrics Committee on Children with Disabilities 2000–2001. Developmental surveillance and screening of young infants and children. *Pediatrics* 108(1):192–196, 2001.

Dixon S, Stein M. *Encounters with Children: Pediatric Behavior and Development*, 3d ed. St. Louis: Mosby, 2000.

Green M, ed. *Bright Futures: Guidelines for Health Supervision of Infants, Children and Adolescents*, 2d ed. Arlington, VA, National Center for Education in Maternal Child Health, 2000.

# CHAPTER 7

# BEHAVIORAL PEDIATRICS

*Gregory Plemmons*

## LEARNING OBJECTIVES

1. Be able to take a thorough, age-appropriate developmental and behavioral history.

2. Describe the typical presentation of common behavioral problems and issues in different age groups.

3. Be able to counsel families about the management of common behavioral problems such as colic, toilet training, and eating disorders.

In few other areas in medicine do human behavior and development overlap as much as they do in pediatrics. Childhood and parenthood are by definition works in progress. When new parents encounter the first-time experience of a colicky infant or the temper tantrum of a willful toddler, often the first person they turn to for guidance is the pediatrician. It is no surprise that Dr. Benjamin Spock's *Baby and Child Care*, first published in 1946, remains the world's best-selling nonfiction publication after the Bible. Parenting is always uncharted territory: Every son or daughter brings unique challenges, and the structures of the family continue to evolve. At times the modern pediatrician is expected to have the assertive objectivity and insight of a Dr. Phil, the medical knowledge of a well-trained physician, the seasoned wisdom of grandparents, and the warmth and demeanor of Mr. Rogers. This section focuses on common behavioral and psychosocial problems that many pediatricians encounter daily in their practice.

## TAKING A DEVELOPMENTAL/BEHAVIORAL HISTORY

Interviewing families or caretakers is crucial to understanding a child's developmental stage, dealing with particular areas of concern, and offering guidance for parents and caretakers. The traditional model has relied on taking a careful, detailed social history (e.g., structure of the family, living arrangements, questions about school and day care) and then offering anticipatory guidance on age-specific behavioral issues. Several resources are available to pediatricians to assist with assessment and guidance during well-child visits. One example is *Bright Futures*, a module produced by the Maternal Child and Health Bureau. Questions typically suggested by *Bright Futures* guidelines are frequently open-ended (not "yes/no"). These types of interview questions promote dialogue between the practitioner and caretakers and often allow for open discussion and voicing of parental concerns. Following are some questions from *Bright Futures*:

- How are you doing as a parent?
- What questions or concerns do you have about your child?
- How would you describe your child's personality?
- Have there been any major changes or stresses in your family since the last visit?
- What do you do when you become angry or frustrated with your child's behavior?
- How are you managing your child's behavior?
- How does your infant or child get along with others?
- How do you think your child is performing or doing in day care or school?
- Does your child talk to you and communicate concerns or fears?

This sounds like a lot to accomplish during a 20-minute office visit, and it is. Historically, reimbursement for identification of and counseling for issues surrounding behavior has been low, and developmental-behavioral issues are often underemphasized during pediatric residency training. Yet almost half of all parents and caretakers report concerns about their children's behavior that may not always be addressed by clinicians. Many experts now advocate the use of standardized screening tools such as the following:

- Pediatric Symptom Checklist
- Eyeberg Child Behavior Inventory
- Parent's Evaluations of Developmental Status (PED)
- Child Behavior Checklist (CBCL)

Standardized screening tools offer the additional theoretical advantage of increasing the detection of significant problems, since it is estimated that clinical judgment alone identifies fewer than 50 percent of children who have serious emotional and/or behavioral disturbances. Although parents and caregivers frequently report the desire for assistance and counseling regarding their children's behaviors, pediatricians often feel ill equipped to offer suggestions. Further, mental health providers and other community resources are often lacking for families, especially those with children who have significant behavioral or developmental problems. However, there is a growing body of evidence that early intervention for some behavioral issues may be effective. It must be remembered that many parents often feel alone and anxious about their parenting skills and may lack knowledge of the wide variations in what is considered normal childhood behavior (e.g., nightmares, temper tantrums, masturbation). These screening tools may provide a venue for effective discussion between parent and provider and strengthen the doctor-patient relationship.

Each developmental age and stage of every child brings unique challenges to both parent and provider. As children develop and interact with their environment, parents frequently ask what is normal or abnormal behavior. This question may be difficult to answer in light of the enormous spectrum of behavior and development seen in each child and across cultures. This section briefly describes some relatively common behavioral concerns and issues specific to various age groups.

## INFANTS

### COLIC

Infant colic is an age-old phenomenon. The strictest definition is the rule of "threes": crying that lasts more than 3 h a day, occurs on more than 3 days a week, and persists for more than 3 weeks for which no other cause is identified. Much of the debate over the last few decades has centered on what is considered normal behavior and crying in infants during the first few months of life. One in four infants cries more than 3.4 hours a day. Indeed, in non-Western cultures, there is frequently no medical terminology to describe an excessively fussy infant; these infants simply are perceived as more demanding rather than having a "disorder."

Colic should always be a working diagnosis and a diagnosis of exclusion. Consideration of other factors that may cause excessive crying should always be in the differential diagnosis, such as gastroesophageal reflux (GER), metabolic and neurodevelopmental disorders, occult fractures, and hair tourniquets, which may cause acute discomfort. Many parents and practitioners frequently ascribe colic to excessive gas or formula intolerance (indeed, the word colic implies gastrointestinal involvement). When infants cry, they flex their legs regardless of the cause, and this often is interpreted as abdominal pain. Gastrointestinal disturbances may play a role in some infants. Other clinicians have proposed differences in temperament or disruptions in maternal-child interaction. The latest theory is that colicky infants lack calming and self-soothing reflexes and may need a "fourth trimester" of the soothing and reduced stimulation that swaddling and other measures sometimes provide.

Little evidence supports the use of antigas medications such as simethicone drops, although this is reportedly harmless. Few dramatic improvements have been reported after a change to a soy-based or hydrolyzed infant formula. Many practitioners recommend soothing techniques such as swaddling, "kangaroo care" (carrying an infant close to the body in a sling), "white noise," and even the time-honored tradition of a car ride around the block to soothe fussy infants. A colicky infant's effect on the household can be substantial, frequently leading to parental exhaustion and marital stress. Colic often is linked to postpartum depression and to child abuse. Mothers of colicky infants frequently report feelings of failure, incompetence, and guilt. Empathy and frequent follow-up from the clinician often are needed to aid new parents during this time. Most colic resolves by 3 to 4 months of age.

## INFANT SLEEPING PATTERNS

Most newborn infants sleep approximately 16 h a day. Usually by 6 months of age, most infants no longer need a nighttime feeding, and so the ritual 3 a.m. feed often is dropped. However, by 9 months of age, as autonomy and separation anxiety increase, it may become much more difficult for an older infant to sleep through the night. Many infants wake on their own during the night and frequently develop dependence on their parents or feeding to return to sleep. Countless books offer assistance to weary and sleep-deprived parents, and frequently camps form around three main approaches to insomniac infants:

1. *The gradual approach.* This approach encourages structured bedtime routines, putting infants to bed while awake, and nonphysical comfort measures. For example, during nighttime crying, the parent may stand at the door and provide comfort verbally but should not respond to the crying infant by picking the infant up and intervening.
2. *The "cold turkey" approach,* or letting infants "cry it out." For many parents this may be unacceptable, or it may be intolerable to other members of the household.
3. *The attachment approach.* The idea that the mother and the baby should be together as much as possible to promote mother-infant attachment and that cosleeping may be acceptable and even advantageous in some instances, particularly among mothers who breast-feed, is accepted in many cultures worldwide.

None of these approaches has been shown to be superior to the others. Recommendations to families regarding sleep management should consider the unique temperament of each child and the culture of each family.

## TODDLERS

### TEMPER TANTRUMS

The majority of toddlers have tantrums weekly, and many have outbursts daily. Many factors may contribute to the frequency or intensity of this normal developmental phenomenon: the child's temperament, the environment, family coping mechanisms, and even physical factors such as hearing loss, otitis, and sleep disturbances. Part of the challenge for both the practitioner and the parents is determining whether this behavior is normal or may reflect potential developmental or psychological problems. Child psychologists historically have proposed that tantrums arise from the internal conflict many toddlers experience betwen newfound autonomy and continued dependence on caregivers or perhaps the inability to express themselves verbally, since language development is just beginning to flourish at this age. As a general rule, tantrums should not be injurious to the infant or others; this may signify more serious behavioral issues.

To manage tantrums, parents may employ a variety of approaches:

- *Positive reinforcement:* rewarding a child for good behavior with frequent praise.
- *Ignoring.* Ignoring tantrums often succeeds in eliminating them but frequently requires strong parental reserve and the possibility that the tantrums will escalate at first.
- *Negative reinforcement,* such as time-out techniques (e.g., having the child sit or stand in a corner for a set amount of time).

Any one or a combination of these approaches may be necessary for the successful elimination of problem behavior; it also may be prudent to avoid situations that frequently trigger tantrums (e.g., trips to the store), offer toddlers some degree of choice among acceptable behaviors (e.g., "You have to wear a shirt. Do you want the red one or the blue one?"), and use distraction or redirection when possible to prevent future "meltdowns."

### TOILET TRAINING

As with sleep and other behavioral issues, the variation in toilet training among children and cultures worldwide is astounding. Although the average accepted age to begin toilet training in most Western cultures is around 18 to 24 months, Digo infants in East Africa are reported to achieve bowel and bladder continence as early as 6 months of age. Less than a century ago, toilet training frequently was achieved at a much younger age than it is today. In the 1960s, a child-centered approach was proposed that emphasizes recognition of the fact that sphincter control and the extrapyramidal tracts of toddlers, as well as the child's ability to communicate effectively, often are not developed before 18 to 24 months of age. The rise of disposable diapers and "pull-ups" has done little to encourage a different approach. The American Academy of Pediatrics (AAP) stresses confirmation of toddler readiness before embarking on training, taking into account the following signs:

- Child can stay dry for at least 2 h or after a nap.
- Bowel movements are regular and predictable.
- Child can communicate via expressions or words when ready to defecate.
- Child can follow simple instructions.
- Child can walk to and from bathroom and help undress himself or herself.
- Child is uncomfortable with soiling.
- Child asks to use potty chair and requests "grown-up" underwear.

Once these milestones have been achieved, many practitioners recommend positive reinforcement (e.g., small rewards and frequent praise) for successful bowel movements on the potty and avoidance of power struggles or negative reinforcement, which may increase resistance to training.

## EATING

Infants typically double their birthweight by 6 months of age and triple it by 12 months. After 1 year of age, growth velocity precipitously begins to plateau. Many new parents interpret the compensatory decline in appetite as "picky eating." A frequent complaint at the 18- to 24-month well-child visit is "My child won't eat anything." If height and weight seem appropriate after plotting on standard growth charts, simple reassurance to families that the child is growing appropriately may be all that is needed. In an era of increasing childhood obesity, clinicians may need to be more emphatic in discouraging frequent snacks or toddler demands for specific foods, since evidence shows that frequent exposure to high-fat foods and increased portion size may reinforce long-term overeating behavior. Rare but significant food behaviors that may require consultation with a pediatrician include *pica* (ingesting inappropriate items such as dirt or paint chips) and *rumination* (frequent regurgitation of food). *Failure to thrive* generally refers to weight loss or slowing of growth parameters and may be multifactorial, but certain developmental or behavioral disorders may also contribute to a child's ability or desire to feed, in addition to medical conditions.

# THE SCHOOL-AGE CHILD

## ENURESIS

Daytime (diurnal) urinary continence usually is achieved by age 4 to 5 years, and nighttime (nocturnal) continence is usually, but not always, achieved by 7 to 8 years. In determining whether enuresis is pathologic or within the realm of normal developmental variability, it is sometimes helpful to classify enuresis into *diurnal* or *nocturnal* since the differential diagnosis for each of these subcategories is quite distinct. It is also useful to determine whether enuresis has been present since early childhood *(primary enuresis)*, which often suggests an underlying pathology or anatomic causes, or whether it was preceded by a brief period of control *(secondary enuresis)*. There may be occasional overlap between these subgroups.

*Nocturnal enuresis* (NE) is the most common subtype. Twenty percent of all 5-year-olds occasionally wet the bed, as well as up to 1 percent of all teenagers. NE predominantly affects males (60 percent), and its cause is multifactorial. A functionally (but not anatomically) small bladder, maturational delay, and sleep disorders all may contribute, as well as heredity. Up to 70 percent of children with NE have at least one parent who had the disorder in childhood. Approximately 15 percent of bed wetters become dry each year after 5 years of age, and so a watch-and-wait approach to management is often acceptable until 8 to 10 years of age, when effects on self-esteem (e.g., at summer camp or sleepovers) may become considerably more problematic.

Treatment for NE may be divided into behavioral and pharmacologic modalities. *Behavioral techniques* include simple household measures such as avoidance of excessive fluids before bedtime and restricting caffeinated beverages (potent diuretics), having the child take an active but nonpunitive role in changing and cleanup, avoidance of pull-ups, and the use of bedwetting alarms or other timed techniques to prompt nighttime voiding.

*Pharmacologic measures* historically have included the following:

- *Desmopressin* (DDAVP), which is available in nasal spray or pill form; risks may include hyponatremia.
- *Tricyclic antidepressants* such as imipramine; mechanism of action is unclear, and side effect profile has significant toxicity.
- *Antispasmodics* such as oxybutynin (Ditropan) and hyoscyamine (Levsin), whose anticholinergic properties may be limiting.

Mounting evidence favors the use of bed-wetting alarms rather than medications because of the large number of children who relapse after the discontinuation of medications and the potential side effect profiles, as well as the considerable expense of desmopressin. Bed-wetting alarms may achieve permanent success in as many as 60 to 70 percent of patients.

In contrast to NE, *diurnal enuresis* often reflects a significant voiding dysfunction and is slightly more common in girls. Although 5 to 10 percent of school-age children may experience occasional daytime accidents, dysfunctional voiding often is accompanied by other symptoms such as dysuria, alterations in frequency, sensations of urgency, incomplete bladder emptying, and constipation. The approach to a child with significant daytime enuresis always should include a careful voiding history, a detailed neurologic examination of the lower extremities to rule out rare causes such as a tethered cord or a central nervous system (CNS) lesion, and urinalysis and urine culture to rule out infection.

## ENCOPRESIS

Encopresis refers to soiling of the underwear or loss of normal continence of stool. Most developmentally normal children achieve bowel continence by 4 years of age. Encopresis frequently is associated with constipation, since chronic distention of the bowel wall from large stools may inhibit awareness of the need to defecate. Indeed, stretch receptors may not alert many children until soiling is nearly complete. In severe cases, stool actually may leak around chronic impaction.

The approach to a school-age child with encopresis always should include a careful and detailed history, including birth information and toilet-training history. Soiling rarely can indicate more serious causes, such as Hirschsprung disease, lower motor neuron disease, anatomic abnormalities, and, rarely, sexual or rectal abuse, particularly if soiling appears to be an acute rather than a long-standing problem (Table 7-1).

The goals of treatment are generally threefold: removal of feces (which may require the administration of enemas, disimpaction, and high-dose laxatives), a retraining period (which may involve daily laxatives, increased fiber, and scheduled "potty times"), and encouragement of self-esteem and autonomy for the child. Although many children with this disorder are referred to pediatric gastroenterologists, the majority can be managed by general practitioners; often frequent follow-up is needed, and one must real-

*Table 7-1* **Encopresis versus Hirschsprung Disease: Clinical History**

|  | **Encopresis** | **Hirschsprung Disease** |
| --- | --- | --- |
| Stool palpated in vault | Very frequent | Rare |
| Large-caliber stools | Frequent | Rare |
| Avoidance of toilet | Frequent | Occasional |
| Constipation in the newborn period | Rare | Frequent |

ize that retraining may take several months and that relapses are quite common for many children.

## ATTENTION DEFICIT HYPERACTIVITY DISORDER

Much attention has been focused on "the hyperactive child." Prescriptions for stimulant medications have risen threefold to fivefold over the last decade. Whether this increase signifies a true increase in prevalence, increasing demands for improvement in school performance, or simply better recognition of atypical presentations [e.g., a primarily inattentive but normoactive child with attention deficit disorder (ADD)] is unclear. Attention deficit hyperactivity disorder (ADHD) remains the most common neurobehavioral disorder of childhood and was described more than a century ago. Approximately 5 percent of girls and 10 percent of boys may have the disorder on the basis of current criteria:

- *Etiology.* No theory has emerged that fully explains the development of ADHD. Heredity plays a role, as ADHD tends to run in families and is more common in males. Emerging studies of brain function have indicated significant differences as well. Theories that have been largely disproved include excessive dietary sugar and specific food additives.
- *Differential diagnosis.* In evaluating a child who presents with symptoms suggestive of ADHD, it is imperative to consider other causes that may manifest as decreased school performance or behavior concerns, including the following:
  - Cognitive impairment, learning disabilities
  - Language disorders
  - Developmental disorders
  - Hearing loss
  - Seizure disorders (e.g., absence seizures)
  - Sleep disorders
  - Depression/mood disorders
  - Anxiety disorders
  - Conduct disorder (CD), oppositional defiant disorder (ODD)
  - Child abuse, neglect

Consideration of these other diagnoses is important in the initial approach. *Up to one-third* of children with ADHD may have other comorbid conditions, with the most common being ODD, CD, anxiety/depression, and learning disabilities.

The AAP published clinical guidelines to assist in the diagnosis of ADHD in 2000, utilizing in part firmly established DSM-IV criteria. Children must manifest symptoms in at least two of the following three areas: *inattention* (frequently fails to follow through on instructions), *hyperactivity* (fidgety, always "on the go"), and *impulsivity* (e.g., blurts out answers before being called on). Children may be classified as primarily inattentive, primarily hyperactive-impulsive, or combined. The symptoms must be present for at least 6 months and must have been present before 7 years of age. To assist in making the diagnosis, input from parents and teachers is frequently obtained in the form of standardized questionnaires as well as direct interviews. It is extremely important when assessing behavior in any child to obtain information from all settings, as environment and social interaction can influence behavior in children greatly.

ADHD remains a clinical diagnosis. Once it is confirmed, management may involve pharmacologic therapy as well as behavioral therapy. Several medications currently are used to treat the inattentive symptoms of ADHD:

- *Stimulants* commonly used include methylphenidate (Ritalin, Concerta) and mixed amphetamine salts (Adderall). Stimulants are thought to activate the brain region responsible for regulatory control and thought processing and enhance concentration rather than exacerbating hyperactive symptoms. The main side effects from stimulants appear to be headaches, abdominal complaints (usually transient), and appetite suppression. There is some evidence that long-term therapy may have a minimal effect on final adult height in a subgroup of patients. Careful monitoring of height and weight as well as side effects is recommended.
- Less commonly used medications include clonidine, atomoxetine, bupropion, and, less commonly, tricyclic antidepressants. Many of these drugs are not U.S. Food and Drug Administration (FDA)-approved for use in children with ADHD but may play a role, especially if there are comorbid conditions.

In addition to medication, many families of children with ADHD clearly benefit from education about the diagnosis and emphasis on the fact that ADHD is a chronic disease whose symptoms may persist into adolescence and adulthood. For a family resistant to medications, behavioral modification therapy may be beneficial in achieving improved outcomes. Positive reinforcement (frequent rewards), time-outs, and "daily report cards" offer the frequent and directed feedback that many children with ADHD often need.

## RECURRENT ABDOMINAL PAIN

Recurrent abdominal pain (RAP) is defined as at least three episodes of *significant* abdominal pain (e.g., leading to the seeking of medical care or disruption of regular activities) occurring over a 3-month period and for which no organic cause can be found. The term *functional abdominal pain* sometimes is used to refer to this syndrome, although paradoxically, RAP often causes significant disruption to daily functioning and school attendance. Various theories abound as to the exact origin.

The approach to a child with chronic abdominal pain always should rule out rare but serious causes of abdominal pain (peptic ulcer disease, gastro-esophageal reflux, inflammatory bowel disease) by including a careful history, growth charts, and appropriate laboratory tests when warranted. Once organic causes are ruled out, practitioners should remain empathetic but firm and should not take the approach that the stomachaches are all "in the child's head," as this may minimize the significant effect RAP can have on the child and the family. A useful analogy for discussion is often comparison to adult headaches, since frequently the causes are unknown but morbidity may be significant. Management is dependent largely on the specific clinical history, but encouraging normal activities is essential. Consultation with a mental health professional may be warranted if there are specific concerns about the child's mood, concerns about conversion reactions, or maladaptive family behaviors.

## ADOLESCENCE

### CONDUCT DISORDER

Adolescence is clearly a time when many teenagers, in an effort to express their individuality, may "take it to the limit." However, a teen who meets the strict DSM-IV criteria for conduct disorder typically must exhibit at least three of the four following behaviors:

1. Aggression toward people and/or animals (e.g., bullying, physical cruelty)
2. Destruction of property (e.g., vandalism, fire setting)
3. Deceitfulness or theft
4. Violation of rules (e.g., school truancy, running away from home)

### OPPOSITIONAL DEFIANT DISORDER

Many teenagers are "oppositionally defiant" at some point in their adolescence, when identity formation and autonomy issues become increasingly important. However, a teen with true oppositional defiant disorder represents the extreme of disruptive negativism. Behaviors include loss of temper, frequent arguments and conflicts with adults, active defiance of established rules, blaming others for one's own mistakes, and being easily annoyed, angry, and/or vindictive. Both conduct disorder and oppositional defiant disorder frequently are linked to school failure and increased chances of dropping out. Improved interventions for both ODD and CD are needed. Pharmacologic therapies may have a role.

## EATING DISORDERS

Trends among adolescents in the United States over the last few decades almost appear to be paradoxical. At a time when more teenagers are considered obese than ever before, there is a growing preoccupation with being thin. In the most recent Centers for Disease Control and Prevention (CDC) Youth Risk Behavior Survey, over one-third of females believed they were overweight and over half were attempting to lose weight. Despite redefinition of the diagnostic criteria for eating disorders in 1996, overlap often still exists between classifications.

### ANOREXIA NERVOSA

Because anorexia nervosa presents with extreme weight loss and often with associated medical complications, it is more likely to be noted than are more covert eating disorders such as bulimia. Revised DSM-IV criteria for anorexia nervosa include the following:

- Refusal to maintain body weight at or above a minimally normal weight for age and height (e.g., weight loss leading to maintenance of body weight < 85 percent of that expected or failure to make expected weight gain during a period of growth, leading to body weight < 85 percent of that expected).
- Body mass index <17.5 kg/m² for older adolescents.
- Intense fear of gaining weight or becoming fat even though underweight.
- Disturbance in the way in which one's body weight, shape, or size is experienced; undue influence of body weight or shape on self-evaluation; or denial of the seriousness of the current low body weight.
- In postmenarchal females, amenorrhea: the absence of at least three consecutive menstrual cycles. [A female is considered to have amenorrhea if her periods occur only after hormone (e.g., estrogen) administration.]

These individuals may present with menstrual irregularity, amenorrhea, cold hands and feet, dry skin and hair, fainting, lethargy, difficulty concentrating, social withdrawal, and depression. Items noted on physical examination and laboratory values may include hypothermia, orthostasis, loss of muscle mass, leukopenia, and hypoglycemia.

Management of an individual with anorexia nervosa must include nutritional support and establishing trust and rapport with patients and their families. Other modalities have included psychotherapy as well as pharmacologic measures, specifically selective serotonin reuptake inhibitors (SSRIs). There have been few randomized trials comparing treatments among adolescents. Family-based therapy appears to offer the most benefit, and there may be a role for SSRI treatment, particularly if there are comorbid conditions (depression, bulimia), in which case SSRIs appear to have more efficacy.

Treatment may involve inpatient hospitalization, particularly if the following criteria are present:

• Weight below 75 percent of ideal body weight or ongoing weight loss despite intensive management
• Refusal to eat
• Heart rate < 50 beats/min in the daytime and < 45 beats/min at night
• Systolic pressure < 90 mmHg
• Orthostatic changes in pulse (> 20 beats/min) or blood pressure (>10 mmHg)
• Temperature < 35.6°C (96°F)
• Arrhythmia

## BULIMIA NERVOSA

In contrast to anorexia nervosa, bulimia may be characterized by weight *gain* as well as weight loss. Binge eating almost invariably is followed by purging (vomiting, diuretic and laxative abuse) or other compensatory behaviors (e.g., excessive exercise, strict dieting, fasting). Bulimia is reported more commonly than anorexia among women, and the true incidence may be even be higher in light of the often covert activities of binging and purging. Current DSM-IV criteria for bulimia nervosa include the following:

• Recurrent episodes of binge eating, characterized by both of the following:
  • Eating, in a discrete period of time (e.g., within any 2-h period), an amount of food that is definitely larger than most people would eat during a similar period of time and under similar circumstances
  • A sense of lack of control over eating during the episode (e.g., a feeling that one cannot stop eating or control what or how much one is eating)
• Recurrent inappropriate compensatory behavior to prevent weight gain, such as self-induced vomiting; misuse of laxatives, diuretics, enemas, or other medications; fasting; and excessive exercise.
• The binge eating and inappropriate compensatory behaviors both occur, on average, at least twice a week for 3 months.
• Self-evaluation is influenced unduly by body shape and weight.
• The disturbance does not occur exclusively during episodes of anorexia nervosa.

In contrast to teens with anorexia nervosa, bulimic individuals may present with weight gain as well as weight loss. The clinician needs to have a high index of suspicion and look for specific physical examination findings and laboratory values that may be associated with purging behaviors:

• Parotid gland enlargement (produced by repeated vomiting)

- Electrolyte disturbances (often a hypokalemic metabolic alkalosis) produced by excessive vomiting or laxative and/or diuretic abuse
- Dental enamel erosion (repeated exposure to acid from vomiting)
- Knuckle calluses (produced by induction of vomiting)

Regarding psychological features, many teens with bulimia may present with depression or anxiety or express guilt over self-induced binging and purging behaviors. Treatment approaches to the bulimic individual often are similar to those for anorexia; they are usually multidisciplinary in nature but frequently involve psychotherapy (usually based on the cognitive behavioral model) as well as the occasional use of SSRIs.

The prognosis for both anorexia and bulimia is generally favorable if the condition is treated. Recent data report a 75 to 85 percent recovery rate for anorexics with hospitalization, with less success reported in those with bulimia nervosa.

## ADOLESCENT MALES AND BODY DYSMORPHISM

Although anorexia, bulimia, and other eating disorders predominantly affect females, there is growing recognition that these disorders also occur in males. Physical appearance is prized more during adolescence than in any other period of childhood and is increasingly valued by adolescent males, as well as females, partly because of media influences and unrealistic portrayals of "six-pack abs." Athletic prowess and performance are emphasized increasingly as well, and the use of performance-enhancing substances such as anabolic steroids has become widespread among adolescents, not to mention adult athletes. As a result, the incidence of both body dysmorphic disorders (a subtype of somatization disorder) and eating disorders is reported to be increasing among male adolescents.

## RISK-TAKING BEHAVIORS

Adolescence is a time when many young adults assert their independence and increasing autonomy; the influence of peers becomes increasingly valued as well. Feelings of invincibility and disconnects between cause and effect often promote risk-taking behaviors in many areas, including automobile safety, experimentation with drugs and alcohol, and sexual activity. Historically, adolescents are the age group least likely to seek regular preventive care from pediatricians. Encounters with teens always should include discussion and anticipatory guidance regarding risk-taking behaviors.

### AUTOMOBILE SAFETY

Motor vehicle accidents are the leading cause of death among the 16- to 20-year-old age group. The number of passengers traveling with teen drivers increases the risk of death; teen drivers are also much more susceptible to crashes caused by alcohol or night driving. Evidence supports graduated driver's license programs and stricter legislation regarding driving under the influence (DUI) as being more efficacious in injury and death prevention than is the time-honored tradition of high school driver's education courses.

## SEXUAL BEHAVIOR

The most recent data from the CDC National Survey of Family Growth indicates that among young adults 15 to 21 years of age, about 47 percent of females and 46 percent of males have had sexual intercourse at least once. Factors associated with the initiation of early sexual intercourse include early puberty, sexual abuse, and poverty. Pregnancy and human immunodeficiency virus (HIV) and other sexually transmitted diseases are all undesired consequences. Practitioners should be able to have frank and unbiased discussions with adolescents; although parental involvement should be encouraged, confidentiality should be assured.

Adolescence is also a time of sexual confusion for some individuals, and many may engage in sexual experimentation that is often poorly predictive of future orientation. At the same time, growing awareness of one's sexual orientation, especially a same-sex orientation, may lead to emotional turmoil. Nonheterosexual youths report verbal and physical assaults, are more likely to engage in substance abuse, and are two to seven times more likely to attempt suicide. The AAP strongly encourages referral of gay youth to other sources if practitioners have personal obstacles to providing care. Clinicians also should be aware that "coming out" often can produce significant family disruption.

## SUBSTANCE ABUSE

More than three-fourths of teenagers have consumed alcohol by high school graduation, and about half of high school youth have tried illicit drugs at least once, according to recent national surveys. The illicit drugs cited most commonly recently (after alcohol and marijuana) include inhalants, LSD, MDMA (Ecstasy), cocaine, heroin, and, most recently, methamphetamine. In most instances (with the exception of high-risk situations or altered mental status), screening for drug use should be carried out only with the individual's consent to maintain the therapeutic relationship and trust between provider and patient. Counseling, support groups, family therapy, and consultation with mental health professionals all may be useful adjuncts in the approach and treatment of youth. Intensive outpatient or inpatient treatment programs may be needed for youth with significant substance abuse issues, recognizing that significant psychiatric illness may contribute to and/or result from drug and alcohol abuse.

## CHALLENGES FOR THE TWENTY-FIRST-CENTURY FAMILY

With the increasing role of women in the workplace, increasing acceptance of single motherhood, and substantial divorce rates, the traditional model of "family" continues to evolve. Many alterations to family structure significantly affect the behavior and mental health of developing children.

### DIVORCE

Children frequently believe that they caused their parents' divorce and may experience feelings of anger, guilt, and anxiety as well as sadness over the loss of the family. Clinicians should be aware that acute, transitional, and long-term adjustments occur and should be advocates for stability and structure whenever possible.

### FOSTER CARE AND ADOPTION

Although orphanages in the United States have largely disappeared from the landscape, many children continue to end up in foster care. "Kinship care"—placement with a family member or relative who has received some parent training—has been emphasized increasingly by the legal system. Abuse and neglect are cited as the most common reasons for removal from the home. Less frequently, children may lose parents to death, mental incapacity, or incarceration. Foster children not only experience many of the issues normally associated with family disruptions but also may develop significant feelings of guilt, separation anxiety, rejection, and abandonment. Attachment disorders also may be common. The increasing number of adoptions overseas (where orphanages are still commonplace) may present significant challenges for many families, some of which remain lifelong. Developmental, behavioral, and mental health disorders are more common among foster care children as well as international adoptees, and clinicians should be familiar with the unique risks and challenges these populations often face.

### FAMILY VIOLENCE

Spouse battering and child abuse often are linked to a spectrum of childhood behaviors ranging from nightmares and frequent somatic complaints to significant psychiatric impairment, including anxiety/depression disorders and posttraumatic stress disorder (PTSD). Primary prevention should be the priority. Screening questions should be asked routinely at health maintenance visits. One author suggests the use of the mnemonic HITS (How often does your partner *h*urt, *i*nsult, *t*hreaten, or *s*cream?).

## BIBLIOGRAPHY

Committee on Adolescence. Policy statement: Identifying and treating eating disorders. *Pediatrics* 111(1):204–211, 2003.

Committee on Quality Improvement and Subcommittee on Attention-Deficit/ Hyperactivity Disorder. Clinical practice guideline: Diagnosis and evaluation of the child with attention-deficit/hyperactivity disorder. *Pediatrics* 105(5): 1158–1170, 2000.

Frazer C, Emans SJ, Goodman E, et al. Teaching residents about development and behavior. *Arch Pediatr Adolesc Med* 153(11):1190–1194, 1999.

Glascoe FP. Early detection of developmental and behavioral problems. *Pediatr Rev* 21:272–280, 2000.

Green M, ed. *Bright Futures: Guidelines for Health Supervision of Infants, Children, and Adolescents,* 2d ed. Arlington, VA: National Center for Education in Maternal and Child Health, 2002. http://www.brightfutures.org.

Lawless MR, McElderry DH. Nocturnal enuresis: Current concepts. *Pediatr Rev* 22:399–407, 2001.

# PREVENTION

*Sandra M. Sanguino*

1. Describe how the risk of injury changes as a child grows.

2. Give examples of age-related injuries.

3. List examples of anticipatory guidance aimed at prevention for children of different ages for motor vehicle safety, falls, firearms, fires, poisoning, and drowning.

## INTRODUCTION

One of the key roles of a pediatrician is the prevention of illness and injury in children and adolescents. The twentieth century saw a remarkable reduction in infant mortality and an increase in life expectancy. Much of this was due to the development of vaccination, antibiotic use, and other public health measures. Although pediatrics has been very successful in preventing many illnesses, there are still numerous challenges. One of the biggest challenges is the prevention of injury. Until relatively recently, injuries were referred to commonly as *accidents*. This term appeared to suggest that these were unpredictable, unavoidable events. Physicians currently prefer to use the term *injury*, indicating that these events can be prevented. Injury prevention is a key component of the anticipatory guidance that pediatricians provide to children and their families.

## EPIDEMIOLOGY

Unintentional injuries are the most common cause of death among children 1 to 19 years of age. In the United States in 2002, 17,589 children from birth to age 19 died as a result of an injury. The types of injury seen vary by age group. The most common cause of injury deaths in children are motor vehicle crashes. In 2003, 1591 children age 14 years and younger died as occupants in motor vehicle crashes and approximately 220,000 were injured. Among children less than 1 year of age, the most common cause of injury death is suffocation. In 2002, 636 infants died as a result of this injury. To help pediatricians implement injury prevention counseling, the American Academy of Pediatrics (AAP) has developed the Injury Prevention Program (TIPP). TIPP consists of a safety counseling schedule, safety surveys, and age-appropriate handouts.

## AGE-SPECIFIC COUNSELING

### INTRODUCTION

This section will discuss specific items for injury prevention counseling. This is not intended to be an extensive review of every safety item that should be discussed. Rather, it is intended to highlight key items. Pediatricians should be reminded to keep up to date on recalled products through the Consumer Product Safety Commission.

### INFANTS AND PRESCHOOLERS

#### SLEEP SAFETY

Parents should be reminded that the preferred position for infant sleeping is the nonprone position. The supine position confers the lowest risk of sudden infant death syndrome (SIDS) and is preferred. If the side position is used, the parents should bring the infant's dependent arm forward to prevent the infant from rolling prone. Infants should not be placed to sleep on soft mattresses, water beds, or sofas. Pillows, quilts, comforters, and soft toys should not be placed in an infant's sleeping environment. If blankets are used, they should be tucked in around the crib mattress so that the infant's face will not become covered. Crib slats should be no more than 2.4 in. apart. Widely spaced slats can trap an infant's head. Bumper pads should be used around the crib until the infant begins to stand. They then should be removed so that the infant cannot use the bumper pad as a step. Hanging crib toys such as mobiles should be kept out of an infant's reach as they can strangle the infant.

## CAR SAFETY

When riding in a car, children should always be placed in a child seat restraint. Children under 20 pounds and 1 year of age may use an infant seat or be placed in a convertible infant-toddler children's restraining device. Infants under 1 year of age and 20 pounds should be placed in the rear seat facing backward; older toddlers and children up to 40 pounds can be placed in the backseat facing forward in a forward-facing convertible or toddler seat. Parents also should be reminded about the importance of their own use of seat belts.

## CHOKING

Household items and foods can serve as choking items for young children. Any small object that can be placed in the mouth is a potential hazard. Before a child begins to crawl, it is important to get down on his or her level to look for potential hazards. Common household items that can represent choking dangers include coins, buttons, batteries, toys with small parts, and latex balloons. Foods that may pose a choking hazard include popcorn, hot dogs, whole grapes, nuts, and hard candy. These foods should not be given to children until age 4. Parents should be reminded that children should not run or play while eating.

## FIRE AND BURNS

Fire and burn prevention also should be discussed. Fires and burns are implicated in approximately 700 deaths among children each year. Smoke detectors should be installed on every floor of the home. Families should be reminded to change the batteries periodically. Hot water heaters should be set at 49°C (120°F) to prevent scald burns. Parents should be counseled not to carry hot liquids when holding a child. Families should have an escape plan in case of a fire in the home. Matches and lighters should be kept out of the reach of children.

## FALLS

Falls account for almost 3 million visits to the emergency department and are the most common cause of injury hospitalization among children. Infants should never be left alone on tables, beds, or other high places, even for a moment. Window guards should be placed on all windows. The window should not be able to be opened more than 4 in. to prevent a child from falling out. Screens are not window guards; they are intended to keep bugs out, not children in. Furniture should be away from windows as it may allow a climbing toddler to have access to the window. The use of walkers should be discouraged.

## POISONINGS

Medicines and household cleaning products should be stored locked in high areas, out of the reach of children. Household products and medicines should be kept in their original containers. Parents should have the telephone number of the local poison control center. The use of syrup of ipecac to induce vomiting after ingestions is no longer recommended.

## DROWNING

Drowning is the most common type of injury death among children less than 5 years of age. Parents should be reminded never to leave children unattended in the bathtub, even for a minute. As children also can drown in buckets, buckets should be emptied as soon as they are used and stored upside down. Swimming pools and hot tubs need to be fenced in on all four sides. Although many children under age 5 take swimming lessons, they should never swim unsupervised.

## FIREARMS

Children as young as age 3 have the strength to pull the trigger on a firearm. Access to firearms in the home is a risk factor for unintentional firearm injuries. Almost one-third of families with children store their guns loaded. The AAP states that the best way to avoid firearm injures is to remove firearms from the environment. If it is necessary to have a gun in the home, it should be stored unloaded in a locked place, with the ammunition locked and stored in a separate place.

## SCHOOL-AGE CHILDREN

### TRAFFIC SAFETY

Children age 4 to 8 who weigh between 40 and 80 pounds should use a belt positioning booster seat. All children age 12 years and younger should ride in the backseat. This eliminates the injury risk of deployed front passenger-side air bags and places children in the safest part of the vehicle if there is a crash. Riding in the backseat is associated with a 46 percent reduction in the risk of fatal injury in cars with a front passenger-side air bag.

Pedestrian safety needs to be reviewed with children and their parents. Children age 5 to 9 appear to be at the greatest risk for pedestrian injuries. All children should learn safe street-crossing skills. Most children do not have the ability to handle traffic situations safely until around 10 years of age.

### BICYCLE SAFETY

Bicycle crashes can result in serious injury and death. Most bicycle-related deaths result from head trauma. The use of a protective helmet is effective in reducing head injuries. Unfortunately, the use of helmets is low among youth. Children always should wear a helmet when riding a bicycle. Parents also should be encouraged to wear bicycle helmets and serve as role models for their children. School-age children also should be reminded not to ride bicycles in the dark. For children who ride scooters, skateboards, or roller blades, helmet, knee, wrist, and elbow pads should be used.

## Water Safety

Children age 5 and older should be encouraged to learn how to swim. Young swimmers should not be allowed to swim unsupervised. For those who are involved in boating, everyone on a boat should use a Coast Guard–approved life jacket. At least one adult swimmer should be present for each child who cannot swim.

### FIREARM SAFETY

Parents should be reminded that if they choose to keep a gun in the home, it should be stored locked and unloaded, with the ammunition stored separately from the gun.

## ADOLESCENTS

### CAR SAFETY

Motor vehicle crashes are the leading cause of death for teens and young adults. More than 5000 young people die every year in car crashes, and thousands more are injured. There are two main reasons teens are at a higher risk for being in a car crash: lack of driving experience and their tendency to take risks while driving. During health supervision visits, it is important to discuss with teenagers the risks associated with driving. Teenagers should be reminded to wear their seat belts at all times. The hazards of drinking and driving also should be discussed. Teenagers should be reminded about the need to remain focused during driving. The use of cell phones while driving and the playing of loud music can be distracting to drivers and should be avoided.

## BIBLIOGRAPHY

Centers for Disease Control and Prevention, National Center for Injury Prevention and Control. US injury mortality statistics. Available at http://wonder.cdc.gov.

Naureckas SM, Galanter C, Naureckas ET, et al. Children's and women's ability to fire handguns. *Arch Pediatr Adolesc Med* 149(12):1318–1322, 1995.

Weil DS, Hemenway D. Loaded gun in the home: Analysis of a random survey of gun owners. *JAMA* 267:3033–3037, 1992.

# CHAPTER 9

# NUTRITION

## M. Robin English

● LEARNING OBJECTIVES

1. Know the dietary requirements for infants and children of all ages.
2. Understand the benefits and challenges of breast-feeding.
3. Know how to counsel parents on adequate nutrition for their children at any age.
4. Understand common nutritional problems in infants and children and be able to identify and counsel patients who are at risk for nutrition-related diseases.
5. Recognize common vitamin and mineral deficiencies in infants and children.

## INTRODUCTION

Proper nutrition is extremely important to the overall health, growth, and development of all pediatric patients, including infants, toddlers, older children, and adolescents. Each age group requires special considerations, however, and these considerations vary from the type of foods given to the amount of calories and nutrients required for growth. The pediatrician plays a critical role in ensuring that his or her patients receive adequate nutrition by providing age-specific counseling at well-child visits.

The infant well visit is especially important in establishing proper nutrition from the very beginning of an infant's life. Parents should be asked whether the baby is fed breast milk, which is the preferred type of nutrition for most infants, or commercially available formula. Questions about urine output and wet diapers, the feeding schedule (including the amount and frequency of feeds), and stool consistency are important to determine whether an infant is receiving the required amount of nutrition. The infant's weight, length, and head circumference are measured and plotted on a growth chart beginning at birth so that the pediatrician can follow growth over time. The growth curve is important in determining patterns of growth, and failure to progress along the curve can be the first clue that an infant's health is declining if, for example, a systemic disease or infection is present.

Toddler nutrition can be a challenging issue for both pediatricians and parents. Many toddlers exhibit difficulty with feeding during this behavioral stage, which is characterized by the development of new language and motor skills and emerging independence. Mealtimes often become a struggle for young children, and many toddlers have a limited diet that does not include foods from all the food groups. Questions about snacks and the structure of mealtimes are important for this age group. The importance of following the growth chart during this time must not be underestimated, as many toddlers will "fall off the growth curve" because of lack of variation in their diets. Other special issues for this age group include the anticipatory guidance given at well-child visits, especially regarding prevention of choking.

Older children and adolescents have other special nutritional issues, including irregular eating habits, increased fast-food consumption, obesity, and eating disorders such as anorexia nervosa and bulimia nervosa. History questions regarding body image, between-meals snacks, and overall diet and exercise habits are important for the pediatrician to explore during well-child visits. Growth curves for older children should be followed at each visit, and counseling should include the child or adolescent as well as the parents.

This chapter highlights the specifics of calorie, vitamin, mineral, and fluid requirements, which vary with age, and discusses several common nutritional problems that pediatricians encounter.

## NUTRITION FOR INFANTS AND TODDLERS

### CALORIC AND FLUID REQUIREMENTS

The amount of fluid required to meet an infant's daily needs changes with the infant's age. Term newborn infants require approximately 120 to 150 mL/kg per day, and preterm infants often require even more fluids because of their increased ratio of surface area to weight and increased insensible losses. The fluid requirement decreases gradually over the next year to approximately 100 mL/kg per day at 1 year of age. Past the immediate newborn period, fluid requirements can be calculated by reference to the infant's weight (Fig. 9-1).

Caloric requirements also vary by age. Term newborn infants require 80 to 120 kcal/kg per day, and this requirement continues until around 3 years

| First 10 kg of weight | 100 mL/kg/day |
|---|---|
| Second 10 kg of weight | 50 mL/kg/day |
| Each additional 1 kg of weight | 25 mL/kg/day |

Example: Weight 10 kg: Daily requirement = 100 mL/kg/day × 10 kg = 1000 mL/day

Weight 15 kg: Daily requirement =  100 mL/kg/day × 10 kg = 1000 mL/day
                                  + 50 mL/kg/day × 5 kg =   500 mL/day
                                                          1500 mL/day

Weight 30 kg: Daily requirement = 100 mL/kg/day × 10 kg = 1000 mL/day
                                + 50 mL/kg/day × 10 kg = 500 mL/day
                                + 25 mL/kg/day × 10 kg = 250 mL/day
                                                        1750 mL/day

*Figure 9-1* **Calculation of Fluid Requirements.**

of age. Preterm and very low birthweight (VLBW) infants often require up to 120 to 150 kcal/kg per day to meet their increased metabolic demands.

Most infants can meet both their fluid and caloric requirements with breast milk or commercially available standard infant formulas, which contain 20 kcal/oz. At times, a formula with higher caloric density (e.g., 24 kcal/oz) is required, especially if an infant has difficulty taking in the necessary amount of fluids. An infant's caloric and fluid intake can be calculated easily (Fig. 9-2).

1 ounce = 30 mL

Breast milk/formula = 20 kcal/oz = 0.67 kcal/mL

Concentrated formula = 24 kcal/oz = 0.80 kcal/mL

Example: 10-kg infant drinks 40 oz/day of breast milk

Fluid intake:        40 oz/day × 30 mL/oz = 1200 mL/day = 120 mL/kg/day
Caloric intake:   1200 mL/day × 0.67 kcal/mL = 804 kcal/day = 80 kcal/kg/day

Example:  6-kg infant drinks 24 oz/day of 24 kcal/oz formula

Fluid intake:        24 oz/day × 30 mL/oz = 720 mL/day = 120 mL/kg/day
Caloric intake:   720 mL/day × 0.80 kcal/mL = 576 kcal/day = 96 kcal/kg/day

*Figure 9-2* **Calculation of Caloric Intake.**

The fluid and caloric intake of an infant should be followed carefully to ensure that the infant gains weight adequately. Most newborns lose up to 10 percent of their birthweight in the first few days after birth because of increased metabolic demands. This weight should be regained by age 2 weeks in term formula-fed infants and by age 3 weeks in term breast-fed infants. After that time, acceptable weight gain for term infants is 20 to 30 g per day for the first few months of life. An infant's weight, as well as length and head circumference, always should be plotted on a gender-appropriate growth chart to ensure proper growth, but *a good general rule is that most infants double their birthweight by 4 to 5 months of age and triple it by around 1 year of age.*

Toddlers in the second year of life continue to require approximately 100 kcal/kg per day. Fluid requirements still are calculated using the formula in Fig. 9-1. As in infancy, the growth chart remains the primary means of determining whether a toddler is receiving adequate calories in his or her diet.

## BREAST-FEEDING

Breast milk is considered optimal nutrition for infants. The pediatrician plays an important role in helping mothers make the decision to breast-feed and to do so successfully. Numerous advantages for breast-fed infants have been identified (Table 9-1). In addition, studies have shown that lactating mothers experience less postpartum bleeding, show improved postpartum bone remineralization, and return to their prepregnancy weight more quickly than do mothers who choose not to breast-feed. Despite these advantages for both the mother and the infant, however, many mothers choose not to breast-feed; this may be due to a lack of education, a lack of paternal support, or perceived or real difficulties with the physical act of

*Table 9-1* **Benefits of Breast-Feeding**

| |
|---|
| Improved maternal-infant bonding |
| Enhanced host defense with decreased incidence of the following: |
|     Gastrointestinal illnesses |
|     Respiratory diseases |
|     Otitis media |
|     Bacterial meningitis |
|     Necrotizing enterocolitis |
| Decreased risk of food allergies and eczema |
| Possible enhanced cognitive development |
| Possible reduced risk of obesity |
| Reduced health-care costs |

nursing. The challenges that a mother may face are discussed later in this section.

A pregnant woman begins to make breast milk at 6 to 7 months of gestation. Several changes in the breast, including distended alveoli, widening and darkening of the areolae, and increased erectile activity of the nipples, take place over the next few weeks. Very little milk is produced, however, until the infant is born. The delivery of the placenta causes decreased estrogen and progesterone levels and a subsequent increase in prolactin, which increases milk production. The sensation created when the infant nurses causes the release of oxytocin, which stimulates contraction of the ducts; this is known as letdown. The milk produced in the first few days after delivery is called colostrum and is yellow-orange in color. Colostrum is higher in protein and antibodies but lower in fat and calories than mature human milk. Transitional milk is produced after colostrum up to around 2 weeks of life. This period is one of markedly increased milk production; this often is referred to as the milk "coming in." Mature human milk is produced after 2 weeks and is white and thin or watery in consistency. The milk produced at the beginning of each feeding is known as foremilk and is high in protein. That produced at the end of the feeding is known as hindmilk and is lower in protein and higher in fat than foremilk.

Human milk contains primarily whey proteins, which are easily digested and promote gastric emptying. These proteins include lactoferrin, $\alpha$-lactalbumin, and secretory immunoglobulin A (IgA), all of which are important for host defense. The fat in human milk is primarily long-chain fatty acids, but very long chain fatty acids—arachidonic acid and docosahexaenoic acid—are also present. It has been suggested that the presence of these very long chain fatty acids increases neural and retinal development. The carbohydrate in human milk is lactose, which is easily tolerated in all infants and is important in the development of lactobacilli in the intestine. Other important and protective factors in breast milk include growth factors, nucleotides, and oligosaccharides. The milk produced by the mothers of premature infants differs in content from term human milk and is more appropriate for a premature infant in several ways, including increased protein content. However, premature human milk is inadequate to meet fully the calcium and phosphorus needs of a preterm infant; therefore, human milk fortifiers can be added for supplementation.

Breast-fed infants should be nursed as soon as possible after delivery to begin the milk letdown process. They should be fed on demand, as soon as signs of hunger, including increased alertness and rooting, appear. This is usually 8 to 12 times per day, about every 2 to 3 h initially. Infants should be nursed until they are no longer actively sucking, usually for 15 to 20 min. Infants can be nursed around 10 min on each breast or can empty one breast fully, switching to the other breast for the next feeding. Both breasts should be offered per feeding in the first few weeks to stimulate milk production, and no more than 4 h should pass without breast-feeding the infant in these first few weeks.

Many mothers may be concerned about the amount of breast milk an infant is receiving. Signs that an infant is receiving adequate milk are a deep, rhythmic suck and regular swallowing. In addition, a mother's breasts should feel softer and less full after nursing. Other signs include frequent soft stools (often after each feed), adequate urine production (six or more wet diapers per day), and infant satiety. One must remember that newborn infants lose 5 to 10 percent of their birthweight in the first days after birth, and breast-fed infants should regain their birthweight by 2 to 3 weeks of life.

Breast-feeding an infant is a rewarding but often challenging experience for mothers. The physical challenges include cracked nipples, clogged milk ducts, mastitis, and engorgement. Cracked nipples may be caused by improper latching on and may result in significant breast pain. This can be treated by improving the latching-on technique, avoiding excessive breast moisture between feedings, and applying breast milk or lanolin to the breasts. A sore breast lump may indicate a clogged milk duct. Frequent nursing or pumping can help drain the breast more effectively, and wearing loose clothing and changing the infant's position during nursing can prevent this from developing. Mastitis develops when an area of the breast fails to drain sufficiently and a bacterial infection subsequently develops. This can be quite painful for the mother, but nursing should continue if possible to help drain the breast fully. Antibiotics and pain medication should be given to the mother. It is important to inform mothers that the infection will not spread to the infant during breast-feeding. Engorgement can occur between feedings as a mother's breasts increase milk synthesis in response to the baby's demand. Frequent feeding, expressing milk between feedings, and warm cloths applied to the breast can alleviate this problem. In general, most of these problems can be prevented or alleviated by increasing the frequency of breast-feeding. Care should be taken to ensure that any medications given to the mother are safe for the infant.

An infant's frequent feeding schedule can be demanding in the first few months of life, and mothers may feel exhausted and overwhelmed. Fathers and other family members can provide important support by helping with positioning the baby during nursing and by performing other tasks, such as dressing and changing diapers. Many mothers are unaware that breast-feeding is the best thing for the baby, and so it is important that obstetricians and pediatricians provide education both before and after the baby is born. Mothers who return to work after a few weeks may pump their breast milk while they are away from the baby, but this is time-consuming and requires the cooperation of the employer. Pediatricians are instrumental in offering support for mothers during these times. Other office staff members, such as lactation consultants and nurses, can be key players in providing counseling and encouragement to mothers during this important process.

## INFANT FORMULAS

For mothers who choose not to or are unable to breast-feed, commercially available infant formulas are acceptable substitutes. These formulas vary by composition primarily, and specialized formulas for infants with unique nutritional needs are often more expensive than standard formulas. Infant formulas are available to parents in three forms: canned powder, which is usually mixed at a ratio of 1 scoop to 2 oz of water; canned concentrate, which is usually mixed with water in a 1:1 ratio; and ready-to-feed, which the parent can give without mixing. Standard infant formulas provide 20 kcal/oz, but formulas with higher caloric density can be purchased pre-mixed or can be mixed at home to a higher concentration. In general, infant formulas can be differentiated on the basis of the protein and carbohydrate composition: cow's milk formula, soy milk formula, protein hydrolysate formula, and elemental formula (Table 9-2). These formulas contain a combination of fats: soy oil, coconut oil, sunflower oil, and palm oleic oil. Some hydrolysate and elemental formulas also contain an increased percentage of medium-chain triglycerides.

Table 9-2 **Composition of Commercially Available Infant Formulas***

| Formula | Primary Protein | Primary Carbohydrate |
|---------|-----------------|----------------------|
| Cow's milk | Casein | Lactose |
| Enfamil | Whey | |
| Similac | | |
| Soy milk | Soy protein | Corn syrup solids, |
| Prosobee | Methionine | maltodextrin, or sucrose |
| Isomil | | |
| Alsoy | | |
| Lactose-free | Casein | Corn syrup solids |
| Lactofree | Whey | Sucrose |
| Similac Lactose Free | | |
| Casein hydrolysate | Hydrolyzed casein | Corn syrup solids, sucrose, |
| Alimentum | | or modified starch |
| Nutramigen | | |
| Pregestimil | | |
| Whey hydrolysate | Hydrolyzed whey | Lactose |
| Carnation Good Start | | |
| Elemental | Free amino acids | Corn syrup solids |
| Neocare | | |
| Elecare | | |

*This table contains brand names of commonly available formulas and is not meant to be all-inclusive.

Cow's milk formulas are generally the first formulas considered when a mother decides not to breast-feed, mainly because their composition is the most similar to breast milk in terms of carbohydrate, protein, and fat. Many cow's milk formulas are supplemented with arachidonic acid and docosahexaenoic acid to imitate human milk further. Cow's milk formulas can be used for most infants. Many parents request a change to a lactose-free formula because of perceived lactose intolerance, such as flatus, bloating, or colic, but primary lactose intolerance is uncommon in infants. Secondary lactose intolerance occurs in approximately 20 percent of infants after diarrheal illnesses, however, and a change to a lactose-free formula may be attempted for a few days after the illness has resolved in this minority of infants. Parental requests for a lactose-free formula should be considered carefully, as there are few true indications for lactose-free formulas and because specialized formulas tend to be more expensive.

Soy milk formulas are also acceptable substitutes for breast milk, although the protein and carbohydrate composition varies from that of breast milk. Soy formulas are completely lactose-free, making them the formula of choice for infants with galactosemia. They are also inexpensive alternatives to lactose-containing formulas after diarrheal illnesses, although, as mentioned above, most infants will tolerate lactose during refeeding. Soy formulas may be chosen by parents who desire a vegetarian diet for their infants. Most infants with documented immunoglobulin E (IgE)-mediated cow's milk protein allergy manifesting as atopic dermatitis can be given soy formula successfully. However, infants with protein-losing enteropathy and enterocolitis from cow's milk protein allergy should not receive soy formula because of the risk of cross-reactivity to the soy protein.

Protein hydrolysate formulas may contain hydrolyzed casein or hydrolyzed whey. The hydrolysis of these proteins decreases antigenicity; therefore, these formulas are indicated for infants with gastrointestinal symptoms of cow's milk protein allergy, which are described in the section on food allergies, below. These hydrolysate formulas are more expensive than standard formulas; therefore, it is prudent to be certain of the diagnosis of true milk protein allergy before considering their use. Most infants with milk protein allergy respond quickly to hydrolysate formulas (within several days) in terms of weight gain and resolution of clinical symptoms.

Elemental formulas are free amino acid–based formulas in which protein is broken down completely to free amino acids. These formulas are even more expensive than hydrolysate formulas and are indicated for infants with severe milk protein allergy and protein-losing enterocolitis, many of whom have demonstrated failure to improve on hydrolysate formulas.

Whole cow's milk should not be given to infants less than 1 year of age. Cow's milk has low iron content, increases the renal solute load for infants, and may cause intestinal blood loss, leading to iron-deficiency anemia.

## SOLID FOODS

The ability of an infant to transition to taking solid foods depends on several factors. To take solid foods, an infant must have good head control and be able to sit, and the tongue extrusion reflex must have disappeared. These milestones occur between 4 and 6 months of age in most infants. In addition, infants need to have normal swallowing function to protect against aspiration. Most infants do not need solid foods before 4 to 6 months, as breast milk or formula alone provides adequate nutrition. An exception is the addition of rice cereal to breast milk or formula to thicken feeds for infants with severe gastrointestinal reflux. Other baby foods should not be added to the bottle.

Infant cereals such as rice and oatmeal are usually the first choice when an infant begins to take solid foods. The cereal should be mixed with a little breast milk or formula and given with a spoon. Pureed fruits, vegetables, and meats then may be introduced, but no more than one should be started at a time, with a period of at least a week before introducing a new food. Pureed baby foods are widely available commercially. Parents may wish to prepare the infant's foods at home; this is acceptable and nutritionally equivalent to commercially available foods as long as care is taken to clean instruments properly. Pureed store-bought canned foods are not acceptable nutrition for infants.

Finely chopped "adult foods" can be given to infants after 10 to 12 months of age. Parents should be sure to chop foods very finely and should be aware of the risk of choking. Foods that never should be given to children under the age of 2 years include hot dogs, peanuts, raw vegetables and fruit, hard candy, and popcorn.

## THE SECOND YEAR

Infants may be transitioned from breast milk or formula to whole cow's milk at 1 year of age. Whole milk should be given until 3 years of age, at which time low-fat milk may be given if desired. The amount of milk given should be limited to 24 oz per day to avoid iron-deficiency anemia.

New foods are introduced at a high rate during the second year of life. Toddlers learn to feed themselves as they reach developmental milestones. Many toddlers become "picky eaters" during this period, and parents should make sure to offer them a wide variety of nutritious foods. Toddlers should eat approximately four to six times per day, including snacks. Many toddlers enjoy fruit juices, which are acceptable in limited quantities. Toddlers who drink an excessive amount of fruit juice are at risk for failure to thrive, which occurs because of inadequate protein and fat ingestion, and diarrhea, which occurs secondary to an increased osmotic load in the intestine. The risk of choking is even higher in toddlers than in infants, and parents should make sure to avoid high-risk foods.

## COMMON PROBLEMS

### FAILURE TO THRIVE

Failure to thrive refers to the failure of an infant to gain weight as expected on the growth curve. Failure to thrive is not a diagnosis in itself; rather, it is a sign of an underlying problem. The differential diagnosis of failure to thrive is one of the longest in pediatrics, but the etiologies generally can be divided into the following categories: inadequate caloric intake, increased metabolic utilization, nutrient malabsorption, and nutrient loss (Table 9-3).

The history is extremely important in determining the cause of an infant's failure to thrive. A detailed history of the type and amount of breast milk or formula that the parent offers as well as the infant's feeding ability should be obtained. If the infant is breast-fed, the frequency and amount of

Table 9-3  **Basic Differential Diagnosis of Failure to Thrive***

| Cause | Examples |
| --- | --- |
| Inadequate caloric intake | Psychosocial issues such as negligence, impaired mother-infant interaction, improper feeding technique |
| | Swallowing or sucking dysfunction, such as neurologic impairment, cleft palate, choanal atresia |
| | Genetic syndromes |
| Increased metabolic utilization | Endocrine abnormalities such as hypothyroidism |
| | Cardiac disease such as congenital heart disease |
| | Chronic systemic infection or disease such as urinary tract infection, HIV, malignancy, bronchopulmonary dysplasia |
| Caloric malabsorption | Gastrointestinal disease such as malabsorption syndromes, pancreatic insufficiency, biliary disease |
| Caloric loss | Gastrointestinal losses such as gastroesophageal reflux, pyloric stenosis, protein-losing enteropathy, other chronic diarrheal diseases |

*This is a generalized approach to failure to thrive and is not intended to be an all-inclusive list of possible etiologies.

time spent nursing should be explored. If the infant is formula-fed, it is important to determine that the parent is mixing the formula properly. Formula that is too dilute offers significantly fewer calories than does properly mixed formula. Questions regarding urine output and stooling patterns will help determine whether the child is receiving adequate fluids. A history of recurrent infections or hospitalizations should be obtained as well as a complete review of systems. A thorough social history, including living and child-care arrangements, and attention to the parent-child interaction are also very important.

The physical examination of infants with failure to thrive should be thorough and should focus on evidence of systemic infection, the presence of dysmorphic features, and developmental progress. Abnormal findings often provide valuable clues to the etiology of failure to thrive, but many infants with failure to thrive actually have normal examinations with the exception of the low weight.

The growth chart is critical in determining the general reason for failure to thrive, and examining the infant's growth curve, with all the previous measurements, is often more important than the actual weight at the time when failure to thrive is recognized. In other words, it is important to know how the infant reached his or her current weight. For instance, an infant who was thriving initially and who has had a dramatic recent decrease in weight gain might warrant an extensive evaluation for systemic infection or another disease process, whereas an infant who has had poor growth since birth might require an evaluation of his or her oral-motor skills or a genetic evaluation. The infant's length and head circumference are also important in determining a cause. For example, if an infant receives inadequate calories, the weight will be affected first and most severely; length and head circumference usually are affected later, in that order. If an infant's growth chart shows that length is affected more than weight or head circumference, an evaluation for an endocrine or genetic abnormality may be indicated.

The degree of failure to thrive will determine the immediate management. Infants who have mild failure to thrive can be managed on an outpatient basis. This requires dietary counseling, frequent visits for weight checks, and compliance on the part of the parents. Infants with severe failure to thrive should be hospitalized both for evaluation and for close monitoring of caloric intake, feeding ability, and weight. Laboratory evaluation generally can be tailored to the patient's history and examination findings. If a clear history of inadequate caloric intake can be elicited, an extensive laboratory workup usually can be avoided. However, if a child appears to take in an appropriate amount of nutrition and still fails to gain weight, the results of laboratory studies may provide clues to the etiology. A complete blood count can give clues to possible infection or anemia. A urinalysis and urine culture often are indicated, as chronic urinary tract infection is a common cause of failure to thrive. Serum albumin may be low and may indicate chronic malnutrition.

Failure to thrive is a common and potentially very serious problem in pediatrics. Prompt recognition and management of this clinical sign are important, as a child's brain growth and immune system are affected by malnutrition. Infants with failure to thrive should be followed very closely, even after good weight gain has been established.

## FOOD ALLERGIES

Food allergies are immunologically mediated responses to the ingestion of specific food proteins. These reactions may be IgE-mediated or non-IgE-mediated and should be distinguished from food intolerance, which is not immunologic in nature. Food intolerance includes adverse reactions to certain components of foods, such as lactose intolerance. Many parents confuse food intolerance with food allergy (hypersensitivity), and a good history and physical examination can be important in helping to differentiate the two entities. The most common foods that induce immunologic hypersensitivity reactions in infants and children are milk, soy, wheat, peanuts, fish, and eggs. It has been suggested that exclusive breast-feeding to 6 months of age helps reduce the incidence of food allergies in children.

IgE-mediated hypersensitivity reactions in infants include atopic dermatitis exacerbations and allergic eosinophilic gastroenteritis, which is actually a mixed IgE-mediated and eosinophilic response. Parents may find that an infant's atopic dermatitis worsens with the ingestion of certain foods. Starting one new food at a time helps identify specific food triggers, and avoiding these specific foods is essential to the proper management of atopic dermatitis exacerbations. Eosinophilic gastroenteritis is a disease that presents in infancy and childhood as abdominal pain, vomiting, failure to thrive, gastroesophageal reflux, or diarrhea. Laboratory evaluation may reveal an increased serum IgE level and positive radioallergosorbent tests (RASTs) to specific food proteins. Skin tests may be performed in older infants. Gastrointestinal biopsy provides a definitive diagnosis but may not be necessary to make the diagnosis. Avoiding specific food proteins by giving affected infants protein hydrolysate formulas is the treatment of choice for this disease.

Food protein–induced enterocolitis is a non-IgE-mediated hypersensitivity reaction that occurs in infants less than 3 months of age. The offending food proteins are usually milk and soy. The symptoms include abdominal distention and pain, bloody or nonbloody diarrhea, and failure to thrive. Serum IgE and skin tests probably will be normal in these infants. Again, avoidance of the food protein is essential to the treatment of this disease, and most infants respond very quickly to protein hydrolysate or elemental formulas. Most of these infants outgrow their hypersensitivity to these food proteins by 2 to 3 years of age.

Food allergies in older children often are associated with other symptoms, such as urticaria, angioedema, and anaphylaxis. Referral to an allergist for skin testing and possible double-blind food challenges is indicated in older children who have hypersensitivity reactions to foods.

## VITAMIN AND MINERAL DEFICIENCIES

Most infants born at term to healthy mothers have sufficient vitamin stores at birth, with the exception of vitamin K, which must be given immediately after delivery to prevent hemorrhagic disease of the newborn. Most of the vitamins and minerals required for infants to maintain sufficient growth and nutrition during the first year of life are present in adequate amounts in both human milk and commercially available formulas. Vitamin D, iron, and fluoride, however, deserve special attention, as supplementation for them may be required.

Formula-fed infants get the vitamin D they require from formula alone. Breast-fed infants, however, are at risk for vitamin D deficiency because breast milk contains a low amount of vitamin D. The American Academy of Pediatrics (AAP) has recommended that *all* breast-fed infants receive vitamin D supplementation regardless of skin tone and sun exposure.

Infants have adequate iron stores until 4 to 6 months of age. Infants who are fed standard infant formulas receive 12 mg/L of iron, which is sufficient to meet requirements. Low-iron formulas have been marketed because of the concern that iron may cause constipation. This has *not* been proven; therefore, low-iron formulas should be avoided to prevent the risk of iron-deficiency anemia. The iron in human milk is readily bioavailable and is present in sufficient amounts to meet breast-fed infants' needs until 4 to 6 months of age. Iron-fortified cereals and foods should be offered at this age to both breast-fed and formula-fed infants.

Most infants do not require fluoride supplementation whether they are breast-fed or formula-fed. The AAP recommends that infants need supplementation after 6 months of age only if the water supply contains less than 0.3 parts per million (ppm) of fluoride.

Several other vitamins and minerals merit mention because some infants may be at risk for a deficiency. Breast-fed infants of strictly vegan mothers may be deficient in vitamin $B_{12}$. Infants who are fed a diet consisting exclusively of goat's milk may become deficient in folic acid. Infants with chronic malnutrition or the autosomal recessive disease acrodermatitis enteropathica are at risk for zinc deficiency, which can have profound effects on the immune system. Other important vitamins and minerals, as well as those mentioned above, and the consequences of both deficiency and excess are discussed in Table 9-4.

A common occurrence in toddlers is the development of iron-deficiency anemia, which is secondary to increased ingestion of cow's milk. These infants often drink more than 24 oz of milk a day, at times up to a gallon of milk every 2 to 3 days. Because their intake of milk is so high, their intake of

Table 9-4 **Common Vitamin and Mineral Deficiencies and Excesses**

| Vitamin | Deficiency | Excess |
|---|---|---|
| A | Xerophthalmia, night blindness | Pseudotumor cerebri |
| B₆ (pyridoxine) | Seizures, peripheral neuropathies | Neuropathies |
| B₁₂ (cyanocobalamin) | Pernicious anemia | — |
| C | Scurvy, bleeding gums | Nausea, abdominal pain |
| D | Rickets, osteomalacia, hypocalcemic tetany | Vomiting, hypercalcemia, polydipsia, polyuria |
| E | Hemolytic anemia (premature infants), neuropathies | Bleeding |
| K | Hemorrhagic disease of the newborn, other clotting disorders | Hyperbilirubinemia (vitamin K analogs only) |
| *Mineral* | | |
| Iron | Microcytic anemia | Hemosiderosis |
| Zinc | Dermatitis, diarrhea, impaired immunity | — |

other important nutrients, such as iron-containing foods, can be very low. Affected infants are often overweight and pale. Treatment consists of limiting milk intake and supplementing with 4 to 6 mg/kg of elemental iron per day.

## NUTRITION FOR OLDER CHILDREN AND ADOLESCENTS

### CALORIC AND FLUID REQUIREMENTS

The daily fluid requirements for older children and adolescents can be calculated according to weight, as shown in Fig. 9-1. Caloric requirements decrease over time; preschool children (age 3 to 5) require approximately 90 to 100 kcal/kg per day, school-age children (age 6 to 10) require 70 to 90 kcal/kg per day, and adolescents require 40 to 55 kcal/kg per day. Children older than 3 years of age should have their weight, height, and BMI plotted on an appropriate growth chart.

## COMMON PROBLEMS

### *EATING DISORDERS*

The pediatrician is often the first person to notice the clinical signs and symptoms of an eating disorder. These disorders include anorexia nervosa, bulimia nervosa, and eating disorders not otherwise specified. The criteria for anorexia nervosa and bulimia nervosa can be found in the *Diagnostic and Statistical Manual of Mental Disorders IV* (see pp. 70 and 71). Many children and adolescents meet some but not all of the criteria for these disorders, placing them in a category of eating disorder NOS (not otherwise specified). Adolescent girls are affected most frequently, although boys and younger girls can be affected as well. All these patients require immediate medical and psychosocial attention. A thorough history, including diet history and adolescent HEADSS (home, education, activities, drugs, sex, safety) assessment, and a thorough physical examination are important in determining the extent of the illness. Affected children should have their weight and height recorded on a growth chart, and calculation of body mass index may be useful in following progress after treatment has been initiated.

Physical examination findings in anorexia nervosa may include hypothermia, bradycardia, and hypotension. Other common findings include lanugo, thin hair, cold extremities, and edema. Adolescent females with anorexia nervosa present with either primary or secondary amenorrhea. Patients with bulimia nervosa also may present with bradycardia and hypothermia, and parotid swelling, knuckle abrasions, and dental erosions are common. Children and adolescents in both groups are at risk for cardiac arrhythmias.

Treatment of eating disorders is a complex process that involves an entire team of health-care professionals. Patients with severe malnutrition and/or vital sign abnormalities should be hospitalized for medical stabilization, and close attention should be paid to electrolyte balance and refeeding syndrome. Feeding the patient with a nasogastric tube is often necessary, sometimes for months after the diagnosis. Once the patient is stabilized and has shown adequate weight gain, transfer to an inpatient psychiatric facility for further therapy is indicated. Adolescents with mild malnutrition and normal vital signs can be managed aggressively on an outpatient basis. It is important to have a psychiatrist, a psychologist, or another counselor involved very early in management regardless of inpatient or outpatient status.

### *OBESITY*

Childhood and adolescent obesity is a growing problem whose scope is beyond this chapter (see p. 48). Several factors are important in the development of childhood obesity, including both genetic and environmental influences. A few different methods for the measurement and/or determination of obesity exist, including weight, weight for height, and triceps or subscapular skin-fold thickness. Skin-fold measurements are the best indications of central adipose tissue and related morbidities.

Obesity in childhood and adolescence may produce significant morbidity. Obstructive sleep apnea, poor ventilation, hypertension, and hyperlipidemia are common cardiorespiratory problems. Insulin resistance and early puberty are well-known endocrine complications. Other morbidities, such as coxa vara and slipped capital femoral epiphysis, occur simply because of increased weight. The negative psychological effects of obesity on children and adolescents cannot be overemphasized.

It is important to identify childhood obesity early and initiate appropriate therapy soon after the diagnosis. The approach should be a multidisciplinary one, including dietary management, exercise, psychological counseling, and family involvement.

## VITAMIN AND MINERAL DEFICIENCIES

Older children and adolescents can be at risk for certain vitamin and mineral deficiencies, but these deficiencies tend to differ from those seen in infants and toddlers. School-age children and adolescents who eat a strict vegan diet are at risk for vitamin D and vitamin $B_{12}$ deficiency and iron deficiency. Adolescent females may be at risk for iron-deficiency anemia because of menstrual blood loss. These children and adolescents should be screened and/or treated for these deficiencies. Many adolescents do not get the calcium required for bone mineralization.

Among those who eat a balanced diet, vitamin and mineral deficiencies are rare and supplementation is not necessary. However, it is common for children in these groups to eat a high percentage of fast food, and many do not get the nutrition required for continued growth. It is important to identify eating habits at well-child visits, as the health consequences of improper diets, such as hyperlipidemia and osteoporosis, may become evident in adulthood. Children and adolescents should be encouraged to eat three meals a day and eat a wide variety of foods, including fruits, vegetables, whole grains, and lean meats. Snacks should be encouraged, but snack foods should be limited in fat and processed sugar content.

## BIBLIOGRAPHY

American Academy of Pediatrics, Section on Breastfeeding. Policy statement: Breastfeeding and the use of human milk. *Pediatrics* 115:496–506, 2005.

Burks W. It's an adverse food reaction—but is it allergy? *Contemp Pediatr* 19:71–89, 2002.

Georgieff MK. Taking a rational approach to the choice of formula. *Contemp Pediatr* 18:112–130, 2001.

Kleinman RE, ed. *Pediatric Nutrition Handbook*, 4th ed. Elk Grove Village, IL: Committee on Nutrition, American Academy of Pediatrics, 1998.

# CHAPTER 10

# IMMUNIZATIONS

*Gregory Plemmons*

## ● LEARNING OBJECTIVES

1. List the immunizations currently recommended from birth through adolescence.
2. Describe the benefits, limitations, adverse side effects, and contraindications of each immunization.
3. Explain how immunizations work.
4. Know the difference between active immunity and passive immunity.

No medical intervention has affected the lives of children over the last century more than immunization. The Centers for Disease Control and Prevention (CDC) cited childhood vaccination programs as one of the top 10 achievements in public health in the period 1900–1999. In less than 50 years, we have witnessed the worldwide eradication of smallpox and a rapid decline in morbidity for at least 14 other childhood diseases in the western hemisphere. A glance at the shot records of many current medical students most likely would reveal only seven vaccines, six of which are routinely combined: DTP (diphtheria-tetanus-pertussis), OPV (oral polio vaccine), and MMR (measles-mumps-rubella). Young adults born before the mid-1980s received fewer than 10 "ouchies" before entering medical school; the average infant today will receive almost twice as many, as vaccines against at least six additional diseases (*Haemophilus influenzae* type B, hepatitis B, varicella, *Streptococcus pneumoniae*, *Neisseria meningitidis*, and influenza) are now available. Still more vaccines are being developed. Despite the success of modern immunization programs, however, concerns over vaccine safety, increasing globalization of diseases, and the specter of bioterrorism continue to challenge the health-care delivery system. Even in the twenty-first century, many of these largely preventable diseases are still very much a part of life for infants born today in the Third World and are only a plane ride away for other infants.

## A BRIEF HISTORY

Medical history largely credits Edward Jenner (1749–1823) with developing the first modern vaccine. In Jenner's era, smallpox was as deadly as cancer or heart disease in today's terms and could kill up to 20 percent of the population during outbreaks in urban centers. Jenner made the simple observation that English milkmaids were rarely susceptible to smallpox (variola), theorizing that their exposure to a similar virus, cowpox (vaccinia), at a young age somehow conferred immunity. He later developed the first widely recognized vaccine, even immunizing his son, although inoculation with smallpox as a means of inducing immunity had been practiced worldwide for hundreds and perhaps thousands of years, though not always successfully. It would be at least another 200 years, however, before scientists were successful at creating vaccines against other diseases, and a scientific understanding of how vaccines work is a relatively recent phenomenon.

## HOW IMMUNIZATIONS WORK

Specific immune responses must always begin with *antigens*. In Jenner's time, antigens might have consisted simply of the unsterile material from an unroofed skin lesion. As recently as 50 years ago, the first vaccines against pertussis were manufactured from the sterilized (but complete) killed cells of *Bordetella pertussis* (the original DTP vaccines sometimes are referred to as *whole-cell*). As microbiologic techniques and assays have improved over time, redefining the pathogenesis of disease-causing organisms, vaccines have followed in consort.

Antigens must be presented to the immune system successfully for each immune cell to produce a unique reaction. Not every cell responds in the same way or even responds at all. B cells, for instance, respond poorly to polysaccharide antigens in children under the age of 2 years. T cells not only respond poorly to polysaccharides but also produce cellular rather than humoral (antibody) immunity against pathogens. A working knowledge of the mechanisms of the body's immune responses can go a long way in helping a person understand the sometimes imposingly rigorous childhood immunization schedule. The most up-to-date immunization schedule can be located at http://www.cdc.gov/nip/recs/child-schedule.htm.

## DIPHTHERIA-TETANUS-PERTUSSIS AND HUMORAL IMMUNITY

The first pertussis vaccine was licensed for use in the United States in 1914. However, widespread immunization did not begin until the 1950s, after an inactivated whole-cell pertussis, along with diphtheria and tetanus toxoid, vaccine was introduced in 1949. Immunity against *Bordetella* infection is thought to be primarily humoral and offers an opportunity to illustrate how immunization works. Although it is still debatable which components of *B. pertussis* are most pathogenic (and which specific antibodies are most protective against disease), for the sake of illustration, one can begin with pertussis toxin. Many pathogens contain toxins that modern medicine has been able to alter into *toxoids*, which retain most of their antigenic properties but little if any of their original pathogenic ability. Tetanus toxoid is one example; it cannot produce paralysis but is still remarkably antigenically similar to the real thing. All current pertussis vaccines contain varying amounts of pertussis toxoid (PT).

## THE IMMUNE RESPONSE

It may be helpful to imagine the human immune system as a military response to understand its particular quirks. If one imagines PT as a terrorist, it first stealthily presents itself to people when they are infants, leaving the nurse's injection syringe and entering the intramuscular space of an infant's thighs. The body's monocytes, dendritic cells, and macrophages are the first responders. They nab the intruders and immediately present them to the authorities: B and T cells. Initially, B cells produce immunoglobulin M (IgM) in response. The IgM response can be quick, but it is not very specific; it often does not do a very good job of recognizing the suspect and is also short-lived. For better defense, the help of the body's own CIA, T cells, is required. T cells not only are able to kill certain infected cells by contact, they are able to signal activated B cells to make IgG. Over time, the B cells that have the best information and the greatest ability to capture the antigen become an elite group of plasma cells that can pour out antibody with each successive invasion. In general, the longer the interval between successive "invasions," the stronger the secondary response. The body's "second responders" are weak or do not respond well if "invasions" are rapid. Therefore, DPT vaccine is repeated at 4 and 6 months as a compromise to provide immunity as soon as possible for infants. Immunity after the 6-month dose is thought to be sufficient to last 12 months; immunity after the booster dose (generally given at 15 to 18 months) is thought to be sufficient to last 4 or 5 years.

## MEASLES AND CELL-MEDIATED IMMUNITY

Measles vaccine was licensed in the United States in 1963. Measles vaccine is a live, attenuated vaccine. Although the body produces both IgM and immunoglobulin G (IgG) in response to measles vaccination, cellular immunity, consisting of cytotoxic T cells and possibly natural killer cells, plays a prominent role in immunity as well as recovery from acute infection. Patients with defects in cell-mediated immunity [e.g., human immunodeficiency virus (HIV)-infected individuals] often have progressive measles infections and have a significantly increased risk of death.

Theoretically, T cells are much more long-lived than B cells, and their memory is longer as well (they sometimes are referred to as "mother-in-law" cells). The body has to see the measles virus (or an altered host cell) only once to remember it. Therefore, most people need a single dose of measles vaccine for lifelong protection, and immunity does *not* rely on the humoral booster response needed for pertussis or *Haemophilus*. Interestingly, about 2 to 5 percent of the general population does not respond to the first dose of vaccine, but the majority of these individuals do respond to a second dose. Maternal antibody also has to be considered when one is immunizing infants, since maternal IgG may linger in babies for up to 6 months after birth. Hence, measles vaccine generally is not given before 1 year of age. If it is given earlier, the mother's residual antibody can inhibit the development of the infant's immunity.

## POLIO AND METHODS OF VACCINE ADMINISTRATION

Historically, all vaccines first were given as injections, either intramuscularly or subcutaneously. In 1952, Dr. Jonas Salk introduced an inactivated polio vaccine (IPV), and mass inoculation of schoolchildren began in 1954. The vaccine was an unqualified success. Another physician-scientist, Albert Sabin, later was able to isolate a rare form of poliovirus that would reproduce in the intestinal tract but not in the central nervous system and helped develop a live attenuated vaccine. Oral polio vaccine (OPV) was licensed in 1963 and quickly became the vaccine of choice, since it was cheaper to make and much easier to administer. Theoretically, OPV should be able to induce immunity after one dose, although it soon was noted that replication of one attenuated strain often interfered with the replication of another strain, and several doses were required for maximum immunity. OPV produces *herd immunity* as well in that vaccinated individuals periodically may shed active attenuated virus, which can immunize unvaccinated household members through fecal-oral transmission.

Unfortunately, because live attenuated viruses may replicate actively, by the law of random mutations, an attenuated strain very rarely may revert to a *wild-type* (disease-causing) strain, and an estimated 5 to 10 cases per year of vaccine-associated paralytic polio (VAPP) were reported annually since licensure in 1963 until recently. Because the risk of VAPP, although incredibly small (an estimated one case per 2.4 million doses), now surpasses the risk of naturally occurring polio disease, the CDC recommended switching to an all-IPV schedule in 2000 in the United States. Polio is being eradicated, although at this writing there are still substantial pockets of epidemics in the Third World, and the ease of administration of OPV and herd immunity induction remain invaluable in eliminating the disease in the rest of the world.

## REFINEMENT OF PRODUCTION AND IMPROVEMENTS IN SAFETY

Despite advances in modern biological technology, in some ways the development of childhood vaccines remained anachronistically crude. MMR and influenza vaccines, for instance, still are produced from cell lines that originally were developed in the 1960s and are grown in chick embryos. Even in the early 1980s, the first hepatitis B vaccine was made by taking blood from people who were infected and purifying hepatitis B surface antigen (HBsAg) from the virus. With advances in recombinant DNA technique, antigen could be manufactured in the laboratory so that there would be no risk of contamination with other bloodborne diseases, and the protein could be made in yeast cells, utilizing plasmid technology.

As former childhood killers such as measles and pertussis began to be eliminated through the use of widespread immunization programs, children still remained susceptible to other serious bacterial pathogens, such as *H. influenzae* type B (HIB), *S. pneumoniae,* and *Neisseria meningitidis.* Unfortunately, young infants remain uniquely susceptible to these bacteria. All three organisms can produce sepsis and meningitis, and their pathogenic capacity for destruction and invasion derives in part from their polysaccharide capsule. The original vaccines against *S. pneumoniae* and *Neisseria* were produced from pure carbohydrate (the outer polysaccharide capsule) but were ineffective in young children. Even in older children and adults, these polysaccharide vaccines induce only short-term immunity; protection wanes rapidly and generally is gone by 2 years.

Immature B cells are unable to mount adequate immune responses to polysaccharides before children reach 2 years of age. To overcome this poor immune response, polysaccharide antigens can be chemically linked to protein carriers to increase the immune response. This was accomplished first with the development of the first vaccine against *H. influenzae* type B (HIB vaccine), which was introduced in 1988. The most recent vaccinations introduced into the childhood schedule, the pneumococcal conjugate and meningococcal conjugate vaccines, rely on this technology as well. The challenge in developing an effective pneumococcal vaccine has been to determine which serotypes are most prevalent and virulent, since there are more than 80 distinct polysaccharide capsules of pneumococcus. The current pneumococcal conjugate vaccine includes seven serotypes and sometimes is abbreviated PCV7; the current meningococcal conjugate vaccine includes four serotypes. Conjugate vaccines also have the added advantage over polysaccharide vaccines of reducing nasal colonization as well.

## PASSIVE IMMUNITY

The preceding discussion focused on the active induction of immunity. Active immunity requires several elements: adequate time for the development of a response, a normal host, and an effective vaccine. When any of these elements is not present, passive immunization also may be employed.

### ADEQUATE TIME

For children traveling abroad and very young children, it may be very difficult to produce an adequate immune response in the time period required. For instance, an infant who has just been born to a mother infected with hepatitis B or a 6-month-old child who is traveling to a measles-endemic area of the world both represent unique circumstances that may benefit from passive immunity. A hepatitis B–exposed infant may receive hepatitis B immunoglobulin (HBIG), a human blood product pooled from various donors that confers antibody against hepatitis B. A 6-month-old traveling to the Third World may not be old enough to complete the routine vaccination series and may receive intramuscular gamma globulin to prevent infection.

### A NORMAL HOST

Many children and adults with a chronic immunodeficiency such as agammaglobulinemia rely on the periodic administration of human gamma globulin to prevent infection.

### EFFECTIVE VACCINE

Respiratory syncytial virus (RSV) remains one of the most common causes of pediatric morbidity worldwide and can be devastating to a very premature infant or an infant with congenital heart disease. However, the development of a safe and effective vaccine has been elusive. In the last decade, advances in both the understanding of immunoglobulins and monoclonal antibody technology have led to the introduction of passive immunoprophylaxis against RSV (palivizumab) and even an effective antidote (Digibind) to digitalis toxicity. Since the half-life of IgG ranges from 7 to 23 days, most forms of passive immunization generally require monthly administration and must be given either intramuscularly or intravenously, substantially increasing the cost of vaccination.

## CONTROVERSIES OVER VACCINE SAFETY AND PRODUCTION

As was discussed earlier with regard to polio vaccine, the road to developing safe vaccines has not been smooth. Probably no vaccine will ever come with a 100 percent risk-free guarantee. Paradoxically, as the incidence of preventable diseases plummets and those diseases disappear from memory, public attention has focused on the safety and potential side effects of vaccines, whether real or imagined.

In some ways, vaccines have become victims of their own success; fear of disease inevitably is replaced by fear of vaccines. During the mid-1970s, legal claims of injury by DTP vaccine were made and damages were awarded despite the lack of scientific evidence. As a result, prices soared and several manufacturers halted production. To reduce liability and respond to public health concerns, the National Childhood Vaccine Injury Act (NCVIA) was passed in 1986.

There are several ways in which vaccine safety is monitored continuously. First, vaccines generally are tested extensively in the laboratory before entering human trials. The U.S. Food and Drug Administration (FDA) requires that all vaccines undergo three phases of trials in humans before consideration for licensure. Prelicensure trials generally involve hundreds to thousands of subjects. After licensure, the U.S. government continues to monitor the safety of a vaccine once it has been introduced into the general population through two main methods: the Vaccine Adverse Effect Reporting System (VAERS) and the Vaccine Safety Datalink (VSD) Project. VAERS is essentially a passive reporting mechanism. Anyone (including parents) who suspects that immunization may have caused an adverse event may file a report, and VAERS data are monitored continuously to look for trends. Since this is a passive system and relies on individual reporting, the CDC also partnered with several large health maintenance organizations (HMOs) in 1990 to form the VSD to monitor actively those rare side effects which might go undetected by VAERS.

## SIDE EFFECTS

The risks of vaccination are generally mild but in very rare instances may be substantial. Redness and soreness at the injection site are fairly common.

Systemic reactions to vaccines are, fortunately, much rarer. Some reactions are unique to the individual vaccine. For instance, MMR may produce a mild rash and/or fever 1 to 2 weeks after the injection; varicella may produce a very slight eruption, often at the site of injection.

## CONTRAINDICATIONS

Allergies to certain trace products that may be unique to each vaccine potentially could produce anaphylaxis. For several years, it was thought that individuals with egg allergy should not receive MMR vaccine since it is derived in part from chick embryos, but recent studies indicate that the risk of anaphylaxis is low, and so egg allergy no longer is considered a contraindication. Each vaccine may have specific contraindications. The recipient and the household always must be considered as well. Live virus vaccines may be contraindicated in certain instances, specifically in immunosuppressed children and in household contacts (e.g., siblings) of immunosuppressed individuals.

## OTHER CONTROVERSIES

Thimerosal is a mercury-containing preservative that has been used in some vaccines since the 1930s to maintain sterility and prolong shelf life. No adverse effects have been reported from the amounts used in vaccine production to date except for minor reactions such as redness and swelling at the injection site. However, in 1999, the Public Health Service (PHS) agencies, the American Academy of Pediatrics (AAP), and vaccine manufacturers agreed that thimerosal should be reduced or eliminated in vaccines as a precautionary measure because of growing evidence that mercury could be more toxic to developing infants and children than had been postulated previously. All immunizations administered to children are now generally thimerosal-free.

Perhaps there has been no greater controversy than that involving MMR and autism. In 1998, the question of a connection between MMR vaccine and autism was raised in a very small study involving only 12 children. In 2004, 10 of the 13 authors of the original study (as well as the *Lancet*) retracted the study's interpretation, and the Institute of Medicine (IOM) and the AAP also have concluded that there was no causal relationship. Some parents may object to vaccination on religious grounds, citing evidence that some of the human cell-line cultures used during the production of vaccines such as varicella, rabies, inactivated polio virus, and hepatitis A originated from fetal tissue obtained from legal abortions in the 1960s, although no additional aborted fetuses have been used since then.

## SPECIFIC VACCINES

### DIPHTHERIA TOXOID, TETANUS TOXOID, AND ACELLULAR PERTUSSIS VACCINES (DTaP)

Two acellular pertussis vaccines are currently licensed in the United States. Two DTaP vaccines are currently available in combination with others (DTaP/HIB and DTaP/IPV/hepatitis B). Seizures, hypotonic-hypotensive episodes, high fever, and prolonged crying episodes have been reported as side effects but are much rarer with the new acellular vaccines. Limb swelling also has been reported rarely with the fourth and fifth dose, although this appears to be harmless and self-limiting.

### INACTIVATED POLIO VACCINE

There is currently one inactivated polio vaccine licensed in the United States. No serious reactions are known to occur after the administration of IPV.

### MEASLES, MUMPS, AND RUBELLA

One MMR vaccine is currently licensed in the United States. MMR vaccine is given after the first birthday, as most infants have passive maternal protection at least until 9 months of age. Transient rashes and, very rarely, transient thrombocytopenia have been reported with measles vaccine. Twenty-five to 50 percent of non-rubella-immune adults have reported mild arthritis after initial vaccination; these symptoms are generally transient and self-limiting.

### HAEMOPHILUS INFLUENZAE TYPE B VACCINE

HIB was the first conjugate vaccine to be introduced into the childhood schedule. The incidence of *Haemophilus* meningitis and childhood epiglottitis has fallen remarkably since its introduction in 1988. Three vaccines are currently available in the United States, one as a combination product (DTaP/HIB). Reported side effects have been exceedingly rare.

### HEPATITIS B VACCINE (HBV)

There are currently two vaccines licensed for use in the United States. One is currently available as a combination product (DTaP/IPV/Hepatitis B). Hepatitis B vaccines have 90 to 95 percent efficacy and may be given as early as birth. Reported adverse effects have been minimal.

### VARICELLA VACCINE (VZV)

Although varicella infection is generally a mild illness, before the introduction of the vaccine, an estimated 50 to 100 children died per year, often from complications of the disease. The vaccine was introduced into the United States in 1996; currently one form is licensed for use. It is a live attenuated virus, but the risk of transmission of vaccine virus appears to be very low.

## PNEUMOCOCCAL CONJUGATE VACCINE (PCV7)

One conjugate vaccine against *S. pneumoniae* is currently licensed in the United States and confers immunity against seven serotypes. Since its introduction in 2000, it has reduced the incidence of serious bacterial illness (pneumonia, sepsis, meningitis) significantly and has had a modest effect on otitis media, particularly chronic otitis, as well.

## INFLUENZA VACCINE

Influenza continues to cause significant morbidity and mortality worldwide, particularly among the elderly as well as the very young (under 2 years). Because of the significant risk to young children, influenza was added to the routine childhood schedule in 2004, unfortunately during a shortage of vaccine in the United States. An intranasal live preparation is available for children over 5 years of age.

## MENINGOCOCCAL CONJUGATE VACCINE

The first conjugated vaccine against *N. meningitidis* was licensed by the FDA in early 2005 and has been recommended for all children beginning at age 11 to 12 years and teens entering high school, as well as college freshmen living in dormitories.

## OPTIONAL VACCINES

## PNEUMOCOCCAL POLYSACCHARIDE VACCINE (PS23)

One vaccine containing 23 polysaccharide serotypes is currently available in the United States and is recommended for individuals at high risk for pneumococcal disease or its complications (e.g., sickle cell disease, immunodeficiencies, asplenia, individuals age 65 years or older).

## MENINGOCOCCAL POLYSACCHARIDE VACCINE

One vaccine containing four polysaccharide serotypes is currently available in the United States. Traditionally, it has been recommended only for high-risk groups as well as individuals such as college students or military recruits who will be living in crowded quarters for the first time.

## PALIVIZUMAB

Palivizumab is a monoclonal antibody product that confers partial immunity against respiratory syncytial virus and is associated with a 40 to 55 percent reduction in RSV hospitalizations. Currently, it is indicated for those infants at highest risk for RSV complications, including premature infants and infants with significant congenital heart disease, and must be administered monthly throughout the RSV season.

## RESPIRATORY SYNCYTIAL VIRUS IMMUNE GLOBULIN INTRAVENOUS (RSV-IGIV)

RSV-IGIV is a human pooled immunoglobulin product that acts against RSV. Like palivizumab, it must be given monthly and additionally must be administered intravenously. It is contraindicated in infants with congenital heart disease.

## HEPATITIS B IMMUNE GLOBULIN (HBIG)

HBIG confers some short-term protection and is indicated in specific post-exposure circumstances (e.g., infants born to mothers who are hepatitis B–positive or whose status is unknown, known exposure). It is a pooled human blood product and must be given intramuscularly.

## ON THE HORIZON

Despite significant progress, several challenges remain in the eradication of disease. Pertussis outbreaks still occur, and the disease remains deadly for the very young. Researchers currently are focusing on introducing pertussis vaccine early in infancy as well as considering booster shots for teens and adults. The continued proliferation of new vaccines has led to the challenge of developing combination vaccines; this often can be difficult, since immunogenicity sometimes is diminished with such products.

Despite better and safer vaccines, the immunity conferred by these miraculous wonders is only as good as the immunization rates and the health-care delivery system. An estimated 25 percent of children in the United States remain either unimmunized or partially immunized according to the recommended childhood schedule. Because well-child care frequently is fragmented, the focus has shifted to the creation of immunization registries and the use of informatics to streamline delivery and boost immunization rates. Finally, misinformation, often derived from the Internet, continues to make parents anxious and threatens to unravel the safety net that childhood immunizations have provided for the last century. Serious outbreaks still occur abroad as well as domestically. For now, the benefits of vaccination far outweigh the risks.

## BIBLIOGRAPHY

Centers for Disease Control and Prevention. *Child and Adolescent Immunization Schedule.* http://www.cdc.gov/nip/recs/child-schedule.htm.

Committee on Infectious Diseases. *Red Book: 2003 Report of the Committee on Infectious Diseases,* 26th ed. Elk Grove Village, IL: American Academy of Pediatrics, 2003.

# CHILD ABUSE

*Aida Yared*

## LEARNING OBJECTIVES

1. List the characteristics of the history that should trigger concern about possible abuse.

2. List the physical and behavioral signs of physical, sexual, and psychological abuse and neglect.

3. Understand the importance of a full, detailed, carefully obtained history and physical examination in the evaluation of child abuse.

## OVERVIEW OF CHILD MALTREATMENT

### INTRODUCTION

Child maltreatment is legally defined as "an act (or failure to act) by a parent, caregiver, or other person as defined under State Law that results in physical abuse, neglect, medical neglect, sexual abuse, emotional abuse or as an act (or failure to act) which presents an imminent risk of harm to a child."

Child maltreatment can take a variety of forms. The most common (60 percent) is child neglect. Less common are physical abuse (20 percent) and sexual abuse (10 percent); other forms (e.g., emotional abuse, bullying) account for the rest of the cases. The children who come to medical attention represent only a fraction of the real problem.

Child maltreatment is a problem of enormous magnitude, spanning all ethnic groups, cultural backgrounds, and social strata. The U.S. government has in place a state agency in charge of Child Protective Services (CPS). The terminology for child maltreatment is standardized by the National Child Abuse and Neglect Data System (NCANDS). It is the duty of anyone suspecting child abuse (neighbor, teacher, health-care professional) to report it. In 2003, CPS received 2.9 million referrals for suspected child abuse involving 5.5 million children; of those referrals, 900,000 were substantiated and 1500 children died. Some 2500 children daily are victims of child abuse, and 4 die of it.

It is the duty of anyone suspecting child abuse to report it to CPS. In the United States, 50 percent of referrals are made by professionals (teachers, health-care workers, or law enforcement officers) and 50 percent by nonprofessionals (friends, family members, or neighbors).

## EPIDEMIOLOGY

### VICTIMS

Victims of child maltreatment span all age groups; however, the risk is highest with younger age, and 10 percent of the victims are infants < 1 year of age. The incidence among children 0 to 3 years of age is 16 cases per 1000 children per year; that number decreases to 6 in 1000 in 15- to 17-year-olds. Victims are equally boys and girls.

Among the 1500 children who die every year as a result of child maltreatment, most are infants, with the majority (80 percent) younger than 4 years, with a slight male preponderance; 10 percent are 4 to 7, 5 percent 8 to 11, and 5 percent 12 to 17 years of age. More than a third of fatalities (35 percent) are due to neglect, 30 percent to physical abuse, and 30 percent to a combination of the two. Half the victims are Caucasian.

Risk factors for being a victim include young age and a vulnerable child; children with an underlying disability (mental or physical) or a behavior problem constitute 6.5 percent of all cases.

### PERPETRATORS

The vast majority (80 percent) of perpetrators are parents (biological, step, or foster parents), 6 percent are relatives, and 4 percent are unmarried partners of a parent. Perpetrators are as likely to be males as females, though the type of abuse varies with the sex of the perpetrator. The mean age of perpetrators is the early thirties. The majority (80 percent) are parents, equally mothers and fathers. Some 75 percent of perpetrators who were friends or neighbors committed sexual abuse.

Risk factors for being a perpetrator include the following:

- Having been abused as a child
- Stress, such as unemployment and poverty
- Drug and/or alcohol abuse
- Social isolation

Münchausen by proxy is an uncommon but an extremely serious form of child abuse in which inflicted injuries are made to mimic medical problems. The variety of injuries is endless, from injection with fecal-contaminated needles to spraying bug spray into a child's eyes, pouring hot water into a cast, reporting high blood pressure readings, and partially smothering a child to induce "apnea." Such injuries can be very difficult to sort out, especially when the inflicting parent has a medical background.

## HISTORY

Most cases of child abuse do not come to medical attention and are handled by CPS. Some cases are referred by CPS for medical evaluation, a child may be brought by a parent or relative for evaluation of injuries, or injuries may be noticed incidentally during a medical visit. If a child has significant bruising on examination, the parents always should be asked how it happened.

The chart in a case of suspected child maltreatment is an important legal document, and medical students in many hospitals are precluded from writing in it. Documentation should be careful, even circumstantial. The place where and time that the history was obtained, as well as listing of all people present and their relation to the child, should be included.

### PRESENT ILLNESS

It is advised to quote verbatim the parent's statements, using quotation marks. It is important to try to obtain a history from both parents separately, if possible, to detect any discrepancies suggesting deception.

In addition to the history surrounding the injuries and the usual review of systems, documentation should include the following:

- Developmental history
- Past medical history of injuries
- Social history, including household composition, employment of parents and their hours, and a list of alternative caretakers

### INTERVIEW OF THE CHILD

An older child may be asked to explain his or her injuries, with "leading" questions avoided. Rather than "Who hit you here?" the child should be asked: "How did that happen?" If the answers raise suspicion of abuse, further interviewing may be assigned to specially trained health-care workers. At times, a child may disclose abuse spontaneously to the physician during a visit. The medical record should clearly document who was present in the room, what prompted the disclosure, and the exact words spoken in quotation marks.

Elements that raise suspicion of child abuse include the following:

- Important injuries of which the parent is not aware
- Important injuries the parent tries to minimize
- A parent who tries to hush or contradict a child
- Injuries that do not conform to the history given
- A history that is vague or changing
- A history that does not match the developmental stage of the infant, for example, a child < 1 year old reported to be running or a toddler tipping over a heavy object

## PHYSICAL EXAMINATION

### GENERAL EXAMINATION

Documentation includes items not usually noted during routine visits, such as the state of cleanliness of the child and the clothes in which he or she is dressed.

#### GROWTH PARAMETERS

The height and weight of a child are general measures of parental attention and growth. Head circumference is important as chronic abusive injuries or a past injury may result in obstructive hydrocephalus.

#### SURFACE INJURIES

The whole body should be examined, and any lesions carefully documented. Abusive injuries can take a variety of forms, including bruises, bite marks, burns, and cuts. A careful description of each lesion (size, shape, and location, as well as the parental explanation of its cause) should be noted. This is most easily done by using a "bodygram." Attention should be paid to possible patterns that suggest abuse, such as hand or finger imprints that would confirm slapping or grabbing, belt buckles, or ropes. Burns that have a clearly defined border ("sock" or "glove") are highly suggestive of abuse.

## LABORATORY EVALUATION

Few laboratory studies usually are required to document abuse. Laboratory data may be useful in cases of malnutrition to rule out an underlying medical condition. In cases of documented sexual abuse, specimens may be obtained; the specimens have to follow a chain of evidence procedure to be accepted as evidence in court.

### LABORATORY AND RADIOLOGIC EVALUATION

Radiologic studies are rarely needed in cases of child neglect or sexual abuse. They are essential in the evaluation of physical injuries.

## MANAGEMENT

The physician should consult with the following professionals:

- A medical team on call for child abuse evaluations if available
- Social worker or Child Protective Services
- In criminal cases, the police or law enforcement agency
- In sexual abuse cases, a rape crisis counselor or other mental health professional

Inpatient care is recommended if the child's safety is a concern or if the child has an acute traumatic injury requiring inpatient treatment.

Regardless of the seriousness of the clinical findings, an important focus is the safety of the child. A "safety plan" may be put in place until a final assessment has been made. Thus, a child with minor injuries may be admitted to the hospital until it is determined whether she or he can be returned safely to the usual caretakers.

After the assessment or investigation, CPS decides on the *disposition*: the determination of whether the available evidence is sufficient to conclude that maltreatment has occurred or is at risk of occurring.

Some children need to be placed in *foster care*, which is defined as substitute care away from parents or guardians for which the state agency has placement and care responsibility. This includes family foster homes, relatives of the child, group homes, and emergency shelters regardless of whether the facility is licensed or financially compensated. All children in care for more than 24 h are considered to be in foster care.

## PREVENTION

The prevention of child maltreatment is a complex social issue. In addition to evaluating suspected or confirmed abuse, CPS provides preventive services to families at risk, such as respite care, family visits, day care, and counseling, as well as "postresponse" or remedial services such as counseling, family support, and at-home services. Among the children not found to be the victims of child maltreatment, some 25 percent receive postresponse services.

## CHILD NEGLECT

### INTRODUCTION

A neglected child most commonly presents to medical attention with failure to thrive (FTT): poor growth or development. FTT that occurs in the absence of an underlying medical problem is termed nonorganic failure to thrive (NOFTT).

## EPIDEMIOLOGY

NOFTT can be due to poverty and lack of resources. Often the family has limited access to social support and resources. Unemployment, drug or alcohol use, and social isolation are often present.

## DIFFERENTIAL DIAGNOSIS

The differential diagnosis of NOFTT includes gastrointestinal problems (severe gastroesophageal reflux disease, chronic diarrhea from maldigestion, and malabsorption, including cystic fibrosis), chronic infections [including urinary tract infections and human immunodeficiency virus (HIV)], neurologic diseases with hypotonia and poor swallowing, renal disease (renal tubular acidosis, chronic renal failure), and endocrine problems (hypothyroidism). An unbalanced diet (typically excessive intake of juices) may result in FTT.

## HISTORY

In addition to the standard history, a detailed nutrition history should be obtained. It includes access to and availability of nutrients. A detailed food diary should be kept, including the types of foods used (ready-made, powdered, or concentrated formula), the method of preparation, and the amount and schedule of feeds.

## PHYSICAL EXAMINATION

### GROWTH PARAMETERS

The hallmark of child neglect is a disproportionate loss of weight compared to height or head circumference growth.

### GENERAL EXAMINATION

The physical examination of a child with suspected neglect or NOFTT should have two foci: identifying whether an underlying medical problem may explain the child's condition and documenting physical findings that suggest neglect.

The clothing of the child should be observed, and note should be made of clothes that are shabby or dirty or incongruous with the prevailing weather. Severe occipital alopecia suggests that a child is seldom picked up. A child whose diapers are changed infrequently may have an unattended diaper rash, often with candidal superinfection.

The physical examination may disclose an underlying medical problem such as a heart murmur in congenital heart disease; adenopathy or hepatosplenomegaly in chronic infection, including HIV; and abnormal muscle tone, which may indicate an underlying neurologic problem.

## FEEDING PATTERN

Observation of feeding helps identify a neurologic problem precluding adequate intake or demonstrates significant gastroesophageal reflux. A child with NOFTT is often an avid feeder.

## PARENT-CHILD INTERACTION

The level of attention of the parent to the child and the parent's willingness to (and effectiveness in) comfort an upset child should be noted. Observations that a parent is withdrawn, unworried, or absent from the bedside may be clues to poor parental bonding.

## LABORATORY AND RADIOLOGIC EVALUATION

Laboratory evaluation may include a complete blood count (CBC) (looking for anemia), a chemistry profile (looking for renal tubular acidosis or chronic renal failure), and albumin level (a low serum prealbumin level indicates chronic malnutrition). Stool examination may be helpful, and sweat chloride may be performed if indicated

Radiologic studies rarely are needed in cases of child neglect but may include a videofluoroscopic swallowing study, upper gastrointestinal (GI) studies, or head imaging. A skeletal survey is not done routinely unless there is suspicion of physical abuse.

## MANAGEMENT

A child with NOFTT often is managed as an outpatient. In unclear cases, a child may be admitted to observe feedings and parent-child interaction. A child with NOFTT will thrive in a hospital or another nurturing environment. Access to ad libitum adequate nutrition often results in "catch-up" growth, which is defined as the crossing of percentiles on growth curves. Rarely, a child with extreme malnutrition (marasmus or kwashiorkor) may need a gradual and careful program of refeeding.

## PREVENTION

The prevention of child neglect may include public health education concerning child nutrition, avoidance of excess juices or junk foods, and a safety net for families with limited resources.

## PHYSICAL ABUSE (SHAKEN BABY SYNDROME)

## INTRODUCTION

Physical abuse is referred to as both nonaccidental trauma (NAT) and battered child syndrome. The best terminology to use may be *inflicted injuries*.

Physical abuse resulting in central nervous system (CNS) injuries often is referred to as shaken baby syndrome (SBS).

## PATHOPHYSIOLOGY

Shaken baby syndrome, first described by John Caffey in 1972, commonly is ascribed to vigorous shaking of an infant or young child who usually is held by the arms or shoulders. Its hallmarks are intracranial bleeding (subdural or subarachnoid hemorrhages) and retinal hemorrhages. A child's brain is vulnerable to injury because the head is large and relatively heavy and the neck muscles are weak. There is ongoing controversy about whether "shaking" is the sole or even a major pathophysiologic mechanism, as isolated "impact," such as slamming down the child against a hard surface, may produce identical findings.

An estimated 1200 to 1400 cases of SBS occur each year in the United States, of which 10 to 25 percent result in death. Most victims are newborn to 5 years old, on average 6 to 8 months old. The helplessness of a young infant, compounded by frustration from a baby's intractable crying, has been described as a common scenario. Thus, "infantile colic" seems to be a situation of risk for inflicted injuries. Frustration over toilet training is an additional risk.

## DIFFERENTIAL DIAGNOSIS

The differential diagnosis of physical abuse includes the following:

- Accidental injuries such as falls. Bruises over the shins or the forehead may be accidental, whereas bruises over the back or buttocks may not.
- Accidental burns such as spilling of hot water and accidentally touching a hot oven. Burns that conform to a "sock" or "glove" pattern suggest forced immersion; hand bruises that involve the palmar creases suggest forcible holding over a hot surface. Significant burns, even if not inflicted by the parents, raise the concern of child neglect or an unsafe environment.
- Folk remedies such as cupping and coining.
- Bleeding diathesis such as thrombocytopenia.
- Impetigo may mimic cigarette burns.
- Cephalohematoma is a common birth injury (a subperiosteal bleed in a cranial bone) that may be accompanied by a linear skull fracture. A cephalohematoma may resolve incompletely with time and raise erroneous concern about child abuse at a subsequent well-child visit.
- Osteogenesis imperfecta often is suggested as an alternative diagnosis in children with multiple fractures. It is an extremely rare genetic disorder of collagen formation that causes fractures with minor injuries.

## HISTORY

Inflicted bruises or fractures often come to medical attention disguised as accidents.

A baby with SBS often is brought in with the chief complaint of a fall, difficulty breathing, seizures, vomiting, altered consciousness, or choking. Severe cases may be lethargic or unconscious, and the parent may report that the child was shaken to try to resuscitate it.

Chronic SBS may be missed or misdiagnosed, and subtle symptoms of poor feeding, episodic vomiting, or fussiness may be attributed to viral illnesses, feeding dysfunction, or infant colic.

The past medical history includes previous injuries and involvement of CPS with the family.

## PHYSICAL EXAMINATION

*Growth parameters.* The height and weight of a child are general measures of growth, reflecting parental care. Head circumference and fontanel size are important parameters, as chronic abusive injuries or a past injury may result in obstructive hydrocephalus. A bulging fontanel indicates high intracranial pressure from intracranial bleeding or brain edema.

*Surface injuries* such as bruises, scars, and burns should be carefully documented, and photographs should be taken for later reference. Special attention should be given to describing their distribution and whether a pattern (e.g., imprints of fingers) can be defined. Some patterns of superficial injuries are highly suggestive of child abuse, including finger marks, burns, and whipping injuries. Burns that have a clearly defined border ("sock" or "glove") or conform to a cigarette tip are highly suggestive of abuse.

*Ophthalmologic examination* may reveal retinal hemorrhages, one of the hallmarks of SBS. Funduscopic examination should be performed by an experienced ophthalmologist, and photographs should be taken for later reference.

*Neurologic examination* includes muscle tone, reflexes, and cranial nerve examination. Mental examination should include a clear documentation of the presence of pain.

*Musculoskeletal examination.* Point tenderness over or reluctance to move an extremity may indicate an underlying fracture.

## LABORATORY AND RADIOLOGIC EVALUATION

The laboratory workup of a child with surface injuries may include a CBC and bleeding studies.

A child with suspected physical abuse requires a skeletal survey, looking for multiple fractures or fractures of different ages that would strengthen the diagnosis of inflicted injuries. Rib fractures suggest forceful grasping of a child.

Spiral fractures indicate a torsional force applied to a bone. They may occur accidentally, but in the right context it indicate a twisting injury.

Computed tomography (CT) and magnetic resonance imaging (MRI) may be indicated in cases of suspected SBS, looking for subarachnoid or subdural hematoma. In chronic SBS, obstructive hydrocephalus may be present.

## MANAGEMENT

Medical management is dictated by the injuries that are present. Often it is advisable to have the managing medical team be separate from the "child abuse" consultants. Medical management may involve orthopedics, neurosurgery, or surgery teams, depending on the injuries present.

Social management was outlined above and may include a criminal investigation, a safety plan, and foster care placement.

SBS results in fatality in 10 to 25 percent of severe cases, and it is estimated that only 10 to 15 percent of shaken babies recover completely. Besides emotional trauma, many surviving children have permanent disabilities that range from feeding disorders, behavior problems, and partial or complete loss of vision to palsies or a permanent vegetative state. Thus, long-term management may include occupational, physical, and speech therapy and special education services.

## PREVENTION

Some experts believe that SBS is primarily the result of anger felt by an adult, culminating in loss of impulse control, and that the perpetrator is aware of the potential harm to the child in that an ordinary person would recognize the action as potentially dangerous. Other experts believe that the perpetrator may be unaware of the dangers of shaking. Thus, the prevention of SBS may include support to high-risk families and the availability of quality child care as well as education of parents and caretakers on the dangers of shaking an infant.

Parents should receive information about SBS prevention in the hospital and/or at well-child visits. Child caregivers, teenage baby-sitters, and respite workers should be aware of the dangers of shaking a child.

Pediatricians should ask parents routinely about the stress of adjusting to a new baby and teach them strategies for comforting a fussy infant. Helpful resources for parents include CHILDHELP (800-4-ACHILD) and the National Child Abuse Hotline (800-422-4453).

## SEXUAL ABUSE

### INTRODUCTION

Child sexual abuse (CSA) is defined by the American Academy of Pediatrics as engaging a child in sexual activities that the child cannot comprehend, for which the child is developmentally unprepared and cannot give informed consent, and that violate social taboos. The legal age of consent varies by state.

CPS receives 80,000 to 90,000 referrals of suspected CSA yearly. The actual number of cases is undeniably higher as many remain unrecognized or unreported. Overall, it is estimated that one in four girls and one in six boys will experience an episode of sexual abuse by the time they become adults.

## EPIDEMIOLOGY

CSA can be "contact abuse," either nonpenetrating (e.g., kissing, fondling) or penetrating (e.g., penile, digital, and object insertion into the vagina, mouth, or anus); it also can involve nonpenetrating injury. CSA also can consist of "noncontact abuse" such as exhibitionism, voyeurism, and sharing pornography. In the majority of cases of CSA, there are no physical findings.

CSA can take place within the family, performed by a parent, stepparent, sibling, or other relative, or outside the home perpetrated by a friend, neighbor, child-care worker, teacher, or adult leader. The perpetrator is rarely a stranger to the child. Female perpetrators are uncommon in this form of abuse.

Risk factors in addition to those outlined above include the following:

- Multiple caretakers for a child
- Caretaker or parent who has multiple sexual partners
- Social isolation and family secrecy

Correctly diagnosing CSA is often complex and difficult. For all these reasons, appropriately trained health professionals always should be consulted.

## DIFFERENTIAL DIAGNOSIS

The following are parts of the differential diagnosis:

- Normal behavior, including age-appropriate masturbation and self-exploration.
- Irritation, including vaginitis resulting from poor hygiene or chemical urethritis (bubble baths). Toilet tissue retained in the vagina may cause discharge or vaginal bleeding.
- Infectious vaginitis (shigella, group A streptococcus, pinworms).
- Urinary tract infection.
- Accidental straddle injury.
- Self-placed vaginal foreign body or retained toilet paper in the vaginal introitus.
- Urethral prolapse.
- Genital warts in a child under age 2 years may be due to acquisition of human papillomavirus (HPV) from the mother during birth.
- Parental false allegations, which are common in custody battles.

## HISTORY

CSA may present in several ways:

The child may disclose information to a child friend, parent or caretaker.
A parent may notice abnormalities in the child's genital area, including injuries, genital warts, or an abnormal vaginal discharge.
With increasing age the child may exhibit unusual behaviors, such as
- Unreasonable fear of a person or place, unusual separation anxiety (refusal to go to day care or school), sleep disturbance or nightmares
- Unreasonable fear of genital contact (e.g., if a parent tries to change or wipe the child) or physical examination
- Sudden unusual interest in sexual matters, including words, drawings, or games
- Overtly sexual or seductive behavior, including attempts to get other children to perform sexual acts
- Secretiveness, depression, or conduct disorders

The most important determinant for abuse is the child's (or a witness's) account of the incident. An interview should be delayed until it can be performed by a specially trained professional. In addition to the child's story, information should be obtained from any other reliable source.

In adolescents, a gynecologic history should be obtained to include last menstrual period (LMP) and the possibility of a pregnancy, history of consensual sexual activity, use of contraception, and prior sexually transmitted disease (STDs).

## PHYSICAL EXAMINATION

The physical findings of CSA are often minimal or absent.

*General physical examination.* Wrists and ankles should be examined carefully for bruises indicating restraint. The examination of the external genitalia should occur as part of the natural progression of the complete head-to-toe pediatric examination. The male genitalia can be examined with the child supine or standing.

*Genital examination.* A genital examination should be performed by a well-trained evaluator for two reasons: to make sure the examination itself is not a traumatic experience and because the examiner needs familiarity with normal variations in the appearance of (female) genitalia versus pathology. Often only an external examination of the genital and rectal area is necessary, looking for trauma or STDs (vaginal or rectal inflammation or discharge).

## LABORATORY EVALUATION

A rape kit should be used if the child presents for an examination within 96 h of a sexual assault. It has a specific protocol, including a chain of evidence procedure.

Cultures for STDs should be obtained if there is any vaginal or penile discharge.

Serology for syphilis [e.g., Venereal Disease Research Laboratories (VDRL), rapid plasma reagin (RPR),] should be obtained at the time of abuse (if the child is at risk) and 6 to 12 weeks later.

Testing for HIV should be considered in areas of high prevalence and if the alleged perpetrator is known to be positive or a drug user. It should be repeated 3, 6, and 12 months later and antiretroviral therapy should be considered.

## MANAGEMENT

Life-threatening physical injuries resulting from CSA are unusual. Most of the morbidity of CSA is psychological. Referral or consultation for mental health or other counseling should be made in almost every case of child sexual abuse.

Prophylaxis usually is not indicated for STDs in prepubertal children but may be considered in adolescents. Children with gonococcal infection or *Chlamydia trachomatis* should be treated for both infections and tested for syphilis, hepatitis B, and HIV. HIV prophylaxis may be required in some cases.

Hepatitis B vaccination or immunoprophylaxis should be given if indicated.

Possible pregnancy and options should be discussed with a pubertal sexual assault victim.

## PREVENTION

Parents can prevent or lessen the chance of CSA by doing the following:

- Teaching children about the privacy of their own bodies
- Discouraging one-on-one adult-child encounters and implementing a "buddy system"
- Teaching children not to keep secrets that make them uncomfortable
- Teaching children that respect does not mean blind obedience to adults and to authority

## BIBLIOGRAPHY

Adams JA, Harper K, Knudson S, et al: Examination findings in legally confirmed child sexual abuse: It's normal to be normal. *Pediatrics* 94(3):310–317, 1994.

American Academy of Pediatrics, Committee on Child Abuse and Neglect. Guidelines for the evaluation of sexual abuse of children: Subject review. *Pediatrics* 103:186–191, 1999.

American Academy of Pediatrics, Committee on Child Abuse and Neglect. Shaken baby syndrome: Inflicted cerebral trauma. *Pediatrics* 92:872–875, 1993.

Houry D. Violence-inflicted injuries: Reporting laws in the fifty states. *Ann Emerg Med* 39:56–60, 2002.

U.S. Department of Health and Human Services, Administration for Children and Families. *Child Maltreatment 2003*. Washington, DC: U.S. Department of Health and Human Services. Administration for Children and Families, 2005.

# CHILD ADVOCACY

## Sandra M. Sanguino

### LEARNING OBJECTIVES

1. Define advocacy.
2. Describe barriers to health care.
3. List the ways in which one can advocate for patients in the office setting.

## INTRODUCTION

The goal of pediatrics is to promote the health and well-being of children and their families. In addition to providing direct clinical care to patients and their families, physicians have a public health role in which they serve as patient and family advocates. Pediatrics is unique in that children are unable to advocate for themselves. Because of this, one of the roles of pediatricians is to advocate for children and families on the individual, community, national, and global levels.

There are many definitions of child advocacy. One definition is that child advocacy is the promotion and protection of the rights of children. The role of advocacy as a key component of the profession of pediatrics has a long history. Abraham Jacobi, one of the fathers of pediatrics, was a leading child advocate in his time. He was the founder of the first free pediatric clinic in the United States and was instrumental in improving the health and well-being of children at that time.

The increasing importance of the role of child advocacy in pediatrics is evident in its prominence in pediatric residency training. The Accreditation Council for Graduate Medical Education (ACGME) has stated that in pediatric residency programs, "[t]here must be a structured educational experience that prepares residents for the role of advocate for the health of children within the community."

The field of pediatrics is filled with numerous examples of successful advocacy efforts. Child restraint laws and the "Back to Sleep" campaign for the prevention of sudden infant death syndrome are two successful examples. Pediatrics continues to advocate for children in many ways. Common advocacy issues include injury and violence prevention, child abuse, obesity, and tobacco use, to name a few. An issue that has a long history of advocacy efforts is access to care for all children. The next section of this chapter outlines some of the barriers that affect care for children.

## BARRIERS TO CARE

### FINANCIAL

There are numerous financial, geographic, and cultural issues that prevent all children from receiving appropriate health care and cause them to have poorer health outcomes. The principal determinant of a child's access to heath care is the ability of his or her family to obtain health insurance. In 2000, approximately 8.4 million children were uninsured. That accounted for nearly 20 percent of all uninsured individuals. Hispanic children (21 percent) were much more likely to be uninsured than were non-Hispanic Caucasian children (7.4 percent), African-American children (14 percent), or Asian children (12.4 percent).

Nearly 30 percent of uninsured children are in families living below the federal poverty level. Another 33 percent of uninsured children are in families with an income between 100 and 200 percent of the federal poverty level. Currently 21.4 million children are covered by a form of public health insurance. Approximately 4.8 million children are insured by the State Children's Health Insurance program (SCHIP). SCHIP was created in 1997 to cover children in families that exceed Medicaid eligibility requirements but cannot afford private insurance. SCHIP is financed by a combination of state and federal funds. Despite the Medicaid and SCHIP programs, approximately 5 million eligible children remain uninsured. The American Academy of Pediatrics continues to advocate for universal health coverage for all children.

### CULTURAL AND LANGUAGE ISSUES

Cultural differences between the patient and the physician can affect the doctor-patient relationship and, consequently, access to health care. Patients and their families have culturally based ideas about health, disease, and illness. Physicians have their own sets of beliefs based on their own culture. Cultural differences may become barriers to access to care. Cultural differences in verbal and nonverbal communication also can present a barrier to care. Verbal language is key to communication. Language often is cited as a barrier to health care. According to the 2000 Census, approximately 45 million people in the United States speak a language other than English at home and approximately 19 million are limited in English proficiency.

Title VI of the Civil Rights Act of 1964 requires that physicians make the best attempt at communicating with patients. Additionally, the federal government requires any health-care provider who receives federal funding from the U.S. Department of Health and Human Services to communicate with patients effectively or risk losing funding. These are referred to as the Culturally and Linguistically Appropriate Services (CLAS) standards. Several of these standards pertain to individuals with limited English proficiency. One of the standards states that "health care organizations must offer and provide language assistance services, including bilingual staff and interpreter services, at no cost to each patient/consumer with limited English proficiency at all points of contact, in a timely manner during all hours of operation." Currently there is no funding to ensure that this standard can be met. In the absence of funding to pay for live or telephonic interpreters, many people rely on bilingual family members or untrained interpreters. This may lead to problems in communication and further barriers to care. Problems in nonverbal communication also may lead to barriers to care. Nonverbal communication may have different meanings in different cultures. For example, in parts of Asia people may nod out of respect, not necessarily because they understand what has been said.

Problems with health literacy may affect a child's ability to receive appropriate care. Individuals with marginal literacy levels may have difficulty reading patient education handouts, prescriptions, or complicated forms that have to be completed for insurance purposes. Approximately 44 million adults are thought to have low literacy skills. Health-care providers can advocate for children by providing culturally sensitive health care to children.

## ADVOCACY IN THE OFFICE

Much of the screening and anticipatory guidance that is provided in the health supervision visit is a form of child advocacy. There are numerous areas in which the pediatrician can intervene and advocate for children in the office setting. This section briefly discusses a few of these issues and ways in which a pediatrician can intervene.

### VIOLENCE PREVENTION

Unfortunately, violence pays a prominent role in the lives of many children. The United States has the highest youth homicide and suicide rate among the 26 wealthiest nations in the world. During the health supervision visit one can encourage and promote care and support systems that will assist families in nurturing their children. Pediatricians can advocate that parents use nonviolent means of disciplining their children and promote the use of praise. In addition, they can discuss the hazards of handguns in the home. If risk factors for violent behavior are identified, it is essential that the physician advocate for the child by referring the child and family to appropriate services. This may involve advocating for the child by interfacing with insurance companies and schools.

## SMOKING

Twenty-five percent of the population regularly uses tobacco. Forty-three percent of children age 2 to 11 are exposed to environmental tobacco. Reducing the use of tobacco should be a health priority for pediatricians. In the office setting there are numerous ways in which a pediatrician can advocate to reduce the use of tobacco. One simple way is to maintain a tobacco-free office environment and try to limit reading materials containing tobacco advertising. One should ask about tobacco use and exposure to smoke at every office visit. The pediatrician should be knowledgeable about tobacco cessation efforts and offer advice on quitting and referrals as appropriate. Anticipatory guidance about tobacco use should begin at age 5.

## DEVELOPMENTAL DISABILITIES

The pediatrician can play a crucial role in advocating for a child with developmental disabilities. It is critical that the pediatrician screen and identify infants with disabilities as soon as possible. Once a disability is identified, the pediatrician can advocate for the child by referring her or him promptly for early intervention services. The pediatrician should continue to advocate on behalf of the child by working with early intervention services and the family to establish an individual family service plan that focuses on medical, developmental, and family services. The physician should be aware of the resources in the community for the child and family and should coordinate the health component of the services. It is also essential that the patient receive access to appropriate medical services.

## BIBLIOGRAPHY

American Academy of Pediatrics, Committee on Children with Disabilities. Role of the pediatrician in family-centered services. *Pediatrics* 107(5):1155–1157, 2001.

American Academy of Pediatrics, Committee on Substance Abuse. Tobacco's toll: Implications for the pediatrician. *Pediatrics* 107(4):794–798, 2001.

Institute of Medicine. *Health Insurance Is a Family Matter.* Washington, DC: National Academy Press, 2002: 111.

U.S. Bureau of the Census. *Profile of Selected Social Characteristics 2000.* Available at http//factfinder.census.gov.

U.S. Department of Health and Human Services, Office of Minority Health. *Final National Standards on Culturally and Linguistically Appropriate Services (CLAS) in Health Care.* Rockville, MD: U.S. Department of Health and Human Services, 2001.

# NEWBORN ISSUES

## Lynn M. Manfred

## LEARNING OBJECTIVES

1. Understand the impact of pregnancy, labor, and delivery on the newborn.
2. Know how to assess the health and transition of the newborn to extrauterine life.
3. Know how to assess and manage the common problems of the newborn period.

## PRENATAL

### FETAL DEVELOPMENT

The first trimester establishes the placenta and the fetus. Most of organogenesis occurs during this period, and so toxins and injuries have the greatest impact on the developing fetus during the first trimester. At the start of the second trimester, all the organ structures exist. These structures, including the lungs, heart, and gastrointestinal tract, all grow in size, differentiate, and develop functionally during the second trimester.

The third trimester of pregnancy is a period of rapid fetal growth and active transport of many necessary nutrients, such as calcium, iron, immunoglobulins, and proteins. At times the immunoglobulins are directed at fetal structures and can attack and destroy those structures. Antibodies to the markers on red cell membranes can cross the placenta and cause a hemolytic anemia and hydrops fetalis if the condition is severe. Thyroid antibodies can attack the fetal thyroid gland, making it unable to release thyroid hormone in the perinatal period.

Intrauterine growth is dependent on a number of factors, including (1) social history, (2) blood flow to the placenta, (3) space availability, (4) toxins and exposures, (5) infections, and (6) family/genetic issues. Most factors other than familial and genetic are maternal factors that can be modified to a greater or lesser degree.

Social issues can pose a threat to the successful growth of the fetus. Pregnant women may not be able to eat regularly or may not get good nutrition. The Women, Infants, and Children (WIC) program was established to address the nutritional factors that contribute to poor infant outcomes. Other social issues that can affect a growing fetus adversely are any risk-taking behavior in the mother or father, environmental toxins at home or work, changing roles with the arrival of the new baby, and domestic violence. Domestic violence is more common during pregnancy as the family tries to address the financial and interpersonal changes that are coming.

Blood flow to the placenta is dependent on the mother's general health and renal and cardiovascular systems. Thus, mothers with major medical issues perfuse the placenta less well, compromising their health and the baby's well being. The baby can receive less nutrition and grow more slowly, and less amniotic fluid can be present. If maternal glucose is elevated, it will cross the placenta, and the baby will produce more insulin. If the mother has an autoimmune problem that causes her to make immunoglobulin to some body tissue, that immunoglobulin is transported across the placenta and may attack the baby's tissue. Autoimmune thyroiditis, lupus, and autoimmune hemolytic anemia are examples.

Depending on maternal body habitus, the uterus can expand to accommodate the growing baby. Multiple-gestation infants are likely to have packaging deformities, many of which will correct in the postnatal period. Feet can be forced into flexion or extreme extension. Amniotic bands can form, cutting off blood supply to the extremities. Multiple-gestation infants are at higher risk of deformities such as molded cranium, dislocated hips, or positional deformities of the foot. Arthrogryposis is an arrest of the developing muscle fibers such that, at delivery, they have been replaced to a large extent with fat and connective tissue. Nowadays, some developmental anomalies detected by ultrasound may be addressed by surgery in utero, and the pregnancy allowed to continue.

Pregnant women ingest a large array of foods, medications, and recreational drugs, all of which are potential toxins for the developing fetus. During organogenesis, many exposures and even temperature changes can affect fetal development. Mothers with seizure disorders often have to take medications, such as phenytoin or carbamazepine, that are known to cause deformations and malformations in the developing fetus. At the right time in development, even small amounts of alcohol can cause problems in the fetus. Vasoconstrictor drugs can cause decreases in blood flow to portions of the developing fetus. These structures then grow slowly or atrophy. Many centrally acting medications can cause withdrawal syndromes in the new-born, including marijuana, cocaine and heroin, as well as antidepressants and caffeine.

Infections during pregnancy can cause a host of problems in the baby. Acute infections can decrease blood flow to the placenta and even cause a miscarriage. Several infectious agents, referred to by the acronym TORCH (toxoplasmosis, other infections, rubella, cytomegalovirus, herpes) (Table 13-1), can cross the placenta and cause congenital syndromes. Febrile illnesses, chorioamnionitis, maternal bacteremia, and sepsis all can precipitate prema-ture delivery. Group B streptococcus, herpes simplex, and hepatitis B infec-tions all can be transmitted to the baby during delivery, and the first two can present as illnesses soon after birth. Sepsis or meningitis with either of these infections has high morbidity and mortality. Pregnant women are immunocompromised during the pregnancy, and that decreases their abil-ity to fight off these infections and limits their ability to keep the infection from the fetus. The pregnancy itself can put the mother at risk for complica-tions such as urinary tract infections, pregnancy-induced hypertension, eclampsia, preeclampsia (abnormal vascular changes and associated hyper-tension), vaginal bleeding (from infection or placenta previa), and preterm labor.

Chromosomal abnormalities of the fetus often cause spontaneous abor-tions or poor growth in utero. Up to a third of first-trimester pregnancies end in early abortion. The mother may have a genetic disorder, such as Marfan syndrome, that makes it hard for her to carry a baby to term and deliver it successfully.

During pregnancy, mothers are screened for many of these prenatal prob-lems by a combination of history, physical examination, and laboratory eval-uation.

Table 13-1 **TORCH Infections**

| Infection | How Acquired |
| --- | --- |
| Toxoplasmosis | Cat feces |
| Rubella | Respiratory/droplet contact |
| Cytomegalovirus | Secretions/day care |
| Herpes | Respiratory/droplet contact |
| Human immunodeficiency virus | Blood/sexual contact/intravenous drugs |
| Syphilis | Sexually transmitted/bloodborne |

## LABOR AND DELIVERY: A TIME OF TRANSITION

### EFFECTS OF LABOR ON THE FETUS

Labor imposes enormous stress on the baby. With each contraction, the blood flow to the placenta is temporarily decreased. The infant already has a PaO$_2$ of only 25 to 28 mmHg, and with the decreased blood flow to the placenta from contractions, this number falls further. The infant's heart rate may slow, and if the fall is severe, the pH may fall. The fetal monitor tells physicians if the variability in fetal heart rate is excessive or if the heart rate stays low, suggesting fetal distress.

Labor also serves to prepare the baby for the first few minutes of life. The contractions of the chest wall seem to stimulate the infant to take his or her first breaths. The slightly lower pH increases oxygen delivery to the tissues, and the slowed heart rate decreases oxygen consumption. These physiologic adaptations and others give the infant time to transition to autonomous breathing outside the uterus.

### EFFECTS OF DELIVERY ON THE FETUS

The stress of being pushed through the birth canal forces some of the amniotic fluid out of the upper airway and apparently stimulates the baby to take its first breaths after leaving the birth canal. These first breaths expand the liquid-filled lungs, increase blood flow to the lungs, and begin gas exchange in the alveoli. Surfactant release from pneumocytes improves the surface tension and allows the alveoli to stay open.

Once delivered, the infant must accomplish all the pulmonary and cardiac tasks. The infant also must maintain its body temperature, send blood to all the tissues, regulate its body functions by using its own hormones, and take in essential nutrients to maintain itself and grow. The stress of delivery helps the infant begin performing these tasks.

### IN THE DELIVERY ROOM

In the delivery room, the pediatrician tries to modify problems for the infant before, during, and after delivery. If the mother is group B streptococcus–positive on her screening vaginal culture at 36 weeks of gestation, she is given antibiotics during labor to decrease the risk of the infant acquiring group B streptococcus infection during delivery. If meconium is present when the membranes rupture, an attempt is made to suction the baby's upper airway once the head is delivered but before the chest is delivered, in order to prevent the aspiration of irritating meconium into the lungs.

Once delivered, infants need to be warmed and dried quickly to prevent hypothermic changes from suppressing respiration and circulation. Then a newborn must have its airway and breathing assessed. If it is delivered through meconium, the infant first should be *suctioned* to remove the thick meconium material from the airway. Other debris also may need to be removed by suctioning the upper airway. Once the airway is clear, the infant must breathe to allow air exchange. Infants who do not breathe spontaneously are *stimulated* to try to increase sympathetic stimulation of the cardiorespiratory system. Frequently, infants do not exchange air well and appear dusky for several minutes after delivery. If they are making adequate respiratory efforts, they can receive supplemental oxygen and generally have a good result. Infants who fail to exchange air sufficiently need to be managed with intubation and ventilation. Once air movement is assured, attention is paid to circulation. Some infants are intravascularly depleted at delivery and require albumin or another colloid to expand their intravascular space. This is similar to the ABCD approach (see Chap. 39) used to assess and manage resuscitation in older children.

At delivery, the Apgar score (Table 13-2) helps predict which infants are most at risk of not making the transition to extrauterine life successfully. A 1-min Apgar score less than 4 identifies an infant who had a very difficult delivery. If the Apgar score at 5 min is not 7, the Apgar is repeated every 5 min until it is above 7 for two consecutive scores. If the Apgar is not above 7 by 20 min, the infant should be monitored in a special care area.

Once circulation has been established, the child is more fully assessed. Some infants have prolonged effects from medications given to their mothers, such as narcotics for pain. These infants are treated. The infant also gets his or her first physical assessment, looking for issues that might hinder the transition to the outside world. A quick gestational assessment is done, focusing on the physical attributes: skin thickness, breast development, genital development, and creases on the feet. A child born prematurely is at

*Table 13-2* **Apgar Scoring System**

| Physical Finding | 0 | 1 | 2 |
|---|---|---|---|
| Heart rate | Absent | <100 | >100 |
| Respirations | Absent | Slow Irregular | Good/vigorous |
| Muscle tone | Limp | Some flexion | Active movement |
| Response to nasal catheter | None | Grimace | Cough or sneeze |
| Color | Blue or pale | Pink body, blue extremities | Completely pink |

increased risk of infection, insufficient air exchange, inability to maintain body temperature, and poor feeding.

The child also is checked for color, traumatic injuries during the birth process, and the appropriateness of his or her size. Infants who are large for gestational age (LGA) have more birth trauma, more low sugars, high hematocrits, and altered calcium levels. Infants who are small for gestational age (SGA) have more difficulty with temperature regulation, more low sugars, and a higher incidence of infection.

## TRANSITIONAL ISSUES

### OVERVIEW

A newborn needs to learn to live in the outside world. An infant must breathe sufficiently to exchange air, maintain a steady body temperature, ingest, digest, and carry nutrients to all the tissues of the body. It must defend itself against the dangers of the outside world and excrete waste products. Literally every organ system is involved.

### CARDIOVASCULAR REGULATION

The heart has been pumping blood around the body for months before delivery. However, the vast majority of the blood has been carrying the nutrients from the placenta to the systemic circulation. Now the infant must make the transition described above and send blood to the pulmonary tree for oxygenation and then send oxygenated blood to the systemic circulation, delivering both oxygen and nutrients. At delivery, the systemic blood pressure rises and the pulmonary pressure falls, and this promotes blood flow to the pulmonary bed. The rising left-sided pressures functionally close the patent foramen ovale. For the first couple of days of life, blood is "shunted" to the pulmonary tree through the open ductus arteriosus. At 24 to 48 h of life, the ductus closes and establishes the final circulatory circuit. When the ductus closes, a previously asymptomatic coarctation of the aorta may become symptomatic.

For most newborns, the parasympathetic tone remains quite high compared with sympathetic tone, making it easy for an infant to become bradycardic and poorly perfused. The infant has been maintained in a uniform temperature environment for the entire pregnancy. Tone in the various vascular beds has been about equal, and blood has flowed to all organs. At delivery the infant must learn quickly to send the right amount of blood to each organ system. Initially this is difficult, and many infants are prone to low body temperatures as they send too much blood to the skin surface and dissipate the heat they are generating. They have blue palms and soles for a few days after delivery. These infants are very volume-dependent since their relatively high vagal tone makes vasoconstriction difficult.

## RESPIRATION

As was noted earlier, the infant now must exchange gas on his or her own and deliver it to the body. The pulmonary pressures fall with the opening of the alveoli, making it easier to send more blood to the lungs. The type II pneumocytes excrete phospholipids in the form of surfactant, which helps the alveoli stay open and grow with each breath. The amniotic fluid is absorbed over the next few hours and the $PaO_2$ rises with improving air exchange to about 80 mmHg. When the amniotic fluid is not absorbed as it should be, the infant develops *transient tachypnea of the newborn.* Persistence of the patent ductus arteriosus (PDA) allows shunting into the low-pressure pulmonary bed and high pulmonary pressures. Infants with PDA tend to have a high respiratory rate and increased work of breathing.

## TEMPERATURE REGULATION

An infant's ability to thermoregulate is determined by its ability to generate heat, insulate against heat loss, and lower blood flow to nonessential skin surfaces to conserve heat. Much of an infant's blood flow goes to its head, which can dissipate heat quickly. Premature infants have little subcutaneous tissue and lose heat easily. Infants who are cold or wet lose heat quickly, and their core body temperature falls, causing cardiac and neurologic decompensation.

## STATE AND METABOLIC CONTROL

Infants need to learn quickly to regulate their state, or orientation to the outside world. They need to move and cry to get warmer. They need to wake to feed. They need to eat to survive and grow, and they must produce the digestive enzymes that assist in the absorption of food. The pancreas must produce insulin and regulate blood sugar levels. Glycogen stored antenatally in the liver is consumed over the first day or two of life, making effective feeding necessary by that time.

Thyroid hormones are made and stored in the thyroid gland for use right after delivery. Parathyroid level in the blood is low at delivery since fetal calcium level is high, but the hormone is available to be released when needed. Adrenal hormones and norepinephrine are also available and contribute to the infant's successful transition to life outside the uterus.

## HEMOPOIETIC AND IMMUNE SYSTEMS

An infant has an ample number of red blood cells (RBCs). In utero, the fetus has a low oxygen concentration, which stimulates erythropoietin release. After delivery, the oxygen concentration in the blood is higher, turning off erythropoietin and shutting down RBC production. Most of the hemoglobin present at delivery is fetal hemoglobin. Many of the now unnecessary RBCs hemolyze in the perinatal period, and the infant's hematocrit falls. The infant's liver then must process the heme degradation products.

The infant's clotting mechanisms are all present at birth but need further maturation before working as they do in older children. At delivery, infants have comparatively reduced platelet aggregation and clotting factors and a low ability to vasoconstrict. The concentration of clotting factors actually falls after delivery. Without vitamin K, the risk of hemorrhagic disease is much higher.

At birth, an infant has cell-mediated immunity and a large load of immunoglobulin G (IgG), which was actively transported across the placenta. Humoral immunity initially develops around the time of delivery but is slow to react to the presentation of new antigen. The infant's experience with antigens in the clean uterine environment is almost nil. The newborn has almost no immunoglobulin M (IgM) or IgA unless he or she has had an in utero infection. All this leaves the infant vulnerable to early infection and slow to fight off infection in the first few weeks of life.

## RENAL FUNCTION

Little blood flows to the kidneys in utero. At delivery, systemic blood pressure increases, more than doubling renal blood flow. The infant has no experience in concentrating urine in utero, and so a large diuresis of the intravascular space that was expanded by amniotic fluid occurs. During this time, there is little glomerular filtration, and so renal perfusion results in the production of urine. Over the first 2 weeks of life, the kidneys mature significantly as renal blood flow increases, glomerular filtration develops, and renal function begins. Function gradually increases, and over several months the kidneys learn to concentrate maximally, excrete optimally, and regulate the baby's fluid and electrolyte status.

## LIVER FUNCTION

The synthetic functions of the liver are largely developed by the time of delivery. Given substrate, the liver can make the necessary blood proteins, complement, clotting factors, and enzymes. The ability of the liver to metabolize waste products and medications is low at birth but quickly develops in the first few weeks of life as the function of the necessary enzymes increases.

## SUMMARY

Most of the organs and systems present in the newborn have some of the function they ultimately will have. Over the first few weeks to months of life, the function of each one grows toward that which it will have when fully mature.

## NEWBORN HISTORY AND PHYSICAL EXAMINATION

### "PAST MEDICAL HISTORY"

The newborn history is that of the pregnancy, labor, and delivery. Therefore, the pediatrician collects information about maternal health before pregnancy, such as age and underlying medical problems, particularly cardiovascular, renal, or autoimmune, as these factors have the greatest potential impact on the newborn. Previous pregnancies and their outcomes, difficulty getting pregnant, and maternal nutrition and medications (vitamins, tobacco, alcohol, prescription and recreational drugs) all are important in assessing possible problems in the newborn.

The expected date of confinement (EDC) is important in assessing the risk for a variety of perinatal conditions. Prematurity is one of the biggest risk factors for infection, respiratory distress, and metabolic problems. Maternal blood tests showing evidence of congenital infections [commonly for syphilis, rubella, herpes, varicella, and human immunodeficiency virus (HIV)] or antibodies to red cells also are checked. Cultures including gonorrhea, chlamydia, and group B streptococcus are done to look for infections that are likely to be transmitted to the baby during labor and delivery. Antenatal testing for spinal closure defects ($\alpha$ fetoprotein), chromosomal abnormalities (amniocentesis or chorionic villus sampling), and prenatal ultrasound results all can give important information about the new baby.

The family and social history are important to the newborn's future. Thus, mothers are screened for substance abuse, domestic violence, poor socioeconomic status, and childhood illnesses or deaths in their families. Preparations for the baby also are checked; the family must have a car seat to transport the baby home from the hospital.

### LABOR AND DELIVERY

Most important is the history of the labor and delivery. How long was the mother in labor? Prolonged labor tires the mother, and there may be decreased perfusion of the placenta for much of that time. When did the mother rupture her membranes? After 18 to 24 h, the risk of chorioamnionitis and sepsis in the infant rises. If the mother had a fever, was she given a dose of intravenous (IV) antibiotics during the labor (this has been shown to decrease the chances of infection in the infant)? Was meconium present when the membranes ruptured? Meconium aspiration can be life-threatening to a newborn.

Delivery, if prolonged, also can limit the infant's oxygen and glucose supply. Hypoxia is quick to set in, and glycogen stores are depleted over a period of hours. Was there any trauma to the newborn? Premature and LGA babies are particularly prone to birth trauma.

## POSTNATAL

The details of how well the infant made the initial transition to life outside the uterus after delivery are very important. What were the Apgar scores? Did the infant cry spontaneously? Was resuscitation necessary? Was oxygen administered? The answers to these questions provide important information about the infant's early transition to the world.

Has the infant voided? As was noted above, if the kidneys are perfused and the collecting system is intact, the baby will make urine. Has the infant stooled? A thick, sticky green substance called meconium constitutes the first infant stool. By 24 h of age, 90 percent of term infants will have voided and stooled. A similar percentage of premature infants will have voided and stooled by 36 h of age. Failure to urinate raises concerns about renal function and the patency of the collecting system. Posterior urethral valves is one of the more common problems that present in this way. Failure to stool raises concerns about intake and the continuity of the gastrointestinal tract.

## NEWBORN PHYSICAL EXAMINATION

The goal of the newborn physical examination is to identify acute illness and important congenital anomalies. Observation of color, posture, work of breathing, and alertness begins the examination. The infant should be pink and in a flexed posture with easy respirations. The infant should cry when stimulated or unwrapped and be quiet when bundled or cuddled. Pallor implies hypovolemia or sepsis or anemia. A ruddy color suggests polycythemia. A floppy infant has neurologic problems or is severely ill. Observation also should include looking for evidence of birth trauma, congenital anomalies, and skin lesions.

The anterior fontanel should be palpable on the top of the head and measure 1 to 3 cm in each dimension unless molding has caused an overriding of the sutures. The head should be palpated for cephalohematoma (bruising over one bone) or caput succedaneum (scalp edema that crosses over a suture line). One should examine the face for congenital anomalies such as pits, widely spaced eyes, and palpebral fissures. The conjunctivae are checked for hemorrhages. Gaze may be intermittently disconjugate for several weeks after delivery. Neonates are obligate nose breathers, and so both sides of the nose must allow airflow. The position of the ears should be noted in relation to the eyes; abnormalities prompt a search for other anomalies, particularly of the renal and collecting systems. The mouth should be checked for natal teeth and an intact palate. Epstein's pearls may be present at the junction of the hard and soft palates.

The examiner then listens to the heart and lungs. Breath sounds should be tubular and equal on the right and the left. The heart rate can be variable for months after delivery, but $S_1$ and $S_2$ should be present. If the baby is in the second day of life, the murmur of a closing ductus may be heard. Brachial and femoral pulses should be palpated simultaneously, and any delay between the two prompts a look for coarctation of the aorta.

The abdomen should be protuberant but not tight. With warm hands, the examiner palpates the abdomen for masses and to feel the liver below the right costal margin and a spleen tip at the left costal margin. The kidneys may be felt on deep palpation. Other masses commonly are associated with kidney malformation and dilation of the bladder or ureters. These masses should be evaluated. The genitals are checked for maturity, symmetry, and proper anatomy. Girls should have a visible clitoris and hood with an opening to a moist, red vaginal mucosa. Males should have bilaterally palpable testes in a well-formed scrotal sac. The urethral opening should be in the middle of the glans, and no openings should be visible on the ventral shaft of the penis over the urethra. The anus should have visible tone and be patent. Either sex may have prominent breasts because of maternal hormone stimulation in utero.

Positional deformities of the lower extremities are common. Positional deformities may be distinguished from skeletal anomalies such as clubfoot by virtue of their mobility. The clubfoot cannot be moved into a neutral position. Hips should be stressed from 90-degree hip–90-degree knee flexion with gentle posterior pressure that produces movement of dislocation. Abduction of the hips from this position (Ortolani maneuver) causes a click in the dislocated hip. Fingers and toes should be counted, and dysmorphic features should be noted. The back should be checked for complete closure of the skin over the meninges.

Primitive reflexes such as the Moro (startle) reflex, palmar and plantar grasp reflexes, and rooting and sucking reflexes should be present and symmetric. The baby should have good tone and be irritated by the examination. The examiner should visualize the posterior pharynx and red reflexes.

Any anomalies noted should prompt a search for other congenital anomalies. About 4 percent of children have some minor anomaly, and less than a tenth of that number have multiple or major congenital anomalies.

## GESTATIONAL AGE ASSESSMENT

The gestational age should be assessed by using a standard evaluation tool such as the New Ballard scale. This instrument checks physical measures of maturity such as skin thickness, size of breast buds, rugae on the scrotum, and relative size of the labia majora and labia minora. It also looks at neuromuscular maturity, checking tone and responsiveness. Physical findings are more reliable in an ill infant than are neuromuscular ones.

## COMMON MALFORMATIONS

As was noted previously, if one congenital anomaly is found, a search for others should be made. A genetic syndrome may be the underlying cause or a cluster of malformations may be the cause. VACTERL is an acronym for one of the more common associations of vertebral, anal, cardiac, tracheal-esophageal fistula; renal collecting system; and radial limb anomalies, which probably are caused by a single problem early in gestation. Spina bifida is a spectrum of problems ranging from a small pit at the base of the spine to a large opening in the skin surface that allows herniation of the meninges and cord. Cleft lip and cleft palate are among the most common congenital lesions, sometimes isolated and at other times associated with multiple anomalies.

## POSTPARTUM CARE

### FEEDING

In the first 12 to 24 h of life, a newborn infant needs to learn to latch on, suck, and swallow a sufficient amount of food to stay hydrated and grow. The decision to breast-feed or bottle feed is up to the parents. There are few circumstances that preclude breast-feeding. They include maternal issues such as HIV and sepsis, severe prematurity, and breast reduction surgery. Infant factors that preclude breast-feeding are hypotonia, oral-pharyngeal problems such as cleft palate, severe developmental delay, and gastrointestinal malformations.

Mothers should be made aware of the advantages of breast-feeding, including the ability to supply all the necessary nutrients to the baby, including a good iron supply, a healthy fat source, and sufficient proteins and fluid for growth. Immunoglobulins are passed to the infant with each feeding. Breast milk is inexpensive, readily available, and always at the right temperature, and it promotes maternal-infant bonding. Breast-fed infants usually do not need to be burped, but some spit up less when they are burped two or three times a feed. Infants should be encouraged to nurse every 2 to 3 h for about 5 min per feeding during the first day of life, 10 min during the second day of life, and 15 min during the third day of life. A healthy infant older than a week can empty the mother's breast in 7 min. Feeding on demand seems to encourage intake of the correct amount of food for normal growth and stimulate sufficient breast milk production. Prolonged sucking is nonnutritive and may cause breast tenderness.

Formula is available in a variety of forms, from powder to concentrate to ready-to-feed. Formula can be cow's milk–based or soy-based. Though rarely necessary medically, a variety of elemental formulas are available, though at a greater expense than the standard formulas. Most infants like formula warmer than room temperature, but care must be taken to heat the bottle uniformly (a microwave does not do that). Formulas are supplemented with the equivalent of a daily dose of vitamins. Iron is added to all the standard formulas.

Infants should be fed on demand, and most breast-fed infants feed slightly more often than do bottle-fed babies. They also stool more frequently. In the first few days of life, infants eat less than an ounce every 2 to 3 h. If they are making urine and stool, they are getting enough fluid and nutrition. As they grow, infants take in more volume with each feed and eat less often. At about 6 weeks of age, their intake increases dramatically and they have a growth spurt. By 2 to 4 months of age, infants take sufficient feeds and have sufficient glycogen stores to be able to sleep 6 to 8 h at night. At 4 to 6 months of age, most infants take in 24 to 32 oz of formula divided into four or five feeds a day as long as they are not taking any solids. As an infant's intake of solids grows, the amount of fluid falls by 40 to 50 percent.

Formula-fed babies should be burped frequently, every ounce or two. This decreases the amount of gas that gets beyond the stomach. They should not be pushed to "finish the bottle," as this encourages overfeeding and ignores satiety signals.

Infants do not need any liquid supplements of either water or juice. They should not receive any solids until at least 4 months of age and preferably not before 6 months. The American Academy of Pediatrics has recommended this to attempt to decrease the number of food allergies in children and promote healthy, appetite-regulated eating.

Some infants are very allergic or have severe digestive problems. These infants are candidates for some of the more specialized formulas, as are extremely premature infants. A premature infant has a less developed digestive system and insufficient stores of the nutrients that are passed through the placenta in the last weeks of pregnancy. The specialized formulas are easier to digest and contain the calcium, iron, and proteins that are missing at delivery.

## ELIMINATION

Infants have very low bladder capacity and therefore urinate frequently and in small amounts. Most infants urinate and stool within the first 24 h of life. Premature infants may not urinate until the second day of life. Infants do not concentrate their urine, and so it is usually clear or light yellow. Occasionally there will be the faint pink color of uric acid crystals in the urine. When they first are born, infants should void at least eight times a day. Over the first year of life, infants gradually develop a bigger bladder capacity and void fewer times a day but in larger amounts.

Breast-fed infants may stool as often as every feed or as infrequently as once every other day. Bottle-fed babies stool once or twice every day or every other day. After the first couple of days, sticky green meconium has all passed, and stools become golden, mushy, and seedy. The stools become more firm after solids are started.

## SLEEP

Newborns can sleep up to 23 h a day. Neonates spend nearly equal time in rapid eye movement (REM) sleep and non-REM sleep. As they grow, an increasing amount of time is spent awake, with frequent naps throughout the day. The amount of REM sleep falls. During the first few weeks, their sleep times consolidate and they develop a pattern in their sleep and wake cycles. Smaller infants should not be allowed to sleep more than 5 h at a time or they are likely to become hypoglycemic.

In 1992, the American Academy of Pediatrics recommended that all infants be placed on their backs to sleep. Once it was demonstrated that the incidence of aspiration is no higher in infants positioned on their backs, this was felt to be the safest sleeping position, especially for very young babies. Since that recommendation was made, the incidence of sudden infant death syndrome (SIDS) has decreased substantially.

## ILLNESS PREVENTION AND IMMUNIZATION

Infants are given a shot of vitamin K in the first couple of hours of life. This increases the precursors available to make the vitamin K–dependent clotting factors and decreases the risk of bleeding caused by hemorrhagic disease of the newborn. Most infants receive erythromycin eye ointment to prevent gonococcal eye disease and blindness; it also may decrease the incidence of chlamydia conjunctivitis.

Children today are immunized for a variety of infectious diseases that once were devastating to young children. Hepatitis B immunization is begun in the newborn nursery and is followed with two subsequent doses at 2 and 6 months of age. The babies of mothers who tested positive for hepatitis B antigen are given hepatitis B immune globulin in addition to the hepatitis B immunization.

## NEWBORN SCREENING

LGA babies, premature infants, SGA infants, and infected infants are at increased risk of hypoglycemia and get bedside glucose monitoring before feeds until they are stable with a safe blood glucose reading. LGA infants and infants of diabetic mothers are at risk of polycythemia, and so a screening hemoglobin and hematocrit may be obtained.

Newborns in all states are screened for a variety of metabolic and genetic conditions via micro blood samples taken after 24 h of age. These tests are designed to detect asymptomatic conditions that have preventive measures or treatments that will improve outcomes. Screens for phenylketonuria are done in almost all states, as are screens for hypothyroidism, galactosemia, maple syrup urine disease, homocystinuria, and hemoglobinopathies. Some states screen for the common varieties of cystic fibrosis.

Hearing is screened in the newborn nursery by means of a short auditory evoked response examination. False positives are common and should prompt rescreening or referral for brainstem auditory evoked response testing.

Car seat testing is done on all small children and hypotonic and premature infants. Those born with these problems have poor head control and can
occlude their airways in standard car seats. Car beds are used until these
infants develop the ability to protect their airways in a car seat.

## SKIN CARE AND PROBLEMS

The skin of newborns is colonized with vaginal flora. Once the infant's temperature stabilizes, the infant is given a cleansing bath to decrease the
amount of bacterial growth on his or her skin. Newborns have sensitive skin
that becomes too dry with excessive bathing. A variety of rashes, such as
milia and miliaria, present in the perinatal period and resolve on their own.

Rashes in the diaper region are common. Newborns are very prone to
irritant and infectious rashes. Rashes on the prominent areas of the skin
probably are a result of irritation from the moisture and pH of the urine.
They should be treated with barrier creams. Bright red rashes with shiny
areas in the skin folds and red satellite lesions are probably yeast infections
that should be treated with topic antifungals. Less commonly, bacterial skin
infections occur around the anus and vaginal opening.

## SAFETY AND INJURY PREVENTION

Infants have heads that constitute a much larger proportion of their body
mass than do those of adults. This makes them more prone to injure their
necks in automobile accidents. Therefore, it is recommended that infants
always ride in rear-facing safety seats in cars.

Infant skin burns more easily than does that of adults, and so it is recommended that hot water heaters be turned down to 49°C (120°F) to
decrease the risk of accidental burns in bathtubs. Children never should be
left unattended near water as they can drown even in very shallow water in
bathtubs.

## CIRCUMCISION OR NOT?

The American Academy of Pediatrics has published a position statement
stating that there is neither medical reason for nor medical contraindication
to circumcision. Male infants who are not circumcised have a slightly
increased risk of urinary tract infections and yeast infections under the foreskin, but not at a rate high enough to recommend routine circumcision.
Therefore, good hygiene is the recommendation.

## WHEN TO CALL THE DOCTOR

Families leave the hospital with many questions about their new babies, and
even more questions arise when they are home. Does his sneezing mean he
has a cold? No, that is how he gets rid of his nasal congestion. Is she having
a seizure if her hand shakes repeatedly? Probably not, but she needs further
evaluation if the shaking does not stop when her hand is held.

Families need to know when to call the pediatrician. They must call if the baby

- Looks sick to them. Parents know the child best, and if they are worried, the pediatrician should know about it.
- Has a temperature of 38°C (100.4°F) or more rectally. In the first month of life, these infants are at risk of overwhelming sepsis and need to be evaluated promptly.
- Becomes limp or cannot be awakened.
- Seems to stop breathing, turns pale or blue, or has difficulty breathing.
- Becomes jaundiced.
- Forcefully vomits for more than one feeding.
- Does not urinate at least once every 3 h in the newborn period and at least six times a day after that.
- Does not stool for 3 days or more.

Many pediatric practices have call-in hours for nonurgent questions or respond to questions by e-mail.

### FAMILY CHANGES

The introduction of a new baby changes the household dynamics enormously. The infant can never be alone. He or she is unable to feed and care for himself or herself and so becomes the focus of the household. The newborn is often in the parents' bedroom and disrupts the parents' sleep. They no longer have privacy and often have less chance to communicate. These changes can be very stressful on even the strongest marriages. Health-care providers should encourage new parents to care for the newborn while simultaneously developing ways to care for themselves and others in the house. Parents should have some breaks from the baby to give them a chance to communicate and relax.

## PERINATAL PROBLEMS

### FEEDING PROBLEMS

In the first day of life, infants have little or no nutritional or fluid needs. They do need to be able to latch on to suck from the breast or bottle. By the second day of life, the child needs to take in small amounts of milk or formula. Observing the infant feeding often tells the physician why the infant is not feeding well. Some infants cannot coordinate their suck and swallow. Other infants do not move the fluid back in their mouth. Still other infants are too ill to generate an adequate suck. Failure to latch on or to get any milk is by far the most common problem, and it can be addressed by lactation consultants.

Infants can have difficulties taking adequate nutrition for a number of reasons. They may have difficulties in sucking or coordinating their swallow. They may have tachypnea from cardiac or respiratory problems that leaves them insufficient time to suck and swallow. Respiratory or cardiac problems also may increase their caloric needs. Others eat enough food but regurgitate or reflux volumes that prevent them from growing. Some do this because of intolerance to one or more of the components of the formula, whereas others have a mechanical obstruction or motor disorder that increases what they reflux. Some just do not burp well and carry their milk up with their burps. Careful observation of the infant's feeding and the child's growth pattern often reveals the cause for feeding problems.

## INFECTION RISK

Maternal infection is one of the leading causes of premature delivery, and these infections can be passed to the newborn during or after delivery. Infants can aspirate organisms during delivery or become infected from organisms deposited on their skin and mucosal surfaces. Mothers who harbor group B streptococcus in their vagina can pass this to their infants during delivery.

Herpes infections, even from asymptomatic women, can present as sepsis or meningitis in an infant shortly after birth. Prematurity and other medical problems make a newborn more vulnerable to infectious diseases.

Newborns can present with congenital infections as well. Syphilis can present with involvement of almost any organ system. Nasal congestion or snuffles; skin lesions, especially on the palms or soles; hepatosplenomegaly; lymphadenopathy; and even bony lesions in an SGA child can be from syphilis. Congenital syphilis, herpes, varicella, and even viral gastroenteritis can be lethal to an infant with an immature immune system.

The TORCH infections (see Table 13-1) present as SGA infants with lymphoid hyperplasia, cataracts, or skin lesions.

## NEONATAL JAUNDICE

Recent guidelines promulgated by the American Academy of Pediatrics (AAP) point out that physicians must pay close attention to infants at risk for jaundice and be aggressive in evaluating and treating it because kernicterus (the chronic sequela of bilirubin encephalopathy) continues to occur. Newborns at increased risk for jaundice are premature infants, infants with large cephalohematomas, infants with blood group incompatibility or other hemolytic disease, infants of eastern Asian descent, siblings of infants treated for jaundice, and infants with polycythemia.

Breast-feeding infants are at increased risk of high bilirubin, particularly if they are losing weight quickly or not feeding well. All breast-fed infants discharged before 48h of age should have a follow-up visit within 48 to 72 h of discharge. Visiting nurses and pediatricians should evaluate the risk of increasing jaundice carefully and check the bilirubin level if there is any question about this.

Bilirubin metabolism is discussed in Chap. 30. Common causes for jaundice include physiologic jaundice resulting from liver enzyme immaturity, infections, autoimmune diseases, hemolytic diseases from red blood cell defects, enzyme abnormalities, and liver disease. Large collections of blood as in cephalohematomas and bruises and certain genetic predispositions all increase a child's chances of having significant jaundice.

Approximately two-thirds of neonates appear jaundiced sometime during the first week of life. Physiologic jaundice typically peaks at 4 days of life and *never* occurs in the first 24 h of life. *All infants who develop jaundice in the first 24 h of life should have a total serum bilirubin level checked.* Infants who develop jaundice within the first 24 h or in whom the cause of the hyperbilirubinemia is unclear should have the following laboratory tests performed to clarify the etiology: total and direct bilirubin level, blood type, direct antibody (Coomb's test), complete blood count (CBC) with differential, smear for red blood cell morphology, and reticulocyte count.

Most infants with hyperbilirubinemia do not need any treatment. Phototherapy is the most common therapy in infants whose bilirubin levels are high enough to require treatment. The AAP has published guidelines for phototherapy that are based on the age of the infant in hours, the total bilirubin level, and whether the infant is at low, medium, or high risk for hyperbilirubinemia. Infants with markedly elevated bilirubin levels who are at risk for kernicterus are treated with exchange transfusion.

## LARGE FOR GESTATIONAL AGE AND SMALL FOR GESTATIONAL AGE BABIES

Infants born at term weighing > 4000 g are designated large for gestational age. Infants of diabetic mothers, postmature infants, and those with Beckwith–Weidemann syndrome are at risk for being LGA. LGA infants are at increased risk for hypoglycemia, polycythemia, sepsis, hypocalcemia, and birth trauma.

The etiologies of being small or SGA are much more extensive and include congenital infection, genetic diseases, maternal illnesses, and premature delivery. SGA infants have more hypoglycemia, anemia, and thermal instability than do appropriate for gestational age (AGA) infants.

## INFANTS OF DIABETIC MOTHERS

Infants born to mothers with diabetes mellitus may have growth problems. Mothers with long-standing diabetes have enough vascular disease to impair the delivery of nutrients to the growing baby. Mothers who have poorly controlled sugars deliver babies who are very large because of the excess calories that cross the placenta. The baby makes lots of insulin and is slow to decrease the amount made when the large placental sugar supply stops at delivery. These babies easily can become hypoglycemic. They are at increased risk of hypocalcemia, polycythemia, and birth trauma. Over the first day of life, most of these infants learn to decrease their insulin production and regulate their glucose appropriately. They need to be fed frequently, and blood sugar should be followed closely until it normalizes.

## LETHARGY

A lethargic infant does not wake to feed or respond to his or her environment. These babies may have had a central nervous system (CNS) insult before or during delivery. They may be hypoxic or hypoglycemic, sedated by a medication given to the mother, or even septic, but there certainly is something wrong. A review of the prenatal history and birth history and a physical examination will uncover most of the problems. Metabolic problems and infectious causes should be evaluated and treated promptly. Any baby in whom the etiology cannot be found readily requires CNS assessment.

## TACHYPNEA AND RESPIRATORY DISTRESS

Newborns have very few ways to show that they are ill. Increases in the respiratory rate or work of breathing usually occur when an infant has an infection, including pneumonia, sepsis, and meningitis. If amniotic fluid is slow to be absorbed as in transient tachypnea of the newborn or if the infant is in heart failure, the respiratory rate may be elevated and the infant may or may not be cyanotic. Congenital heart lesions that cause shunting or increase pulmonary blood flow all can cause increases in the respiratory rate.

Tachypnea also can result from withdrawal from street drugs, alcohol, or even prescription medications that the mother has been taking.

## CYANOSIS

Poor color can have a variety of causes, from being unwrapped or cold to shunting unoxygenated blood to the systemic circulation. Heart failure can cause cyanosis as the tissue extraction of oxygen can be quite high when oxygen delivery to the tissues is low. The first decision to be made is whether this is central cyanosis, which probably has a cardiac or pulmonary etiology, or whether it is peripheral cyanosis, which has a more local cause. Evaluation follows from this decision.

## PREMATURITY

Prematurity affects almost every organ system in the body. The body is still developing, and delivery disrupts the nutrient flow that allows continued growth. Skin is thinner, making the infant more vulnerable to infection. The CNS is less mature, and intraventricular or intracerebral bleeding is more common. The suck is not mature, neurologic tone is low, and the liver is still developing its enzymes and proteins. The gastrointestinal tract cannot digest many foods and is at risk for necrotizing enterocolitis (NEC). The respiratory system does not exchange gases as it will later since the pneumocytes are just beginning to make surfactant. Even the respiratory center is immature, leaving a premature infant at risk for apnea. Most of all, a premature infant has a high likelihood of infectious complications from the immature immune system, poor skin and mucosal barriers, and undernutrition.

## DEVELOPMENTAL DYSPLASIA OF THE HIP

The acetabulum of the hip joint is formed in response to the close proximity of the femur to the pelvic bones. If the femur is not present or moves about too much, the stimulus for normal hip development is not present and the hip is dislocatable. Risk factors for developmental dysplasia of the hip (DDH) include being the first child, being female, a breech presentation, and a positive family history. Hips should be examined in the nursery, and if a click or laxity is found and persists, an ultrasound of the hip should be performed to check for acetabular development. Infants with DDH are treated with a Pavlik harness, which holds the femoral head in place to stimulate joint growth. Persistent abnormalities of the hip should be followed by a pediatric orthopedic surgeon.

## SUMMARY

The health of a newborn infant is dependent on many maternal factors in the prenatal period, labor and delivery, and postnatal care. An infant is at risk for many infectious complications as well as congenital anomalies. Many of an infant's organ systems do not yet have full function and put the child at risk of infections, thermal injuries, and circulatory problems.

## BIBLIOGRAPHY

Ballard/Dubowitz Scale. Available at www.neonatology.org/ref/dubowitz.html.

Seidel HM, Rosenstein BJ, Pathak A. *Primary Care of the Newborn*, 3d ed. St. Louis: Mosby, 2001.

# CHAPTER 14

# ADOLESCENT ISSUES

### Lynn M. Manfred

● LEARNING OBJECTIVES

1. Describe the physical, cognitive, emotional, and sexual changes that constitute puberty.

2. Be able to do a health maintenance visit that screens adolescents for risk-taking behaviors such as drug use and early sexual activity as well as common problems of adolescence.

3. Know how to evaluate some of the common problems of adolescence, including menstrual disorders, eating disorders, depression, substance abuse, and sports injuries.

## INTRODUCTION

Adolescence is a time of enormous growth and change that can be confusing and difficult for both teens and the adults around them. Physical growth and pubertal development occur along a predictable and visible continuum. Cognitive, emotional, moral, and sexual developments occur concurrently but are much more difficult to assess. Consciously attempting to evaluate the developmental progress of adolescents in each of these areas will assist the student in providing adolescent care. An adolescent's ability to participate in evaluation and treatment is determined in part by his or her developmental progress and prior health-care experiences.

## ADOLESCENT DEVELOPMENT

Most developmental specialists divide adolescence into early, middle, and late phases. These phases represent markers on a continuum, not steps with clear divisions. Although it is rare to have adult development in one area and childlike development in another, an individual usually is in different places in the various domains of development. Progress in each of these areas of development can be uneven. Attention to these domains of development can be very helpful in the assessment of adolescent health.

*Early adolescence* typically occurs at 10 to 14 years of age. Physical growth and sexual changes occur at a rapid pace. Body image is of paramount importance, and there is much self-preoccupation. There emerges a conflict over independence from parents, and a struggle to establish independence begins. The peer group assumes an important role. Concrete thought patterns are still dominant, and the long-range consequences of actions and decisions are not anticipated.

*Middle adolescence* typically occurs at 15 to 17 years of age. Body changes slow down during this time, and secondary sexual characteristics are well developed. Decreased preoccupation with these changes turns the focus of the adolescent toward establishing new relationships with same-sex and opposite-sex adolescents. Romantic relationships and sexual experimentation occur. The peer group becomes of paramount importance, and further steps are made toward becoming independent from parents. Feelings of invincibility may lead to risk-taking behavior. The ability to think abstractly becomes more developed. This is often the stage of greatest turmoil.

*Late adolescence* typically occurs at 18 to 21 years of age. A late adolescent with growing independence from parents, a more adultlike body, and a more mature style of relating to peers and adults looks toward the future. These adolescents develop their own sense of personal values and are more likely to seek and accept advice from their parents. They are more comfortable with their body image and develop a sense of self identity. Intimate relationships and close friendships begin to develop. Risk-taking behaviors decrease as thought processes become more abstract. Educational and/or occupational goals are established. A young adult is able to see more clearly the implications of decisions and actions.

## ADOLESCENT HEALTH MAINTENANCE VISIT

### HISTORY

Like health maintenance visits in other age groups, the adolescent well visit is used to screen for the problems and asymptomatic diseases that are most likely to harm the individual. The major causes of morbidity and mortality in adolescents are accidents, homicide, and suicide. These three causes often have their roots in developmental problems, early sexual activity, and substance use. Therefore, the adolescent visit focuses on the evaluation of the young person's development, warning signs of problems, and risk-taking behaviors.

The provider must take into account the adolescent's cognitive developmental stage when asking questions and doing evaluations. In early adolescence, a teen is likely to be concrete in his or her responses: "I am not sexually active; I just lie there." The adolescent may not use words the same way adults do. He may interpret petting or wet dreams as sexual activity; she may interpret kissing as oral intercourse. Therefore, try to be certain that you understand what the teen is telling you.

A teen is also likely to be fearful that normal physiologic changes are abnormal but not report them. Many teens are certain that the leukorrheic discharge before the initiation of menses represents an infection even though they have never been sexually active.

The health maintenance visit is structured the same way as for other age groups. For most school-age children, part of the visit should be done with the parent and part should be done separately. *Privacy* and *confidentiality* should be discussed with both parent and teen. The provider often elicits any concerns from the parent or teen. Next, *old problems and illnesses* should be reevaluated and any new family issues should be assessed. Providers should continue to ask about eating, sleeping, urination, and defecation. Many adolescents have a very poor diet, skip, meals or make bad nutritional choices. Few teens have enough calcium or iron in their diets. A large percentage of teens have dieted or are dieting to lose weight or increase muscle bulk. Urinary problems can arise with the growth spurt, and constipation is common as teens rarely have enough fiber in their diets.

Increasing evidence suggests that much of the population of the United States is sleep-deprived, and adolescents are particularly sleepy. Teens usually need a fair amount of sleep, but school starts earlier than it did in the elementary school years. More homework is assigned. More activities are available, and each one takes more time than it used to. Also, many teens have difficulty settling down to sleep and more trouble getting up; their biological clock prefers a later schedule.

## HEADSSS SCREEN

The social history is often gathered by using the HEADSSS (Home, education/employment, activities, drugs, sexual activity/orientation, suicidal ideation, and sexual/physical/emotional abuse) screen (Table 14-1). The screen has been added to over time, but the goal has remained the same: to assess the major areas of a teen's life and functioning. For middle and late teens, this information comes from the teen alone. Developmental domains merit particular attention throughout this evaluation.

*Table 14-1* **HEADSSS Screen**

| | Sample questions: Tailor to the developmental stage of the person. |
|---|---|
| Home | Where do you live? |
| | Who lives at your house? |
| | Do you spend overnight anywhere else? |
| | Do you have your own room? |
| | Do you have privacy? |
| | Are there any guns in the house? |
| |   Who do they belong to? |
| |   How are they stored? |
| |   Are they loaded? |
| Education/employment | Where do you go to school? |
| | What grade are you in? |
| | Are you in any special classes? |
| | Have you ever repeated or skipped a grade? |
| | Do you earn money or do you have a job? |
| |   How many hours a week? |
| |   Does it interfere with getting your schoolwork done? |
| |   Does it interfere with your social activities? |
| Activities | Do you have friends? |
| |   Who is your best friend? |
| |   What do you do together? |
| |   What do you do for fun? |
| | Do you have activities after school or outside of school? |
| |   Do you sing or play an instrument? |
| |   Do you play any sports? |
| Drugs | Have you ever tried drugs, alcohol, tobacco, steroids? If yes, how much? How often? You may consider asking, "Do your friends . . ." or "Do you know anyone who . . ." |
| Sexual activity/ orientation | Are you sexually active? |
| |   If yes, with men, women, or both? |
| |   What sorts of sexual activity? |
| |   Do you use protection? If so, what? |
| |   Should we talk about protection for you? |

*(continued)*

*Table 14-1* **HEADSSS Screen (continued)**

|  |  |
|---|---|
|  | If no, are you interested in anyone sexually? Men, women, or both? Are you worried that you might be gay or straight? Are you having wet dreams or fantasies about someone? |
| Suicidal | How is your mood? What would your friends say? What would your parents say? Are they correct? Have you ever thought about hurting yourself? Have you ever tried? |
| Sexual/physical/ emotional abuse | Have you ever been hurt in a relationship? Physically/emotionally? Have you ever had sex when you did not want to? Have you ever felt unsafe in a relationship? |

Teens often are concerned about these areas. Giving factual and normative information to a teen during the course of asking the HEADSSS questions can be very helpful. For example, telling a teen that many people his or her age have sexual thoughts about someone of the same sex and that this does not mean that a person is gay can be helpful. Similarly, telling a teen that at least half of his or her classmates are not sexually active can help support a teen who has decided not to be sexually active.

## PHYSICAL EXAMINATION

The physical examination should be done in privacy as soon as the child requests it. During this time, the provider should comment on the normal aspects of the physical examination since teens often worry that they are not normal. Adolescents are particularly modest, and so the clinician should try to uncover only the area being examined. Shorts and a loose T-shirt are more acceptable than hospital gowns to teens and should be considered for some examinations.

Growth should be plotted on growth curves through the completion of physical growth and genital maturation. The provider should comment on normal growth and the expected changes that will happen in the next year.

New findings in the physical examination are unlikely except in a few areas. Known prior problems should be reevaluated, such as obesity, asthma, and murmurs. Growth can change visual acuity and blood pressure, and so both should be tested at each health maintenance visit. Puberty can be associated with thyroid disease, and so palpation should be done as soon as the child enters puberty. The musculoskeletal system should be screened carefully for injuries, overuse syndromes, and developmental changes. Examine any area with a reported injury or pain or stiffness. An annual scoliosis screen from the preadolescent growth spurt until the completion of Tanner stage 4, when most growth is complete, should be performed. A careful skin examination should be done annually, with comments on sun protection and the development of moles.

Sexual maturation should be documented for breast and female genital development or male genital and testicular development. Again, the provider should comment on the reassuring progression through puberty. The clinician also should inquire about any changes that are of concern during the course of the examination. Many early adolescents are concerned or frightened by the development of genital hair or the growth of genitals. It is also appropriate to tell an early teen that he soon may experience wet dreams or that she may have clear vaginal discharge as a result of the progression through puberty.

## HEALTH MAINTENANCE ASSESSMENT AND PLAN

The assessment for an adolescent visit includes assessing the teen's development in the cognitive, physical, emotional, and sexual areas and whether it is progressing appropriately. A plan should be made to reduce risk and promote a healthy lifestyle and the emotional development of the teen.

As noted above and in the paragraphs that follow, adolescents progress from concrete, factual knowledge and following the rules to beginning to operationalize and deal with uncertainty and make conditional decisions. Where the teen is on this continuum should be noted.

Tanner staging should be documented and used to counsel the adolescent on her or his activities. Physically less mature adolescents should not play contact sports with more physically mature adolescents. Overuse injuries are more common in less skeletally mature adolescents. Pitcher's elbow and rotator cuff injuries are common problems. Assessment of the appropriate progression of skeletal maturity should be made, and an evaluation should be performed if it is not going as expected. Teens should be told what to expect over the coming year, particularly in the area of genital growth and changing function.

In regard to immunizations, most adolescents will have their primary series and a hepatitis B series of three shots. They need a diphtheria-tetanus (Td) booster 10 years after the last tetanus shot. The meningococcal vaccine was approved for use in 2005 and is recommended for patients 11 to 12 years of age. Varicella vaccine should be considered if a patient has not received the vaccine and has not had chickenpox. Those more than 13 years of age should receive two doses given at least 4 weeks apart. One should consider their activities in regard to whether they may need rabies vaccination (if they work with a vet or in a pet store). Hepatitis A vaccine should be given if they are traveling to areas of the world where the water is not treated, and they should receive other vaccinations that are specific to the region they may travel to or work in.

Emotional development also should be assessed and commented on. Does the teen have friends? Is she developing self-control? Does he moderate his mood appropriately? Advising adolescents and their families of the changes to come is good practice as well.

As was noted above, the most likely causes of morbidity and mortality in the teenage years are accidents, homicide, and suicide. Therefore, counseling to modify risk-taking behavior is the most important aspect of the plan for this visit. Adolescents often believe that risk does not apply to them. To be successful in effecting change, the provider needs to find a reason why that particular teen should change that behavior. For many girls, the reason they may quit smoking is that it gives them bad breath and wrinkles. For some young men, the reason not to drink is that it impedes their ability to have intercourse or impairs their athletic performance. Neither group is worried about the risk of cancer or liver disease; they have only short-term concerns.

Teens who drink or use illicit drugs are vulnerable because of the judgment-altering effects of alcohol and drugs. They may be forced to have unwanted intercourse, or they may ride in a car with someone who is impaired. Helping teens develop a safety plan is the most effective way to keep them from being victims.

For teens whose employment or activities put them at risk, it is often helpful to point out that the "heroes of the game" use protective equipment. For those who are drinking alcohol or smoking, one must recognize that these may be "gateways" to using illegal drugs as well as putting a teen in a vulnerable position.

There is a large overlap between teens who drink or smoke and those who are sexually active. Most teens do not use contraception correctly, if at all. The result is increases in sexually transmitted diseases (STDs), pregnancy, and human immunodeficiency virus (HIV). Thus, the physician must look for signs and symptoms of STDs. Screening for these diseases is a must. For females, a genital examination may reveal swollen lymph glands, venereal warts, vaginal discharge, or a red cervix. For males, lymphadenopathy, visible warts, and a penile discharge should be looked for. Urine tests are available to screen for gonococci (GC) and chlamydia. For males, a urinalysis by dipstick that reveals leukocytes constitutes evidence that cultures for STDs should be performed. Blood must be obtained if syphilis, HIV, hepatitis C, or hepatitis B are suspected. The various contraceptive methods, including abstinence, barrier methods (condoms, vaginal diaphragms), oral contraceptives, and contraceptive injections, should be explained and discussed to determine which would work best for the patient. Teens need to be asked about sexuality, sexual orientation, and sexual behavior, because they are not always congruous. A male may consider himself gay but be having intercourse with women. This apparent contradiction should be clarified and discussed.

Pointing out the consequences of any of the problems the clinician finds can help alter the teen's behavior. Statements such as "You have chlamydia, and no one can know how long you have had it or who you shared it with. It can cause scarring and infertility" can help a teen look ahead and modify his or her behavior.

Personal safety is an important topic to cover with teens since lack of safety is one of the most common causes of death and disability in this age group. Teens are more independent than children and also do more independent thinking. Therefore, the interview of an adolescent must include screening for these safety issues and concomitant counseling for self-protection. Asking about firearms and insisting on locking up the bullets and the gun or other weapon is good practice. Far more adolescents and children are hurt by guns than are hurt by home intruders.

Providers need to ask adolescents how they will protect themselves in different situations. What if their friends or acquaintances are doing unsafe things? How will they handle the situation? What will they do if someone picks a fight or bullies them? Having an action plan for safety can be literally lifesaving.

One of the biggest risks to teens is their newfound mobility in bigger and faster vehicles. Discussing with the teen and parent a safety plan for getting to and from the teen's activities is helpful. Teens may find themselves unexpectedly with someone who is supposed to transport them, and that person is intoxicated or cannot provide transportation. Unless there has been a previous discussion, the teen knows that his parent will be upset about being awakened to drive him or her home. However, no parents would want their children to place themselves knowingly in an unsafe position and ride home with a stranger or someone who is intoxicated.

Adolescents often do not take into account the risks they take. They drive fast without considering the consequences or what could appear around the corner. They experiment with drugs and alcohol because they do not think that what they have been warned about will happen to them.

## PREPARTICIPATION SPORTS PHYSICAL

The preparticipation sports physical has the threefold purpose of screening participants for *increased risk* of injury or death with participation, *preventing injuries*, and advising about the care and *rehabilitation* of prior injuries. This may be done by the team physician or by the primary care provider. In either situation, all three areas must be addressed. Part of the risk of participation depends on the activity. Any activity that taxes the cardiovascular system increases the risk of sudden death from asthma, arrhythmias, or cardiac outflow tract obstruction. Contact sports such as football and lacrosse and high-impact sports such as gymnastics and baseball have the highest risk of traumatic injuries, whereas noncontact sports such as volleyball and swimming have a higher risk of overuse injuries. The history portion of the assessment often is obtained in a questionnaire to give the participant a chance to inquire about some of the areas addressed.

### INCREASED RISK

Increased risk of injury or death should be assessed by history and physical examination. Participants should be queried about any episodes of syncope or near syncope, seizures, chest pain during participation, known murmur and its evaluation, family history of sudden death, palpitations or known arrhythmias, and known medical problems such as asthma and Down syndrome. Any positive responses should receive a full evaluation before participation. All persons with Down syndrome need a neck radiograph looking for odontoid ligament laxity.

The physical examination portion of the evaluation should document symmetric and correctable visual acuity, good dental health without loose teeth, good air movement, and absence of pathologic murmurs or heart sounds. Symmetric muscle bulk and reflexes help assure that protective mechanisms are in order. Physical development must be documented for all contact sports and most high-energy-using sports. Early pubertal patients who participate in contact sports with late or postpubertal participants are much more prone to musculoskeletal injuries.

Any syncope or chest pain during exercise or immediately afterward should preclude participation until a thorough cardiovascular and neurologic evaluation is completed. A family history of sudden death mandates evaluation for arrhythmias, such as prolonged QT syndrome, and hypertrophic cardiomyopathy (HCM). Murmurs need to be explained before participation. Most murmurs in this age group are innocent flow murmurs, but ones from outlet flow tract obstruction are also systolic and flow type, and this obstruction can cause sudden death during exercise. Asthma must be well controlled, and the athlete must have a plan for prevention and early recognition of poor control. Athletes should be encouraged to participate in contact and team sports with others of similar size and musculoskeletal development to minimize the risk of injury.

### INJURY PREVENTION

Injury prevention should be done in two areas: developmental and paired organs or senses. A musculoskeletal system that is changing rapidly during adolescence can be more prone to injury and disability in situations of overuse or undue stress. Young pitchers whose tendons and ligaments have not developed fully easily can injure their elbows if they are encouraged to throw too many innings or throw in positions that are stressful to the elbow or throw "sidearm." Young dancers can injure their feet and ankles if they are encouraged to spend too long "on toe" before their skeletons have matured adequately and they have sufficient muscle strength to support their weight. Female soccer players are prone to anterior cruciate ligament (ACL) tears from planting their feet and pivoting before they have sufficient quadriceps strength to change the body's momentum.

Every effort should be made to prevent injuries to the paired organs and special senses. For example, if an athlete is competing in a contact sport and has little or no use of one eye or ear, special protection should be mandatory for all practices and games to prevent blindness or deafness. Athletes who have lost one testicle to torsion or injury should wear special protection to prevent injury to the remaining organ.

The provider also should encourage every athlete to comply with the personal protection recommendations for his or her sport. Snowboarders, bikers, and skaters should wear helmets, and soccer players should wear shin guards and mouth guards. Each of these protective devices is effective only if the athlete wears it and it fits correctly.

## INJURY REHABILITATION

Musculoskeletal injuries are common in most sports. Ankle sprains, broken fingers, callus formation, and falls are the most frequently reported injuries, but each sport has one or more frequently seen problems that are specific to it. Ask about injuries from the patient's sport or other activities. Check that the injury is fully healed and that there is no residual muscle weakness from the inactivity required for healing. Recommend muscle strengthening or other rehabilitation to prevent a recurrence.

## CLOSED HEAD INJURIES

Closed head injuries are common in some sports, but head injuries can occur off the field as well. Football and hockey players are particularly prone to injury on the field, but these injuries can happen on or off the field.

Immediately after the injury, players who have been unconscious or who have residual headache or tinnitus, dizziness, or neurologic problems should be evaluated by a medical professional and must not be allowed to return to the activity.

More commonly, an athlete reports having had a "concussion." He or she must not be allowed to return to practice or competition until all the symptoms have resolved completely for at least a week. Premature return to activity can cause prolonged or permanent neurologic problems such as headache, weakness, dizziness, and tinnitus.

## MEDICAL ISSUES

Medical problems in adolescence are similar to those which occur in childhood and adulthood. The social and cognitive changes of puberty can make managing these problems more difficult. Often a well-controlled diabetic patient becomes poorly controlled as he or she takes increasing responsibility for managing the diabetes in adolescence. The teen wants more autonomy and the responsibility for taking his or her medicine. However, he or she faces the pressures of conforming with the peer group. Many times the pressure to fit in wins out and the teen skips medication, physical therapy, or eating, with results that compromise her or his health. The practitioner must find strategies for helping the teen fit in while caring for medical issues as well.

Chronic illnesses can delay the onset of puberty and the growth spurt that an adolescent's friends are experiencing. When this happens, an adolescent can feel left out and childish. The better managed and the less severe the illness is, the less impact there is on the teen's growth. The physician should watch for signs that this is happening and discuss it with the chronically ill patient, allowing the teen to take as much responsibility as is feasible and maximizing the teen's understanding.

Some medical problems are ameliorated by puberty. When asthmatics grow, that growth gives them better lung function. Some diabetic patients have better control with the easier to measure higher doses of insulin.

Other medical problems worsen through adolescence. The growth spurt demands increased oxygen delivery to tissues. To accomplish that, the heart needs to increase cardiac output, the lungs need to increase their ability to oxygenate the blood with increased surface area, and the kidneys need to excrete more waste. The way the body manages medication changes over the course of puberty.

### THE MENSTRUAL CYCLE

One of the most common reasons for a young woman to visit the doctor is to discuss menstrual problems. Puberty causes changes in many hormones, including estrone, estradiol, testosterone, dihydrotestosterone, androstenedione, progesterone, and dehydroepiandrosterone. As one might expect, these hormones rarely get to the levels at which they need to be at the same time. This lack of coordination creates a variety of problems, including irregular menses, amenorrhea, and dysfunctional uterine bleeding.

Girls begin to have breast buds that develop into breasts under the stimulation of estrogen. They develop some fine genital hair. They also have a growth spurt during Tanner stage 2. During Tanner stage 3, most girls begin to menstruate. Frish has developed tables of percentage of body fat that girls must achieve in order to menstruate. For girls the percentage of body fat rises with the growth spurt of puberty, whereas for boys it falls (see Table 3-2).

Girls develop an areola and a nipple. Genital hair becomes curly. Tanner stages 4 and 5 include progressive maturation of the breast and genital structures. A small percentage of girls ovulate during the early Tanner stages, but the majority do not until they enter Tanner 4. Early on only a few cycles each year are ovulatory, but more and more become ovulatory with time. By their twenties, most women ovulate in 8 to 10 cycles of the year.

Periods do not become regular for the first couple of years for most girls. In some months periods are very heavy, and during others quite scant. The first reason for amenorrhea to be ruled out in every girl is pregnancy. Some girls get pregnant before they realize that they have started to menstruate.

Primary amenorrhea—never having had a period—usually is due to hormonal abnormalities, but it also can be due to structural congenital anomalies. If growth also is impaired, chromosomal abnormalities may underlie the problem. More common is the delayed onset of puberty as a result of other medical problems, such as thyroid disease, renal failure, and eating disorders. Therefore, a careful history and physical examination together with screening laboratories should uncover the etiology of the amenorrhea.

Secondary amenorrhea is very common. After having three or more periods, the adolescent then misses two or more. The cause for this is most frequently stress, whether physical or psychological. Illnesses and injuries can cause amenorrhea, as can depression, anxiety, and nutritional deficiencies. Severe weight loss, as with inflammatory bowel disease or anorexia, also can lead to menstrual irregularities or amenorrhea.

## PREGNANCY

Teens are very likely to get pregnant when they start having intercourse. Many of their cycles are ovulatory, and the egg can be fertilized for a few days. Teens are not well developed for pregnancy; many have very low iron stores, poor nutrition, and low body fat. They must receive good prenatal care and emotional support. They may not be emotionally ready for the responsibilities of parenting. A teen should be given as much responsibility for her child as is possible without endangering the baby. Repeat pregnancies are much less common when a teen is responsible for her child.

## GENITAL INFECTIONS

Many teens who are sexually active do not practice safe sex. The result is unintended pregnancies and sexually transmitted diseases. Common presentations for STDs are vaginal discharge or abdominal pain and fever. When girls become sexually active, it is common for them to develop a urinary tract infection (UTI). Thus, when a teen comes in with a UTI, it is prudent to screen her or him for STDs.

## SCHOOL ISSUES

School is the work of children and teens. A change in their ability to function at school is a marker of problems. Social issues are the most common, including fights, truancy, and difficulty with friendships. Some indications of new social problems are depression, anxiety, and substance use. A good history and physical examination usually will uncover the cause and suggest a treatment plan. Academic issues also come to light during the teenage years. Some are due to previously undiagnosed learning disabilities, and others come to light only when students are asked to do higher-order thinking such as explaining, finding patterns and associations, and applying information in a variety of settings. Educational testing helps distinguish an educational problem from a medical or psychiatric one.

## PSYCHIATRIC PROBLEMS

Adolescents have a high incidence of psychiatric problems. Attention deficit disorder (ADD) usually is well managed with classroom methods in the early grades. As adolescents have more teachers, take on increased amounts of independent work, and have to do more organizing of their time, behavioral methods have to be augmented or complemented with specialized strategies. A teen who is newly having trouble in school or recently has started getting into fights or resists going to school should be evaluated. Note that although distractibility, fidgeting, and impulsivity are seen commonly in adolescents with ADD, they also can be seen in teens with other conditions. Other psychiatric problems seen in adolescents include eating disorders, depression, suicide, and substance abuse.

## EATING DISORDERS

Eating disorders are a cause of morbidity and occasionally mortality in adolescents. Bulimia nervosa occurs in 1 to 5 percent of adolescents, and anorexia nervosa occurs in 0.5 to 1 percent. Although they occur more commonly in females, males also can develop eating disorders. Both disorders stem from a distorted body image ("I'm too fat"), leading to an obsession with becoming thin. A number of individual, familial, and societal factors play a role in the development of these disorders. The DSM IV (*The Diagnostic and Statistical Manual of Mental Disorders*, 4th edition) lists the criteria for both illnesses. Some of the criteria for anorexia nervosa include low body weight (less than the 15th percentile for age), intense fear of gaining weight, a disturbed body image, and absence of three consecutive menstrual cycles. Adolescents with bulimia nervosa often have recurrent episodes of binge eating and lack of control during the binges. They also have a disturbed body image and may attempt to prevent weight gain by means of purging (using vomiting or lax-atives) or nonpurging (fasting or excessive exercise).

## HISTORY

When one is obtaining a history, questions about the patient's diet and exer-cise routine should be asked. In females, a menstrual history should be obtained. Many adolescents with eating disorders are depressed, and so questions about mood are important. The family members may suspect an eating disorder if they report binge eating in an adolescent without any apparent weight gain. Patients should be asked if they are happy with their bodies. The family history may reveal family members with psychiatric dis-orders such as depression and obsessive-compulsive disorder. The social his-tory may reveal a chaotic, dysfunctional family.

## PHYSICAL EXAMINATION

Growth parameters are especially important in patients with suspected eat-ing disorders. Those with anorexia nervosa typically have a weight less than the 15th percentile for age, and that may give them an ill-looking appear-ance, whereas those with bulimia nervosa often have normal weight and appear healthy. In reviewing vital signs, physicians find that patients with anorexia nervosa and bulimia nervosa who have excessive purging may have hypothermia, hypotension, and bradycardia. The general affect of the patient may be depressed or anxious. As a result of weight loss, those with anorexia nervosa have a malnourished appearance, with fine lanugo hair, brittle hair and nails, dry cold skin, and dependent edema. Patients with bulimia nervosa who purge have findings that result from excess vomiting (trauma to the palate and hands, loss of dental enamel, parotid swelling).

## LABORATORY EVALUATION

Eating disorders usually are diagnosed on the basis of the history and phys-ical examination. Laboratory abnormalities occur as a result of malnutrition and purging. Electrolyte abnormalities such as low potassium, low chloride, and high blood urea nitrogen may be present in those with excessive vomit-ing. If electrolytes are abnormal or an arrhythmia is suspected, an electro-cardiogram should be obtained. A complete blood count (CBC) may reveal anemia and leukopenia. Thyroid function tests are important if symptoms of hypothyroidism are present.

## MANAGEMENT

The management of a patient with an eating disorder requires a multidisci-plinary team approach that includes the family. Normal eating habits and nutrition must be established. Nutritional counseling and individual and family therapy are necessary. Most patients are treated on an outpatient basis. Hospitalization may be required if there are severe electrolyte abnormalities, dehydration, arrhythmias, depression or suicidal ideation, and/or failure to gain weight.

# DEPRESSION

It is estimated that up to 9 percent of all adolescents have a major affective disorder. Up to 20 percent of those patients have suicidal ideation. Depression seems to affect females more than males.

DSM-IV outlines the criteria for major depression and dysthymic disorder. Some of the criteria for depression are a depressed or irritable mood, insomnia or hypersomnia, fatigue or energy loss, decreased interest or pleasure in activities, weight gain, and weight loss.

## HISTORY

Adolescents with depression may have a wide range of physical, behavioral, or psychological symptoms. Physical complaints may include abdominal pain, headache, decreased appetite, overeating, insomnia, and fatigue. Behavioral symptoms include school difficulties or missing school, acting-out behavior, change in eating or sleep habits, loss of pleasure in daily activities, desire to be alone or withdrawal, and substance abuse. Psychological symptoms include low self-esteem, feelings of worthlessness, sadness, and feelings of hopelessness. The past medical history is important. Patients with chronic medical conditions or learning disabilities are more prone to be depressed. Family dysfunction may be present, and there may be a family history of depression or other psychiatric disorders.

## PHYSICAL EXAMINATION

The physical examination is typically normal. Weight loss may be present in depressed patients with decreased appetite. The patient may have a flat affect during the history and physical examination.

## LABORATORY EVALUATION

No laboratory tests typically are done in patients with suspected depression.

## MANAGEMENT

Management typically consists of some combination of educational, psychological, and psychiatric counseling and medication. The counseling may involve only the patient or may include the family.

# SUICIDE

Suicide is the third leading cause of death in adolescents, after accidents and homicide. Although adolescent females attempt suicide more often than males do, males are more successful in their suicide attempts. A suicide attempt is often an impulsive response to what appears to be a minor problem that is compounded by enormous societal and family unrest. It is not the result of a few isolated events but rather the end of a process of extremely frustrating situations. Just as in depression, a suicidal individual is trying to deal with some sort of personal conflict, loss, or major perceived change in his or her life. There are a number of risk factors for suicide. The more common ones include a family history of depression or suicide, a previous suicide attempt, and physical, sexual, or substance abuse.

## EVALUATION OF SUICIDAL INTENT

At least two-thirds of suicidal persons communicate their intent. This communication can take many forms, direct or vague. Many suicidal communications are "calls for help." People who have made the decision to kill themselves are not calling for help; they are convinced that there is no help to be found and that no hope exists. The absence of an external purpose for making a suicidal attempt is an ominous sign. More commonly, however, an attempt is a way to say "listen to me." Who is serious about suicide and who is not? There are no hard and fast rules, but the following factors are seen in those who are serious: The attempt is made in isolation with precautions taken to avoid discovery, preparations are made in anticipation of death, others are informed beforehand, a suicide note is written, and extensive planning has taken place.

## HISTORY

Asking an adolescent patient about suicidal ideation or intent does *not* plant or reinforce the idea, and so such inquiries should be part of the routine adolescent history. Most patients will be relieved that you brought up such a delicate topic; in fact, three in four persons with serious thoughts of suicide will be willing to discuss it candidly with you. Start by asking a wide range of general questions in a conversational manner. Listen and be nonjudgmental. Eventually hone in on questions specific to depression and suicide. Do use the word *suicide* in your questions and discussions. Accept every suicidal thought as serious.

## PHYSICAL EXAMINATION

The abnormalities on the physical examination of an adolescent patient who has attempted suicide depend on the method used. Those who ingested a toxin or overdosed may have findings specific to the toxin or drug. Descriptions of the physical signs of various drug ingestions are given in Chap. 39. Scars, especially on the wrists, may be due to a previous suicide attempt or physical abuse. Most often the physical examination is normal.

## MANAGEMENT

A multidisciplinary team approach, including social workers, psychologists, and/or psychiatrists, is involved in the care of these patients. In general, all adolescent patients who have attempted suicide should be hospitalized.

There is no guarantee that a patient who has attempted suicide will follow through on recommendations for outpatient treatment. Education, counseling, and pharmacotherapy, if necessary, can be started during the hospitalization.

## SUBSTANCE ABUSE

The majority of adolescents have experimented with alcohol, tobacco, and/or marijuana by the time they are high school seniors. Adolescents use alcohol and drugs for a variety of reasons, including social acceptance by peers, use by family members or peers, experimentation, low self-esteem, and acting-out behavior. The levels of drug use vary. Some teens may experiment with drugs to experience a new phenomenon. Others may engage in recreational or circumstantial use to achieve a specific desired effect under limited conditions. The more serious cases of abuse or dependent use involve adolescents who have compulsive drug use that interferes with biologic, psychological, or social function.

### HISTORY

School-related problems (decreased attendance or a decline in grades or performance) are often important clues to the possibility of substance abuse. Recent changes in friends or family stressors such as divorce and death can lead to substance use. Parents may notice mood swings, which may be related to drug use or may be a sign of an underlying psychological problem such as depression. Suggestive behaviors such as running away, poor grooming, sloppy dress, and increased attention to the drug culture should raise suspicion for substance abuse. Some adolescents have overt signs of drug or alcohol use or may have legal involvement (e.g., driving while intoxicated) as a result of substance abuse.

### PHYSICAL EXAMINATION

Although a complete physical examination should be performed, physical findings related to substance abuse or withdrawal are rare in adolescents.

### LABORATORY EVALUATION

Urine and blood can be screened for drug metabolites, with urine testing the more commonly used of the two. False positives and false negatives are associated with both tests. Random drug screening of adolescents is a controversial topic. The American Academy of Pediatrics does not support random drug screening. A drug screen should be performed without the adolescent's consent only when the adolescent is mentally incompetent to make an informed decision or if there is a medical or legal reason to perform the test.

## MANAGEMENT

Management is based on the reason for and degree of drug use. Those who are experimenting with drugs may benefit from education and anticipatory guidance. Others may require individual counseling. Adolescents with serious substance abuse problems may benefit from an ambulatory drug treatment program such as Alcoholics Anonymous. The most severely affected may need some type of residential treatment program.

## BIBLIOGRAPHY

Rudolph CD, Rudolph AM, Hostetter MK, et al. *Rudolph's Pediatrics*, 21st ed. New York: McGraw-Hill, 2003: 2094.

# CHIEF
# COMPLAINTS/
# COMMON ACUTE
# ILLNESSES

# COUGH

## Stephanie Starr

### LEARNING OBJECTIVES

1. Describe the pathophysiology of cough.

2. Summarize general differences in approaching cough in children as opposed to adults.

3. Specifically define *bronchitis* and explain the pathogenesis and treatment of this entity in children.

4. List the differential diagnosis for acute cough and chronic cough in children, paying attention to differences based on age.

5. Describe the pertinent historical and physical examination information in caring for children with cough and explain how it helps narrow the differential diagnosis.

6. State the most common diagnoses as well as the diagnoses not to miss for acute and chronic cough in children.

## INTRODUCTION

Cough is one of the most common pediatric chief complaints encountered in the outpatient setting. The most common etiology for cough in children is viral upper respiratory tract infection, and supportive measures are all that is required. However, cough also may herald a serious acute disease (lobar pneumonia with pleural effusions) or be the initial manifestation of a chronic disease (cystic fibrosis) in a pediatric patient. It is important to understand the pathophysiology, differential diagnosis, and management of cough not only to optimize patient management and comfort but also to ensure the judicious use of antibiotics and avoid the use of unnecessary therapies.

There are several issues particular to children that must be taken into consideration in evaluating children with cough:

1. As with most other chief complaints, the differential diagnosis of cough can vary greatly on the basis of the patient's age. An adolescent with recurrent cough and wheezing is likely to have asthma, but an anatomic anomaly such as a vascular ring or sling should be considered in an infant with recurrent cough and wheezing.
2. Infants typically have physical examination findings that are very different from those of adults, such as the lack of a productive cough and reliable ausculatory findings on lung examination.
3. Among children who experience cardiopulmonary arrest, the large majority do so because of respiratory distress or dehydration and shock rather than primary cardiac pathology (such as acute myocardial infarction) as in adults. Therefore, it is critical that those caring for children be able to recognize the symptoms and signs of impending respiratory failure so that they can prevent cardiopulmonary arrest and effectively treat the underlying disease process.
4. Some therapies that are effective in adults (e.g., over-the-counter cold preparations) have no advantage over placebo in children studied to date.
5. Foreign bodies and toxic ingestions are common in children and always should be considered in working through the differential diagnosis of any chief complaint in a pediatric patient. Cough is perhaps the most common chief complaint associated with inhaled foreign bodies in children.

It is also worthwhile to understand the use of the term *bronchitis* as it relates to diagnosing and treating pediatric patients with cough. Bronchitis is defined as inflammation of the bronchial respiratory mucosa. The clinical definition of bronchitis in children is not well established, and several studies have concluded that this self-resolving illness is usually viral in origin. It is important to keep in mind that pediatric patients with chronic lung disease (e.g., cystic fibrosis or chronic tracheobronchitis secondary to tracheostomy) should be excluded from this general discussion, as these patients may benefit from antibiotics to treat presumed lower respiratory tract infection in the absence of documented pneumonia. Despite the nebulous clinical definition of bronchitis in children, the diagnosis is made frequently by some practitioners, and antimicrobials frequently are prescribed. Pediatric patients with recurrent diagnoses of bronchitis often in fact have asthma, which is one of the most common chronic diseases in childhood. Many pediatricians avoid the diagnosis of bronchitis entirely as it is often synonymous with bacterial infection in the minds of parents. In this chapter, the term *bronchitis* thus is avoided. Treatment of a pediatric patient with a prolonged acute cough when pneumonia, asthma, and other diagnoses have been excluded is discussed later in the chapter.

## PATHOPHYSIOLOGY AND ANATOMY

To be an effective diagnostician, one must understand the basic science behind the chief complaint. The chief purpose of any cough is to remove secretions and inhaled foreign material. A cough occurs either because the patient coughs voluntarily or through an involuntary cough reflex. Mucus or foreign material initiates this reflex by stimulating cough receptors throughout the respiratory tract (the nose, sinuses, pharynx, larynx, trachea, large bronchi, and/or terminal bronchioles). Afferent impulses from these receptors travel via cranial nerve pathways to the medullary cough center. In the medulla, efferent impulses stimulate coordinated closure of the glottis and contraction of diaphragmatic, chest wall, abdominal wall, and pelvic floor musculature.

The anatomy of a cough also can be viewed as consisting of three phases: inspiratory, compressive, and expiratory. During the inspiratory phase, the glottis closes after deep inspiration. The compressive phase is brief and is defined by an increase in intrathoracic pressure generated through contraction of the expiratory muscles. In the expiratory phase, the glottis opens and air is propelled forcefully out, clearing the respiratory tract of mucus and foreign material.

## DIFFERENTIAL DIAGNOSIS

Educators have observed that seasoned "master" clinicians approach diagnostic dilemmas (chief complaints) by generating an early differential diagnosis. The clinician then uses the history and physical examination to "rule in" or "rule out" the diagnoses on the list. Laboratory and radiographic studies then are used to confirm or refute the final diagnoses on the list. Earlier learners in medical education often find that general categories are useful in organizing their differential diagnoses until they have more patient experience and have read more extensively about the chief complaints they encounter. As one sees more patients and reads about chief complaints, one comes to rely less on lists and tables to come up with the differential diagnosis.

There are many possible approaches to thinking about the differential diagnosis of cough in children. First, it is important to consider whether the patient has a medical condition that increases the risk of a more serious or uncommon diagnosis. For example, patients with chronic immunosuppression (malignancy, systemic lupus erythematosus, specific immunodeficiency) or diabetes mellitus are at higher risk for infectious diseases. Children with chronic lung diseases, as was mentioned above, are also at higher risk for lower respiratory tract infections. Next, one should consider how to organize the differential diagnosis. The list of possible diagnoses can be classified on the basis of acute (< 3 weeks) versus chronic cough, anatomic location (nasal etiologies, below the nose but above the vocal cords, between the vocal cords and the bifurcation of the trachea, etc.), characteristics of the cough, and the age of the patient. Another approach would be to consider the types of stimuli that could trigger a cough (mechanical, inflammatory/infectious, chemical, heat/cold, psychogenic, toxins).

One practical approach is to start by considering the most common etiologies and the etiologies not to miss (those which have the potential for high morbidity and mortality) and then consider the age-appropriate differential diagnosis for acute (< 3 weeks) or chronic cough. It is helpful to remember that at least 90 percent of cases of cough in children are caused by a respiratory tract infection [upper respiratory infection (URI), croup, pneumonia, bronchiolitis, whooping cough], but noninfectious etiologies should be considered in children with markedly prolonged cough. Tables 15-1 and 15-2 list the most common and less common diagnoses that can present as acute or chronic cough. Table 15-3 lists the diagnoses not to miss in children with cough. (For more detailed information on URIs, see Chap. 20.) Benign chronic cough without wheezing appears to be a different disorder from asthma, as chronic cough without wheezing in children who are otherwise well-appearing and without risk factors for asthma does not respond to asthma therapy and spontaneously resolves.

## HISTORY

As was discussed above, the history is essential in narrowing down the differential diagnosis. In the HPI (history of present illness), start by asking the questions that describe the chief complaint: When did the cough start (duration)? This will clarify whether you are formulating the differential for an acute (< 3 weeks) versus chronic cough. What is the frequency? Timing? A chronic cough that occurs at night suggests asthma or postnasal drip as with allergic rhinitis or sinusitis. Are there aggravating and/or relieving factors? Cough associated with meals suggests gastroesophageal reflux disease or aspiration, whereas cough triggered by exercise or cold weather is suspicious for asthma. What is the quality of the cough? A barky cough suggests croup, whereas a spasmodic cough should alert the practitioner to the possibility of pertussis. Is the cough dry and "hacking" in nature, as is seen frequently in asthma? A throat-clearing sound suggests postnasal drip, whereas a "honking" or "foghorn" cough (especially one that disappears at

*Table 15-1* **Differential Diagnosis of Acute Cough (< 3 Weeks)**

| | Infants (0–12 Months) | Young Children (1–5 Years) | Older Children and Adolescents (5–18 Years) |
|---|---|---|---|
| Most common | Infections<br>✓ Viral (influenza, RSV, parainfluenza, adenovirus, rhinoviruses)<br>✓ URI<br>✓ Croup<br>✓ Bronchiolitis<br>✓ Viral pneumonia<br>✓ Bacterial<br>✓ Bacterial pneumonia<br>✓ Other infections<br>✓ *Chlamydia pneumoniae*<br>✓ Pertussis<br>✓ Anatomic/ingestion<br>✓ Foreign body | Infections<br>✓ Viral<br>✓ URI<br>✓ Croup<br>✓ Pneumonia<br>✓ Bacterial<br>✓ Pneumonia<br>✓ Sinusitis<br>✓ Other<br>✓ *Mycoplasma pneumoniae*<br>✓ Pertussis syndrome<br><br>Anatomic/ingestion<br>✓ Foreign body | Infections<br>✓ Viral<br>✓ URI<br>✓ Pneumonia<br>✓ Bacterial<br>✓ Pneumonia<br>✓ Sinusitis<br>✓ Other<br>✓ Atypical pneumonia (e.g., Mycoplasma) |
| Less common | Anatomic/ingestion<br>✓ Caustic ingestion<br><br>Infections<br>✓ Tuberculosis<br><br>Other<br>✓ Gastroesophageal reflux disease | Infections<br>✓ Bacterial<br>✓ Bacterial tracheitis<br><br>Anatomic/ingestion<br>✓ Caustic ingestion<br><br>Infections<br>✓ Tuberculosis<br><br>Malignancy<br>✓ Acute lymphoblastic leukemia (infection overlying relative immunodeficiency) | Malignancy<br>✓ Lymphoma (mediastinal mass causing compression)<br>✓ Acute lymphoblastic leukemia (infection overlying relative immunodeficiency) |

RSV = respiratory syncytial virus; URI = upper respiratory infection.

Table 15-2 **Differential Diagnosis of Chronic Cough**

| | Infants (0–12 Months) | Young Children (1–5 Years) | Older Children and Adolescents (5–18 Years) |
|---|---|---|---|
| Most common | Infections<br>✓ Viral<br>  ✓ Prolonged cough from URI<br>  ✓ Bronchiolitis<br>  ✓ Pneumonia<br>✓ Bacterial<br>  ✓ Pneumonia<br>✓ Other<br>  ✓ *Chlamydia pneumoniae*<br>  ✓ Pertussis<br><br>Inflammatory<br>✓ Asthma<br><br>Irritants<br>✓ Passive smoke<br><br>Anatomic/ingestion<br>✓ Foreign body<br><br>Other<br>✓ Gastroesophageal reflux disease | Infections<br>✓ Viral<br>  ✓ Prolonged cough from URI<br>  ✓ Pneumonia<br>✓ Bacterial<br>  ✓ Sinusitis<br>  ✓ Pneumonia<br>✓ Other<br>  ✓ *Mycoplasma pneumoniae*<br>  ✓ Pertussis<br><br>Inflammatory<br>✓ Asthma<br>✓ Allergic rhinitis<br><br>Irritants<br>✓ Passive smoke<br><br>Anatomic/ingestion<br>✓ Foreign body<br><br>Other<br>✓ Benign persistent cough without wheeze | Infections<br>✓ Viral<br>  ✓ Prolonged cough from URI<br>  ✓ Pneumonia<br>✓ Bacterial<br>  ✓ Sinusitis<br>  ✓ Pneumonia<br>✓ Other<br>  ✓ *Mycoplasma pneumoniae*<br>  ✓ Pertussis<br><br>Inflammatory<br>✓ Asthma<br>✓ Allergic rhinitis<br><br>Irritants<br>✓ Passive smoke<br>✓ Tobacco use<br><br>Other<br>✓ Benign persistent cough without wheeze |
| Less common | Anatomic/ingestion<br>✓ Congenital malformation<br>  ✓ Vascular ring or sling<br>  ✓ Cystic adenomatoid malformation<br>  ✓ Bronchogenic cyst | Anatomic/ingestion<br>✓ Congenital malformation<br>  ✓ Vascular ring or sling<br>  ✓ Cystic adenomatoid malformation | Irritants<br>✓ "Huffing"<br><br>Compression<br>✓ Malignancy (e.g., lymphoma causing mediastinal mass)<br>*(continued)* |

*Table 15-2* **Differential Diagnosis of Chronic Cough (continued)**

| | Infants (0–12 Months) | Young Children (1–5 Years) | Older Children and Adolescents (5–18 Years) |
|---|---|---|---|
| Less common | ✓ Tracheomalacia<br>✓ Tracheoesopha-<br>  geal fistula<br><br>Congestive heart failure<br><br>Genetic disorder<br>✓ Cystic fibrosis<br><br>Recurrent aspiration<br><br>Infections<br>✓ Tuberculosis | ✓ Bronchogenic<br>  cyst<br>✓ Tracheomalacia<br>✓ Tracheoesopha-<br>  geal fistula<br><br>Compression (e.g.,<br>  mediastinal mass)<br><br>Genetic disorder<br>✓ Cystic fibrosis<br>✓ $\alpha_1$ antitrypsin<br>  deficiency<br><br>Immune deficiency<br><br>Recurrent aspiration<br><br>Primary ciliary<br>  dyskinesia<br><br>Infections<br>✓ Tuberculosis<br><br>Cough tic | Genetic disorder<br>✓ Cystic fibrosis<br>✓ $\alpha_1$ antitrypsin<br>  deficiency<br><br>Immune deficien-<br>  cies<br><br>Recurrent aspira-<br>  tion<br><br>Primary ciliary<br>  dyskinesia<br><br>Infections<br>✓ Tuberculosis<br><br>Psychogenic cough |

URI = upper respiratory infection.

night) suggests psychogenic cough. Note that although identifying sputum production may be helpful in the differential diagnosis in adult patients, in children it is less helpful as young patients frequently swallow any sputum that is present.

Next, inquire about associated respiratory symptoms. Is there stridor? If you identify both cough and stridor, this will help narrow the differential diagnosis significantly (to include croup and bacterial tracheitis). Hoarseness also suggests croup. Asking about wheezing can be helpful when a parent or older adolescent has some knowledge about what is meant

Table 15-3  *"Don't Miss" Diagnoses of Cough*

|  | Acute Cough (< 3 Weeks) | Chronic Cough (> 3 Weeks) |
|---|---|---|
| Infants (0–12 months) | Foreign body | Asthma<br>Cystic fibrosis<br>Congenital anatomic abnormality<br>✓ Vascular ring/sling<br>✓ Tracheoesophageal fistula<br>✓ Tracheobronchomalacia<br>✓ Laryngeal cleft<br>✓ Hemangioma |
| Young children (1–5 years) | Foreign body<br>Caustic ingestion | Asthma<br>Foreign body<br>Cystic fibrosis |
| Children and adolescents (5–18 years) |  | Asthma<br>Foreign body |

by wheezing. To a provider, wheezing suggests airway obstruction, but this history should be interpreted with caution as some parents describe noisy upper airway breathing from nasal congestion as wheezing as well. Ask specifically about symptoms or signs of increased work of breathing with exertion (exercise in children and feeding in infants). In infants and very young children, the parents may describe fast or labored breathing; they may observe chest retractions or even cyanosis. An older child or adolescent can describe the sensation of breathlessness (dyspnea). Historic or physical examination findings of respiratory distress should alert the practitioner to a more serious illness. Chest pain in the setting of an acute cough frequently is seen with asthma as well as chest wall pain from coughing and referred pain from pleural effusions. Hemoptysis, which is relatively uncommon in pediatric patients, may suggest epistaxis or a more serious pulmonary disease such as tuberculosis, cystic fibrosis, and other etiologies of bronchiectasis. It can occur with foreign body aspiration and can be mistaken for blood arising from the gastrointestinal tract.

The next portion of the HPI should help the clinician "rule in" or "rule out" the possibility of a generalized infection. Is there fever? Change in the level of activity or alertness? An infant or child who is not interacting with his or her environment (not playful or active, not making eye contact with providers) and is excessively somnolent or irritable has a serious infection such as meningitis until proven otherwise. For this reason, pediatricians use the term *lethargic* only to refer to patients in whom they suspect altered mental status that requires investigation for meningitis. Headache and sore throat alone without cough suggest pharyngitis such as strep, but the triad of cough, headache, and sore throat suggests influenza. Rhinorrhea may suggest a generalized infection but also can be seen in allergic rhinitis. Children with recent illness exposure (at home, at school, or in day care) are more likely to have an infection. Consideration of the season (bronchiolitis is more common in January and February, whereas croup is more common in the autumn) is helpful in narrowing the list of infectious possibilities. A vaccine history is important to identify infants and children who have not been immunized against pertussis. A travel history is not always necessary but may reveal the risk for tuberculosis in a child with chronic cough and recent travel to a tuberculosis-endemic region.

In addition to travel, consider asking about environmental exposures, such as passive tobacco smoke. Sometimes a clear history for foreign body ingestion is easy to obtain; if there is no such history, ask about access to small toys, parts, or foods, or an older sibling who may have innocently "fed" his or her brother or sister an object that presents a choking hazard.

As part of the HPI, remember to obtain other historical information that will assist in the management of a child with cough. In infants and children, it is particularly important to identify patients who are dehydrated, as this will affect patient management. Is the patient drinking fluids? Is he or she losing fluids to emesis or diarrhea? In children who are still in diapers, parents can easily estimate changes from baseline urine output. Parents may note the absence of tears when crying, which also suggests dehydration.

It is important to include at least a brief past medical history, even for patients with an acute cough. Is the cough recurrent? This may suggest asthma, cystic fibrosis, or allergic rhinitis. In young infants, a pregnancy and birth history can be helpful in identifying infants at risk for bronchiolitis (premature infants and those with chronic lung disease), chlamydia pneumonia (mother treated for chlamydia during pregnancy), or bacterial pneumonia (mother colonized with group B streptococcus). Does the child have a history of cardiac disease? If so, consider congestive heart failure. As was mentioned above, it is important to know if the child or adolescent may be immunosuppressed [human immunodeficiency virus (HIV) infection, primary immunodeficiency, chemotherapy, and steroids or antirejection drugs for patients with solid organ transplants] and therefore at increased risk for infection. Does the child have a history of recurrent bacterial or opportunistic infections? Consider the possibility of a previously undiagnosed immune deficiency. A family history of atopic disease (asthma, allergies, atopic dermatitis) can be helpful in making the diagnosis of asthma or allergies. It is important to ask about a family history of cystic fibrosis if a child with chronic cough has poor weight gain, recurrent wheezing, and/or chronic diarrhea. A family member with active tuberculosis or undiagnosed cough and fever may point to tuberculosis as the diagnosis.

## PHYSICAL EXAMINATION

It is necessary to obtain the pertinent physical examination information to narrow the differential diagnosis further as well as to aid in patient management. The importance of observing pediatric patients with any chief complaint cannot be overestimated. It is helpful to think of general appearance in three broad categories: well-appearing, sick but nontoxic, and toxic or "lethargic." These descriptions aid the provider in identifying a seriously ill child and correctly documenting the child's status in the medical record. Avoid "well-developed, well-nourished" as this is a general descriptor only. Consider describing a child as "smiling" or "playful." Most commonly, children who are ill appear uncomfortable, tired, and perhaps "clingy" with regard to their interaction with their parents in the office. However, these patients will interact briefly with the parent and examiner and will be consoled easily in a parent's arms. Children who are seriously ill (from shock, meningitis, severe dehydration, and other etiologies of altered mental status) do not interact with their environment. Observation is also important to identify cyanosis and respiratory distress (discussed in more detail below).

Vital signs and growth parameters are equally important in diagnosing and treating pediatric patients with cough. Respiratory rates should be measured by observing chest wall movement over one 60-s or two 30-s periods and compared with normal values. *The best single finding for ruling out pneumonia in infants and young children is the absence of tachypnea.* Fever, if present, suggests infection. Tachycardia may signify dehydration, fever, and/or pain. Pulse oximetry should be used in patients with cyanosis, tachypnea, and/or other evidence of respiratory distress. In infants and small children, the percentage of weight loss from baseline may help determine the severity of dehydration. A pattern of poor weight gain in a patient with chronic cough or recurrent wheezing should raise suspicion for cystic fibrosis.

The respiratory examination starts with the respiratory rate and includes both the lung examination and an assessment of the patient's work of breathing. To do this, infants and young children are best examined at a distance, with the chest fully exposed, to measure the respiratory rate and look for increased work of breathing. It is important to remember that a sleeping child may not manifest respiratory distress but that the same child may work harder to breathe when awake and active. In addition, infants and children with croup may exhibit stridor when active or agitated but not when they are at rest.

Stridor merits special discussion. The most common diagnosis of childhood that presents with cough and stridor is croup (viral laryngotracheobronchitis). Stridor can be inspiratory, biphasic, or expiratory, depending on the location of the airway narrowing. For example, in croup, stridor can be biphasic as the narrowing occurs at the vocal cords. A foreign body below the cords (e.g., in the trachea itself) can present as expiratory stridor; obstructions above the cords can present with inspiratory stridor alone.

Grunting, nasal flaring, and retractions are all manifestations of increased work of breathing (respiratory distress) in infants and young children. The costal margin typically does not move much during normal breathing (if it does move, it moves upward and outward because the normal diaphragm lifts the costal margin outward). In airway obstruction, the depressed diaphragm may apply an inward traction on the chest, resulting in paradoxical movement of the chest wall during inspiration. Paradoxical breathing or abdominal breathing is seen when the abdomen moves outward while the chest moves inward during inspiration.

The lung examination is the final portion of the respiratory examination. Although this is the portion of the examination that most early clinicians prioritize in patients with respiratory disease, infants can present with a significant respiratory illness without abnormal auscultatory lung findings. For a novice examiner, it can be difficult to distinguish upper airway sounds that are transmitted into the chest in infants and small children from true adventitial lung sounds. The easiest maneuver is to place the stethoscope over the child's nose and mouth; if the sounds are louder there than in the chest, they are upper airway sounds. It is helpful to gauge the amount of air movement; patients with a severe asthma exacerbation may have no wheezes on examination because there is essentially no air movement. A prolonged ratio of the I (inspiratory) phase to the E (expiratory) phase suggests airway obstruction.

There is some confusion about the nomenclature of some of the adventitial lung sounds. The terms *crackles* and *rales* are used synonymously to describe the "popping" sound that occurs at the end of inspiration. *Wheezes* are continuous sounds that can occur during both inspiration and expiration; they can be musical and are high-pitched. Wheezes often can be appreciated by listening to the sounds of breaths from infants' and small children's mouths (audible wheezing). Wheezing is seen most commonly in asthma, foreign bodies (typically unilateral wheezing), and bronchiolitis in infants. The term *rhonchi* typically refers to low-pitched continuous sounds that sound like snoring or rattling. Tubular breath sounds (when listening over the lungs, sounds as if the examiner is listening directly over the trachea) suggest a consolidative process such as pneumonia.

The HEENT (head, ears, eyes, nose, and throat) examination can be helpful in determining the etiology of the cough. In younger patients, it is wise to consider examining the tympanic membranes and the throat at the end of the examination, as these are more invasive than other maneuvers. Injected conjunctivae may suggest allergic conjunctivitis with allergic rhinitis as the etiology of cough. They also may signify a viral conjunctivitis, giving the diagnosis of viral syndrome. Periorbital swelling may suggest ethmoid sinusitis. Swollen nasal mucosa is a nonspecific finding and may be seen in a viral URI, bacterial sinusitis, and allergic rhinitis, although the mucosa is typically more pale and boggy in allergic rhinitis. Nasal polyps should alert the examiner to the possibility of cystic fibrosis. A nasal crease and dark discoloration or "shiners" under the eyes are common in allergic rhinitis. Evidence of fluid in the middle-ear space suggests a viral process or allergic rhinitis. Middle-ear fluid with tympanic membrane inflammation suggests acute otitis media, which can be seen either as a primary viral or as a secondary bacterial process. Both occur frequently in the context of a child with a cough from a viral URI. Dry oral mucosa suggests at least mild dehydration, as does the absence of tears, which will affect patient management. Posterior pharyngeal wall cobblestoning (hypertrophied lymphoid follicles seen in chronic postnasal drainage) can be seen in allergic rhinitis.

Many items in the pediatric physical examination can provide clues to the etiology of cough besides those listed above. Lymphadenopathy generally is evaluated by palpating for anterior or posterior cervical and submandibular nodes during the neck examination and is seen most frequently in URIs. Keep in mind that although regional lymphadenopathy is common, generalized lymphadenopathy (such as large nodes in the inguinal or axillary region) should raise suspicion for malignancy. A rash may signify a viral syndrome (viral exanthem) or may alert the examiner to atopy (atopic dermatitis or eczema) and suggest allergic rhinitis or asthma. Growth failure and clubbing are signs of recurrent or chronic processes such as cystic fibrosis and congenital heart disease.

## LABORATORY AND RADIOGRAPHIC EVALUATION

Most infants, children, and adolescents with cough do not require laboratory studies, as those studies do not aid in diagnosis or management. Chest radiographs are unlikely to be positive for pneumonia if all clinical signs (respiratory rate, auscultation, and work of breathing) are negative.

Children with acute cough who are ill-appearing (to include the presence of respiratory distress) or have a chronic cough may benefit from further evaluation. Chest radiographs should be considered in children with respiratory distress and those in whom pneumonia is suspected on the basis of other examination findings. An opaque foreign body may be seen on airway or chest films. A complete blood count may identify a patient with a bacterial process based on leukocytosis with a shift toward more immature cells. It also may identify a patient suspected of having leukemia based on extreme leukocytosis, leukopenia, and one other cell line down (anemia or thrombocytopenia). Eosinophilia may suggest atopy.

Viral antigen studies may be useful in both the diagnosis and the management of acute cough. Nasal secretions may be obtained for respiratory syncytial virus (RSV) (causing bronchiolitis) or influenza (causing bronchiolitis or classic influenza syndrome) by trapping the secretions with a suction device. To confirm the diagnosis of influenza, a Calgi swab touched to the nasopharynx may be sent as well. Children over 2 years of age with the triad of cough, fever, and sore throat presenting in the first 48 h of illness should be tested for influenza, as antiviral medications may shorten the course of illness. Children and adolescents with a history suggestive of pertussis should be tested, as treatment may limit the symptoms and decrease the likelihood of spread of the disease.

In chronic cough, spirometry is helpful in school-age children and adolescents with chronic cough when the diagnosis of asthma is suspected but first-line treatment does not result in improvement. Other "second-line" tests also may be indicated. A sweat chloride test is the first-line test in ruling out cystic fibrosis, but as there are many genetic mutations that cause cystic fibrosis, a negative sweat test does not rule out the diagnosis. Bronchoscopy is used to look for an inhaled foreign body, investigating persistent collapse, confirming anatomic malformations, or obtaining tissue from children who have undiagnosed infiltrates or suspected ciliary dyskinesia syndrome. A barium swallow study revealing esophageal compression may be diagnostic in identifying vascular rings and slings that are causing chronic cough with or without wheezing in infants; pH probe testing may be helpful in linking symptoms with gastroesophageal reflux. Otolaryngology referral may be helpful in children with suspected upper airway abnormalities such as an upper airway mass or significant laryngotracheomalacia. Immunodeficiency and $\alpha_1$ antitrypsin testing also may be indicated.

Sputum is difficult to obtain from young children, but it is important to send it for culture and sensitivity in patients known to have cystic fibrosis. Sputum for acid-fast bacilli (AFB) should be sent for stain and culture if pulmonary tuberculosis has been diagnosed on the basis of a positive purified protein derivative (PPD) test and consistent chest radiograph findings.

## MANAGEMENT

Acute cough is usually the result of a viral illness, and supportive measures are typically all that is indicated. It is sometimes helpful to reduce parent anxiety by defusing concerns about cough. In mild nonspecific cough, parents should be reassured that cough is a normal part of the disease, that it is protective, and that it is self-limited. Randomized controlled trials do not suggest that over-the-counter cold medications (antitussives, antihistamine-decongestant combinations, other fixed drug combinations, and antihistamines) are more effective than placebo in treating acute cough in children.

There is also no evidence that narcotics such as codeine are more effective than placebo in treating acute cough in a pediatric patient.

The most important consideration in treating acute cough in children is the judicious use of antibiotics. Antimicrobials should not be prescribed in otherwise healthy children unless a bacterial infection (such as pneumonia) is diagnosed. Children with underlying lung disease (chronic tracheobronchitis from tracheostomy, bronchopulmonary dysplasia, lung hypoplasia, cystic fibrosis) may benefit from treatment directly specifically at *Bordetella pertussis, Mycoplasma pneumoniae, Chlamydia pneumoniae, Pseudomonas aeruginosa,* or other specific infections.

Children with chronic cough should have a thorough investigation, as was discussed above, with a management that is tailored to the disease. Bronchospasm should be an early consideration in children with chronic cough and wheezing; in this case, a trial of albuterol may be both diagnostic and potentially therapeutic.

## BIBLIOGRAPHY

De Jongste JC, Shields MD. Cough: 2. Chronic cough in children. *Thorax* 58(11): 998–1003, 2003.

Durbin WJ. Cough. In Hoekelman RAMD, ed., *Primary Pediatric Care*. St. Louis: Mosby, 2001: 1012–1015.

Faniran AO, Peat JK, Woolcock AJ. Persistent cough: Is it asthma? *Arch Dis Child* 79(5):411–414, 1998.

Friedman MJ, Attia MW. Clinical predictors of influenza in children. *Arch Pediatr Adolesc Med* 158(4):391–394, 2004.

Hay AD, Schroeder K, Fahey T. Acute cough in children. *BMJ* 328(7447):1062, 2004.

Margolis P, Gadomski A. The national clinical examination: Does this infant have pneumonia? [comment]. *JAMA* 279(4):308–313, 1998.

O'Brien KL, Dowell SF, Schwartz B, et al. Cough illness/bronchitis—Principles of judicious use of antimicrobial agents. *Pediatrics* 101(1):178–181, 1998.

Schroeder K, Fahey T. Should we advise parents to administer over the counter cough medicines for acute cough? Systematic review of randomised controlled trials [comment]. *Arch Dis Child* 86(3):170–175, 2002.

Subcommittee on Management of Sinusitis and Committee on Quality Improvement. Clinical practice guideline: Management of sinusitis. *Pediatrics* 108(3):798–808, 2001.

# FEVER

*Stephanie Starr*

## LEARNING OBJECTIVES

1. Define fever as it relates to infants and children.

2. Summarize general differences in approaching fever in children as opposed to adults.

3. Describe the pathophysiology of fever.

4. Describe different methods of recording temperature and list the advantages and disadvantages of each one.

5. Describe the differential diagnosis for fever in children, paying attention to differences based on age.

6. List the pertinent historical and physical examination information in caring for children with fever and understand how it helps narrow the differential diagnosis.

7. State the most common diagnoses as well as the diagnoses not to miss for fever.

8. Briefly discuss the evaluation and treatment of fever in infants and children, paying careful attention to the approach to young children with fever without an obvious source.

## INTRODUCTION

Fever is one of the most common chief complaints in infants and children in pediatric practice. Some estimate that as many as 30 percent of all pediatric office visits are secondary to fever, and countless phone calls are made to primary care providers and triage nurses by anxious parents. Physiologically, fever is beneficial, is rarely harmful, and does not need to be treated routinely. Although most febrile illnesses are viral syndromes, a small proportion of these illnesses are serious bacterial infections (bacteremia with or without sepsis, meningitis, urinary tract infection, septic arthritis, osteomyelitis). These infections can cause significant morbidity and mortality.

Caring for infants and children with fever presents some challenges. Febrile infants with a serious bacterial infection may appear well and have no other evidence of infection besides the fever. Localized bacterial infections in young infants may disseminate quickly to cause bacteremia and sepsis. In an era of increasing antimicrobial resistance, judicious use of antibiotics is more important than ever. As providers seek to differentiate febrile children with significant illness from those with benign viral illness, it has become increasingly important to provide both evidence-based and cost-effective health care. Concerned parents also present with "fever phobia," or the perception of fever as dangerous. It is the responsibility of the clinician to educate the family in this regard. Because of these challenges, it is critical that pediatric providers be knowledgeable about fever and skilled in obtaining the appropriate history, performing the physical examination, and choosing the appropriate diagnostic studies to identify and appropriately treat children with serious illnesses.

## PATHOPHYSIOLOGY

Fever is a disorder of thermoregulation and occurs when the hypothalamic "set point" is adjusted to a higher level. The body then works to raise its core temperature (defined as pulmonary artery temperature) to the new set point. An initial trigger (such as a viral infection) causes macrophages to release cytokines such as interleukin 1 and interleukin 6. These chemicals act on the anterior hypothalamus to increase local levels of prostaglandin $E_2$ and increase the thermostat or set point to a new higher level. Some evidence suggests that vasopressin and melanocyte-stimulating hormone may play a safety role in limiting the height fever can reach. The body works to raise its core temperature to the new set point through a number of mechanisms, including shivering (skeletal muscle movement increases heat), peripheral vasoconstriction, and inhibition of sweat production (both prevent heat loss).

Unlike fever, which is defined by abnormal thermoregulation, hyperthermia occurs in the face of excess heat production despite normal thermoregulation. Forces such as inappropriate heat generation (as in thyroid storm), inability to dissipate heat (excessive clothing or coverings), high environmental temperature, and/or strenuous exercise result in more heat than the body can dissipate through normal mechanisms. One or several of these forces cause the body's temperature to exceed its hypothalamic set point. Whereas fever causes the body to increase its temperature to meet the higher abnormal set point, hyperthermia causes the body to decrease its temperature to return to its normal set point. Flushing, peripheral vasodilation, and sweating occur to lose as much heat as possible and lower the body's core temperature. Hyperthermia can result in dangerously high temperatures, and although it is uncommon in children, it is associated with significant mortality (80 percent).

Fever is part of the body's natural defense against infections. This favorable effect has been attributed largely to interleukin 1. Fever increases leukocyte bactericidal activity and mobility, enhances the effects of interferons, and decreases the availability of some trace metals (particularly iron) that are required by some bacteria. Some animal evidence suggests that organisms that are unable to mount a fever experience increased mortality.

A variety of methods are used to measure body temperature in infants and children, and it is important to understand the advantages and limitations of each method. The gold standard for measuring temperature is to sample pulmonary artery blood, but this requires significant intervention. Rectal temperature is the next best method for approximating core temperature. Glass thermometers (with alcohol or mercury) have been used traditionally, but digital thermometers are used increasingly. The thermometer is lubricated and then inserted 3 to 7 cm into the anal canal. The peak rectal temperature will register in 2 to 3 min when using a glass thermometer and in 30 s when using a digital device. Rectal temperatures are the preferred method of measurement in children because they estimate core body temperature most closely and are not affected by environmental temperatures. They are avoided in older children for comfort reasons and should not be obtained in pediatric patients in whom minor rectal trauma is a significant concern (e.g., in neutropenia). Some parents are concerned about harming a child by measuring temperature rectally, but in a 30-year review, only 30 cases of rectal perforation were reported, all in newborns during the first week of life.

Tympanic thermometers are a common means of measuring temperature in children. They estimate body temperature by measuring the thermal infrared energy emitted from the tympanic membrane, which shares its blood supply with the hypothalamus. There is evidence that shows a good correlation between core temperature and tympanic temperature in older children and adults. Advantages include speed (temperature measurement takes only 1 s) and comfort. They can be used safely in neutropenic patients. However, variables such as inaccurate placement within the ear canal and fever in young infants < 3 months of age can cause inaccurate estimation of core body temperature. Tympanic temperatures also can be affected by environmental temperature.

Many parents ask if they may measure axillary temperature in their children and then add a degree to estimate rectal temperature. Unfortunately, axillary temperatures are affected by environmental temperature, correlate poorly from infancy though adulthood, and can vary as much as 3°C from the rectal temperature. Accordingly, there is no standard to convert axillary to rectal temperatures consistently. The only group of patients in whom good correlations between axillary and rectal temperatures have been identified consists of premature infants under radiant warmers.

Oral temperatures can be used reliably after 4 or 5 years of age. The temperature will be approximately 0.5°C below the rectal temperature in 1 min. Children should not eat or drink cold or hot foods 1 h before measuring oral temperature as this may cause a falsely low or high reading. Newer, less invasive means of measuring temperature, such as plastic strips placed on the forehead and pacifier-type thermometers, have not been shown to measure temperature accurately.

Traditionally, "normal" temperature has been defined as 37°C (98.6°F). Of note, this value was derived from a study of over 1 million axillary temperatures measured in adults. Many children have higher core temperatures than does the average adult. In addition, there is normal diurnal variation of body temperature, with temperatures rising in the evening and decreasing in the morning. Many pediatric clinicians define fever in children (and especially young infants) as a rectal temperature greater than or equal to 38°C (100.4°F).

## DIFFERENTIAL DIAGNOSIS

Benign viral infections cause the majority of fevers in children. However, as with other chief complaints, clinicians are encouraged to consider a broad differential diagnosis when evaluating infants and children with fever. A systematic history and physical examination will enable the clinician to narrow the list of possible etiologies further. It is particularly important to remember that younger infants require a more careful approach to diagnosis and management because rapid dissemination of local bacterial infection from the lungs, meninges, bones, and joints can lead quickly to bacteremia and sepsis.

The approach to evaluation and management discussed in the remainder of this chapter applies to fever of less than 2 weeks' duration in otherwise healthy children. Individuals with congenital or acquired immunodeficiency, immunosuppression, functional or surgical splenectomy, and nephrotic syndrome require special consideration. Fever of unknown origin (FUO) is defined as daily rectal temperature exceeding 38.3°C (101°F) that lasts > 2 weeks whose cause has not been determined by thorough history, physical examination, and simple diagnostic tests. The differential diagnosis of FUO is broad and is beyond the scope of this chapter. Children with heat-related illness must be identified early, as heatstroke is associated with an 80 percent mortality. Heatstroke is associated with temperatures > 42°C

(107.6°F) and presents with anhidrosis and coma. The associated mortality is 80 percent.

The differential diagnosis for fever is lengthy. It is helpful to start by considering which diagnoses occur most commonly and by considering those serious diagnoses which are less common but carry increased risks for significant morbidity and mortality. Clinicians also may start by considering broad diagnostic categories such as infection, inflammatory disease, neoplasm, metabolic disease, hematologic disorder, drug reaction (including immunizations), and toxic ingestion. Infectious possibilities include viral and bacterial infections as well as less common infections such as tuberculosis. Urinary tract infection (UTI) is the most common bacterial infection in children 0 to 3 months of age. Kawasaki disease is an inflammatory disorder that typically presents with 5 or more days of high fever. Transfusion reactions commonly present with fever. Many drugs taken at therapeutic or toxic doses (e.g., aspirin overdose) may cause fever. Live vaccines such as varicella may cause fever as late as 30 days after immunization; inactivated vaccines such as the 7-valent pneumococcal vaccine also may cause fever.

In addition to serious bacterial infections such as bacteremia, meningitis, and UTI, there are a number of etiologies for fever in children that must not be missed because of the associated morbidity and mortality. Febrile children presenting with petechiae should be evaluated expeditiously. Although viral infections such as enteroviruses can cause both fever and petechiae, meningococcemia (overwhelming infection with *Neisseria meningitidis*) often presents with fever and petechiae. Although *N. meningitidis* can cause significant invasive infections such as meningitis and bacteremia, meningococcemia is a separate and rapidly evolving entity. Children with meningococcemia may progress from general malaise, fever, and early rash to fulminant infection, shock, and loss of a limb (as well as death) in as little as 24 h. Herpes simplex meningoencephalitis is another serious infection seen in febrile infants that may have an insidious onset. Herpes simplex virus (HSV) meningoencephalitis can cause neurologic devastation in young infants. Young infants with an HSV central nervous system infection may present with a vesicular rash, fever, and neurologic symptoms, such as seizures and irritability. Clinicians treating febrile infants less than 2 months of age should have a high index of suspicion for this disease.

Bacterial tracheitis is another infection that requires a low index of suspicion. Patients with bacterial tracheitis initially may resemble those with viral croup, often appear more toxic, and have higher fever. The tracheitis can form a membrane in the trachea; if the membrane is sloughed, the child may have an acute airway obstruction. Appendicitis frequently presents with low-grade fever, anorexia, and abdominal pain. Whereas adolescents may present with a classic history and physical examination, young children with appendicitis are at higher risk for perforation before diagnosis, as the history and physical examination are often more subtle in this age group.

Febrile children 2 to 36 months of age who appear well and have no identified source for their fever after the history and physical examination have
been done merit special mention. Historically, occult bacteremia (bacterial
blood infection in febrile children who appear well and have no focus such
as osteomyelitis or cellulitis to suggest the initial source of bacterial infection) has been a serious diagnostic possibility in these febrile children. With
the success of *Haemophilus influenzae* type B (HIB) vaccine and the increasing
use of the 7-valent vaccine against *Streptococcus pneumoniae*, the incidence of
occult bacteremia has decreased significantly. Historically, infants age 0 to 2
months with fever (defined in this group as rectal temperature equal to or
greater than 38°C (100.4°F) are presumed to have a serious bacterial infection
until proven otherwise. Table 16-1 shows a differential diagnosis for fever in
infants and children; see Table 16-2 for diagnoses not to miss in febrile children.

## HISTORY

As discussed in previous chapters in regard to other chief complaints, the
history of present illness should start with a description of the chief complaint. How high is the fever? Parents may be describing a temperature of
37.2°C (99°F) as a fever. How was the temperature measured? As was noted
above, temperatures taken rectally, for example, more closely approximate
core temperature than do other noninvasive modes of measurement. Neither
the magnitude of the fever nor the response of fever to antipyretics specifically predicts whether the illness is viral or bacterial in nature. What is the
duration of fever? A consistent daily fever for 7 days should prompt a thorough evaluation, whereas a one-time fever in an older infant or child is less
worrisome for significant bacterial infection. As was noted above, the age of
the patient is critical in determining the extent of both evaluation and management.

Next, inquire about general and specific associated symptoms. Is the
child febrile but intermittently playful? If so, meningitis is less likely. Is the
child truly listless and not responding well to his or her environment?
Children have generalized signs and symptoms when the fever peaks, such
as malaise, chills, and listlessness. However, a child who is truly lethargic
(has no interaction with the environment and/or appears toxic) should be
presumed to have meningitis until proven otherwise.

Specific symptoms can help narrow the differential diagnosis significantly. A febrile child with vomiting and no other symptoms still may have
a myriad of etiologies for the fever, such as central nervous system (CNS)
infection, UTI, or viral syndrome. A febrile, nontoxic child with vomiting
and nonbloody diarrhea is more likely to have a viral gastroenteritis. A

**Table 16-1 Differential Diagnosis of Fever (< 2 Weeks' Duration)**

|  | Infants 0–2 Months | 2–36 Months | 3+ Years |
|---|---|---|---|
| Most common | Infection<br>✓ Viral URI<br>✓ Viral gastroenteritis<br>✓ Bronchiolitis<br>✓ Urinary tract infection<br>✓ Pneumonia | Infection<br>✓ Viral URI<br>✓ Viral gastroenteritis<br>✓ Otitis media<br>✓ Croup<br>✓ Bronchiolitis<br>✓ Urinary tract infection<br>✓ Pneumonia<br><br>Immunization reaction | Infection<br>✓ Viral URI<br>✓ Viral gastroenteritis<br>✓ Urinary tract infection<br>✓ Pneumonia<br>✓ Strep pharyngitis<br>✓ Sinusitis |
| Less common | Infection<br>✓ Meningitis<br>✓ Bacteremia<br>✓ Osteomyelitis<br>✓ Septic arthritis<br>✓ Meningococcemia<br>✓ Bacterial colitis<br>✓ Tuberculosis<br><br>Malignancy | Infection<br>✓ Meningitis<br>✓ Bacteremia<br>✓ Bacterial tracheitis<br>✓ Osteomyelitis<br>✓ Septic arthritis<br>✓ Meningococcemia<br>✓ Bacterial colitis<br>✓ Tuberculosis<br><br>Inflammatory<br>✓ Kawasaki disease<br><br>Malignancy<br>✓ Acute lymphoblastic leukemia<br><br>Ingestion<br>✓ Aspirin | Infection<br>✓ Otitis media<br>✓ Croup<br>✓ Meningitis<br>✓ Bacteremia<br>✓ Osteomyelitis<br>✓ Septic arthritis<br>✓ Meningococcemia<br>✓ Tuberculosis<br><br>Malignancy<br>✓ Acute lymphocytic lymphoma<br>✓ Lymphoma<br><br>Inflammatory<br>✓ Juvenile rheumatoid arthritis<br>✓ Inflammatory bowel disease |

URI = upper respiratory infection.

Table 16-2 *"Don't Miss" Diagnoses for Fever (continued)*

| Infants 0–2 Months | 2–36 Months | 36+ Months |
|---|---|---|
| Meningitis | Meningococcemia | Meningococcemia |
| Bacteremia/sepsis | Meningitis | Appendicitis |
| Herpes simplex virus | Bacteremia/sepsis | Meningitis |
| Meningoencephalitis | Bacterial tracheitis | Tuberculosis |
| | Appendicitis | Acute lymphocytic lymphoma |
| | Tuberculosis | |
| | Kawasaki disease | |

febrile infant with cough should prompt investigation for respiratory infections, including pneumonia and bronchiolitis.

There are other questions that aid in the diagnosis. The season (spring, summer, autumn, or winter) can provide a clue to possible viral agents (influenza and respiratory syncytial virus occur commonly in the winter months, parainfluenza in the spring and autumn, and enterovirus in the summer months). It is helpful to inquire about illness exposures at home, in school, and at day care. Has the patient recently traveled outside the country? A sexual history is necessary in evaluating adolescent females with fever and abdominal or genitourinary complaints as pelvic inflammatory disease should be considered. As with all pediatric patients, information regarding hydration status (amount of vomiting and diarrhea, urine output, fluid intake, tear production) is vital to diagnosing and appropriately treating associated dehydration. A parent who brings a well-appearing child with mild fever in for evaluation may have specific concerns and may benefit from additional education about fever and its treatment.

Immunization and past medical histories are important in determining the etiology of fever. A 6-week-old with fever and coughing spasms should be evaluated for *Bordetella pertussis* infection. Children with surgical splenectomy, functional splenectomy (sickle cell disease), or active nephrotic syndrome are at increased risk for infection by encapsulated bacteria such as *S. pneumoniae*. Children who have primary or secondary immunodeficiencies should undergo more aggressive evaluation; specific recommendations for evaluating febrile, neutropenic children are beyond the scope of this chapter. In infants less than 2 months of age, the mother's prenatal group B streptococcus status must be clarified, as late-onset group B streptococcus infections in this age group are not affected by maternal antibiotic prophylaxis at delivery.

## PHYSICAL EXAMINATION

The general appearance of a febrile child is of supreme importance. Observation is a critical part of examining pediatric patients; noting the child's overall appearance may enable the examiner to identify more quickly a child with a serious bacterial infection. Historically, pediatricians use the term *lethargic* when recording the physical examination only when there is true evidence of altered mental status. Young children who are febrile but smile at the examiner or are playful in the office are unlikely to have meningitis, but an irritable or inconsolable infant may have such an infection. Most pediatricians do not use the term *lethargic* unless they have decided already that the child's general appearance is worrisome enough to proceed with a thorough evaluation to include cerebrospinal fluid studies.

Febrile children may have abnormal vital signs for a number of reasons. A febrile child may be tachycardic because of the fever or because of dehydration. Generally, the pulse is elevated by 10 to 15 beats per degree Celsius of fever. Tachycardia and poor perfusion (prolonged capillary refill, decreased urination, altered mentation) even in the face of a normal blood pressure suggest shock, as children can maintain cardiac output [CO (cardiac output) = SV (stroke volume) × HR (heart rate)] by increasing contractility of the heart for a long time. Once hypotension occurs, these children progress rapidly to cardiopulmonary arrest. Tachypnea can result from fever alone, but significant tachypnea should alert the examiner to a lower respiratory tract infection. In this case, pulse oximetry can be helpful in determining poor oxygenation. The child's weight is important both for diagnosis (dehydration) and for management (dosing of fluids and medications).

A child with an open fontanel should have a brief head examination, looking for a significantly sunken (in dehydration) or bulging (with increased intracranial pressure) fontanel. The eye examination can reveal conjunctivitis, which is seen in adenoviral and some bacterial infections. Ipsilateral conjunctivitis and otitis media should suggest *H. influenzae* infection. Nonexudative conjunctivitis with sparing around the limbus is one finding in Kawasaki disease and can be seen with toxic streptococcal and staphylococcal infections. Nasal inspection may reveal thick rhinorrhea. Ear examination may reveal otitis media. The diagnosis of viral infection is made easier by identifying lesions in the posterior oropharynx (hand-foot-and-mouth disease) or the gingiva and lips (herpes gingivostomatitis).

A febrile child with a stiff neck should be assessed carefully and evaluated for meningitis. Torticollis is not uncommon in the setting of a retropharyngeal abscess. Bilateral anterior cervical lymphadenopathy is seen commonly in streptococcal pharyngitis and is less impressive in nonspecific viral upper respiratory tract infections. Bilateral posterior cervical lymphadenopathy (as well as hepatosplenomegaly) should raise suspicion for infectious mononucleosis. A single, large, tender, and mobile cervical lymph node may represent a bacterial lymphadenitis, a mycobacterial infection, or cat-scratch disease. A large, nontender fixed supraclavicular node is suspicious for lymphoma. Generalized lymphadenopathy in multiple locations (cervical, axillary, inguinal, etc.) may represent generalized infection, lymphoma, or leukemia.

The cardiovascular examination may aid in the diagnosis if a new murmur is auscultated, suggesting the possibility of infective endocarditis. An examination suggestive of congestive heart failure (muffled heart sounds with hepatosplenomegaly) with supportive features in the history may point to a viral myocarditis. Although tachypnea and retractions are more specific than is chest auscultation in predicting pneumonia, focal inspiratory crackles (also called rales) typically distinguish older children and adolescents with pneumonia from those with viral respiratory infections. Infants with bronchiolitis may have a combination of bilateral inspiratory crackles and expiratory sounds suggestive of wheezes.

The abdominal examination is critical in a child who presents with fever and abdominal pain. Diminished bowel sounds, right lower quadrant tenderness, peritoneal signs (rebound tenderness, guarding, positive iliopsoas sign, localized right-sided tenderness on rectal examination) should make appendicitis the primary diagnosis to rule out. Young children are less likely to have classic examination findings and older children can have more subtle findings early in the progression of the disease, and so a low index of suspicion must be maintained so that appendicitis is not missed.

A child with fever and extremity pain requires close scrutiny. Joint swelling suggests septic arthritis, a diagnosis that requires urgent surgical intervention. Children with septic arthritis at the hip may present with fever and limp or refusal to walk, and limited range of motion at the hip may be the only significant clue. Tenderness to palpation over a long bone suggests osteomyelitis. Children with acute lymphoblastic leukemia often present with fever and nonspecific lower extremity pain because of marrow infiltration. Cellulitis should be ruled out. A febrile child with restricted flexion of the back suggests diskitis, osteomyelitis of the spine, or a malignant process causing marrow infiltration. A child with urinary symptoms, fever, and costovertebral angle tenderness is likely to have pyelonephritis.

A febrile child should be completely undressed, as the skin examination may provide significant clues to the etiology of the fever. The presence of a vesicular rash may suggest varicella, whereas a fleeting maculopapular rash suggests other viral syndromes. Coxsackie virus can cause papulovesicular lesions of the palmar and plantar surfaces, locations where rashes typically are not seen. A number of viral infections can cause urticaria. Children who receive measles-mumps-rubella (MMR) vaccination can have a febrile illness with rash; this typically occurs 6 to 12 days after vaccine administration. Fever and petechiae (macules that do not blanch) should cause the examiner to entertain meningococcemia as a potential diagnosis, but this also can be seen in enteroviral infections. Erythema marginatum is associated with rheumatic fever.

The pediatric neurologic examination is critical if a CNS infection is suspected. Most of the neurologic examination in children is done by observation, and some assessment of mental status is made during assessment of the child's general appearance. Classic signs of meningismus such as the Brudzinski and Kernig signs are often absent in children younger than 24 months of age.

## LABORATORY AND RADIOGRAPHIC EVALUATION

Viruses cause the vast majority of febrile illnesses in children; thus diagnostic studies are not required for most of these patients. When pediatric patients present with fever with a source that suggests bacterial infection other than otitis media, the diagnostic approach should be tailored to the suspected disease. This includes obtaining chest radiographs to confirm pneumonia, a white blood cell count with an absolute neutrophil count and blood cultures in suspected sepsis, and urine culture when urinary tract infection is suspected.

Febrile infants and children who appear toxic on examination but have no clear infectious etiology should undergo a comprehensive diagnostic evaluation and be treated empirically with broad-spectrum antibiotics. A comprehensive evaluation should include a white blood cell count with absolute neutrophil count, blood culture, urinalysis, urine culture, and cerebrospinal fluid evaluation and culture. Chest radiographs should be considered in children with respiratory symptoms (cough, tachypnea, increased work of breathing, rales, and/or decreased breath sounds). Stool Gram stain should be obtained if there is a history of diarrhea. A white blood cell count > 15,000 should prompt a blood culture specimen to be sent, as these children are five times more likely to have bacteremia than are those with normal counts. Before the 7-valent pneumococcal vaccine, an absolute neutrophil count > 10,000 correlated with an 8.2 percent increased risk of pneumococcal bacteremia. Urine samples should be obtained by catheter in infants and young children who are not toilet trained, as a bag urine specimen frequently is contaminated by skin flora.

Numerous studies over the last decade have addressed the diagnostic dilemma of well-appearing infants and toddlers (children 0 to 36 months of age) with fever and no obvious source despite a thorough history and physical examination. For many years, the approach described by Baraff and colleagues has been accepted as a consensus guideline. In this approach, infants less than 28 days of age were recommended to undergo a comprehensive evaluation, be admitted to the hospital, and receive parenteral antibiotics (or, alternatively, observation alone) pending cerebrospinal fluid, blood, and urine results. Low-risk febrile infants 28 to 90 days old (defined as previously healthy, white blood cell count 5 to 15,000/mm$^3$, normal urinalysis or urine Gram stain, and < 5 white blood cells per high-power field in the stool if diarrhea is present) were recommended to undergo urine culture with careful observation. Alternatively, clinicians could choose to obtain blood, urine, and cerebrospinal fluid cultures; deliver an intramuscular dose of ceftriaxone; and ensure patient follow-up within 24 h.

More recent studies in neonates (infants 0 to 28 days of age) suggest that perhaps some of these young infants do not require empiric antibiotics. In 1997, a study concluded that many febrile neonates categorized as low risk can be identified and managed safely as outpatients without antibiotic therapy. Neonates at low risk were defined as appearing well, previously healthy, without a focus of infection, with a white blood cell count 5000 to 15,000/mm$^3$, a spun urine specimen with < 10 white blood cells per high-power field, and a C-reactive protein value < 20 mg/L. Despite these new data, there is no current consensus regarding the management of well-appearing febrile neonates. In light of this, infants 0 to 2 months of age with rectal temperature $\geq$ 38°C (100.4°F) should undergo a prompt and thorough evaluation, be categorized as high- or low-risk, and be treated individually based in part on the reliability of follow-up and adequate interval observation. Regardless of the approach chosen for a specific infant, it is critical that febrile infants less than 2 months of age have cerebrospinal fluid sent for examination and culture before any empirical antibiotic therapy is initiated.

Children 2 to 36 months who have a documented temperature $\geq$ 38.3°C (101°F) and have no focus of infection have posed a challenge: to identify those children with serious bacterial infection while minimizing unnecessary procedures and antibiotics. Many researchers have attempted to determine factors that can differentiate those with serious bacterial infection accurately from those with benign viral illnesses; studies have focused on children 2 to 36 months of age because of the frequency of fever and because assessment is more difficult in this age group. Response to antipyretics has been shown not to be helpful in differentiating children with serious bacterial infection from those with viral syndromes.

There is no consensus regarding the approach to a febrile, nontoxic child 2 to 36 months of age with no focus of infection. In 1993, Baraff and others described a consensus approach to these patients by conducting a meta-analysis of 85 earlier studies. Diagnostic strategies were aimed at identifying children with occult bacteremia (bacteremia in a nontoxic child without an identifiable source such as osteomyelitis, pneumonia, or cellulitis) and UTIs. Since that time, invasive H. influenzae type B has been nearly eradicated with the use of HIB vaccine (licensed in 1987). The largest recent study of over 5000 nontoxic, febrile [temperature $\geq$ 39°C (102.2°F)] 2- to 24-month-olds demonstrated a 2 percent prevalence of occult bacteremia; 83 percent of these infections were caused by *S. pneumoniae*. The study was conducted before the 2000 licensure of the 7-valent pneumococcal vaccine (PCV-7) for children less than 2 years of age. Subsequent rates of invasive infections caused by *S. pneumoniae* are on the decline, causing some experts to wonder if providers should continue to screen nontoxic, febrile 2- to 36-month-olds for occult bacteremia, particularly if they have had at least one PCV-7 vaccination.

## MANAGEMENT

Febrile illnesses that have proved to be a serious infection should be treated promptly with the appropriate therapy. Similarly, febrile children who are toxic-appearing and do not have an obvious focus of infection should have a thorough diagnostic evaluation and be treated with broad-spectrum parenteral antibiotics until the cause of fever is identified. Because most febrile illnesses in children are viral, the most important step in managing fever is typically to educate the parents that fever plays a positive role in fighting infection and does not necessarily need to be treated.

When, then, should a fever be treated? There are three general indications for fever treatment. First, if the infant or child is at increased risk from complications associated with fever. Keep in mind the fact that direct complications of the high temperature are unusual if the temperature is below 41°C (105.8°F) unless the child has a history of febrile seizures or a history of epilepsy with a decreased seizure threshold when febrile. Unfortunately, antipyretics have not been shown conclusively to prevent recurrence of febrile seizures. Second, patients with increased metabolic demands (congenital heart disease and cardiac infections, cystic fibrosis, acute brain injury) should have their fever treated promptly as they are at increased risk for decompensation. Third, fever treatment should be considered if a febrile infant or child is uncomfortable. Parents with an active, playful febrile child should be reassured and educated on the benefits of fever rather than focusing on the use of antipyretics.

There are two primary methods for treating fever. Physical maneuvers may be used to aid in heat dissipation. Methods that have been used traditionally include tepid baths, tepid sponging, and cooling blankets. A 2003 Cochrane Database review concluded that there was limited evidence that sponging has an antipyretic effect, and this small effect was seen in children already given an antipyretic. No other methods were demonstrated to lower temperatures in febrile children. Temperatures are more likely to climb after physical maneuvers because the abnormal set point has not been altered. Antipyretics work by lowering the temperature set point and are the mainstay of fever treatment.

There are several practical rules for the use of antipyretics in children. In the United States, acetaminophen and ibuprofen are used most commonly.

Aspirin is avoided in children (especially in cases of influenza and varicella), as there remain concerns for a potential relationship between Reye syndrome and aspirin use in febrile children. Antipyretics are avoided in infants younger than 2 months because acetaminophen and ibuprofen have longer half-lives in this age group and because of the potential to mask serious bacterial infections. Because very young infants have a higher surface area for their weight than do older children and adults, physical maneuvers such as unbundling, increasing air circulation, and decreasing the environmental temperature are more likely to provide relief.

Acetaminophen has been used for many years and, when given in therapeutic doses (10 to 15 mg/kg), can be quite effective in treating fever. Liver toxicity, the major concern in acetaminophen use, is unlikely to occur at doses lower than 140 mg/kg, and liver destruction is less likely in children below 6 years of age. Ibuprofen has several advantages over acetaminophen, including less frequent dosing (every 6 to 8 h compared with every 4 to 6 h for acetaminophen) and anti-inflammatory properties. Side effects, including gastritis and platelet function inhibition, are more common than they are with acetaminophen. There is no evidence that alternating acetaminophen with ibuprofen is more effective than using acetaminophen or ibuprofen alone in lowering temperatures in febrile children.

## BIBLIOGRAPHY

Alpern ER, Alessandrini EA, Bell LA, et al. Occult bacteremia from a pediatric emergency department: Current prevalence, time to detection, and outcome [see comment]. *Pediatrics* 106(3):505–511, 2000.

Baraff LJ, Bass JW, Fleisher GR, et al. Practice guideline for the management of infants and children 0 to 36 months of age with fever without source. Agency for Health Care Policy and Research [see comment] [erratum appears in *Ann Emerg Med* (9):1490, 1993]. *Ann Emerg Med* 22(7):1198–1210, 1993.

Chiu CH, Lin TY, Bullard MJ. Identification of febrile neonates unlikely to have bacterial infections. *Pediatric Infect Dis J* 16(1):59–63, 1997.

Meremikwu M, Oyo-Ita A. Physical methods for treating fever in children. *Cochrane Database Syst Rev* 2:CD004264, 2003.

Stoll, ML, Rubin LG. Incidence of occult bacteremia among highly febrile young children in the era of the pneumococcal conjugate vaccine: A study from a children's hospital emergency department and urgent care center. *Arch Pediatr Adolesc Med* 158(7):671–675, 2004.

Van der Jagt EW. Fever. In Hoekelman RAMD, ed., *Primary Pediatric Care*. St. Louis: Mosby, 2001: 1085–1092.

Van der Jagt EW. Fever of unknown origin. In Hoekelman RAMD, ed., *Primary Pediatric Care*. St. Louis: Mosby, 2001: 1093–1096.

# SORE THROAT

*Stephanie Starr*

● LEARNING OBJECTIVES

1. List the differential diagnosis for sore throat in children, paying particular attention to differences based on age.

2. List the pertinent historical and physical examination information in caring for children with sore throat and understand how it helps narrow the differential diagnosis.

3. State the most common diagnoses as well as the diagnoses not to miss for sore throat in children.

4. Explain when and why sore throat should be treated with an antimicrobial.

## INTRODUCTION

Sore throat, or odynophagia (pain with swallowing), is a common chief complaint in the pediatric outpatient setting. Typically, children who complain of sore throat have pharyngitis, or inflammation of the pharynx, but this may not be the main focus of the illness. By far, the majority of cases of pharyngitis in children are viral, but there is significant parental and patient concern about the possibility of missing "strep throat." As with other acute respiratory illnesses, judicious use of antibiotics is critical to minimize the incidence of antimicrobial resistance as well as unnecessary costs.

There are some differences in caring for children with sore throats. Group A streptococcal pharyngitis is most common in children 3 to 18 years of age and accounts for about 15 percent of cases of pharyngitis in this age group. Adults with pharyngitis are diagnosed with streptococcal pharyngitis in approximately 5 to 10 percent of cases. Adults with streptococcal pharyngitis are unlikely to have an initial case of rheumatic fever, but the incidence of this is significantly higher in children. In fact, the primary reason for treating strep throat in children (in addition to shorter duration of symptoms and decreased communicability) is to prevent rheumatic fever, as the pharyngitis is a self-limited disease.

The importance of parent and patient education in caring for children with a sore throat is difficult to overstate. Parents understandably are concerned about missing streptococcal pharyngitis but are often unaware that a throat swab for rapid antigen or culture does not have to be obtained in every child with a sore throat. In fact, a culture positive for group A streptococcus obtained in the absence of true pharyngitis (no significant erythema) probably represents a carrier state and does not require treatment (as there is no increased risk for rheumatic fever).

The signs and symptoms of group A streptococcal pharyngitis and nonstreptococcal pharyngitis overlap so broadly that an accurate diagnosis on the basis of the history or physical examination is usually impossible. For example, adenovirus can cause a purulent pharyngitis, and palatal petechiae are not specific for *Streptococcus pyogenes* pharyngitis. Group A streptococcal pharyngitis is the only bacterial pharyngitis (except for rare bacterial etiologies of pharyngitis such as *Corynebacterium diphtheriae* and *Neisseria gonorrhoeae*) in which antimicrobial therapy is of proven benefit. Therefore, the primary consideration in diagnosing and treating children with a sore throat is to determine whether group A streptococcus is the cause.

## PATHOPHYSIOLOGY

Pharyngitis is inflammation of the pharynx. Patients with a sore throat typically present with odynophagia. Sore throat should be differentiated from isolated dysphagia, or difficulty swallowing without pain. The term *trismus* refers to difficulty opening the mouth fully and is suggestive of a more significant illness, such as a retropharyngeal or peritonsillar abscess.

## DIFFERENTIAL DIAGNOSIS

As was noted in previous chapters, seasoned clinicians typically start with a differential diagnosis and then rule out possible diagnoses by a process of elimination with pertinent positive and negative historical and physical examination data. Diagnostic testing is used to confirm or refute the remaining possible diagnoses. As novice clinicians see more patients and read about chief complaints, they come to rely less on lists and tables to come up with the differential diagnoses. By far the majority of children presenting with sore throat have symptoms lasting < 2 weeks and pharyngitis, and so the remainder of this chapter addresses acute sore throats only. As with other chief complaints, the differential diagnosis should be broadened for patients with immune deficiency (acquired or secondary).

Viral pharyngitis accounts for the large majority of cases of acute sore throat in children and adolescents. A number of viruses can cause pharyngitis (see Table 17-1 for details). Epstein-Barr virus can present with pharyngitis in children and in teens with infectious mononucleosis; this syndrome is common in older children and adolescents but has a less prominent presentation in younger children. Influenza merits special mention, as newer antiviral medications may be efficacious if the disease is identified early in its course. Adenovirus can cause both an exudative pharyngitis and conjunctivitis (pharyngoconjunctival fever). Coxsackie A virus can cause stomatitis or discrete palatal lesions (hand-foot-and-mouth disease) in addition to pharyngitis. Herpes simplex viruses can cause gingivostomatitis.

Group A streptococcus, or *Streptococcus pyogenes,* is not the only bacterial etiology of pharyngitis. Group C and G streptococci may be identified on throat cultures but are self-limited and do not progress to rheumatic fever. Diphtheria is uncommon in the United States. *Neisseria gonorrhoeae* is an uncommon cause of tonsillopharyngitis. The potential roles of *Mycoplasma pneumoniae* and *Chlamydia pneumoniae* are unknown. They typically occur with cough, and the pharyngitis alone has not been proved to benefit from antibiotics. See Table 17-2 for common syndromes with other infectious agents in pharyngitis.

Children and adolescents with acute sore throat may have conditions more serious than pharyngitis. Peritonsillar and retropharyngeal abscesses are suppurative complications of group A streptococcal pharyngitis. Epiglottitis represents a true respiratory emergency. Kawasaki disease is an acute febrile illness that causes a severe vasculitis. The exact etiology is unknown. Children with Kawasaki disease present with at least 5 days of high fever and a combination of other signs [bilateral bulbar conjunctivitis, a solitary enlarged anterior cervical lymph node, oral mucosa changes (cracked lips, strawberry tongue) and peripheral extremity changes (swollen hands or feet with eventual desquamation), and maculopapular rash]. This disorder is important to recognize because approximately 20 percent of affected children develop coronary artery abnormalities such as aneurysms.

Occasionally children present with a sore throat in the absence of pharyngitis (i.e., no evidence on examination of pharyngeal inflammation such as erythema); typically, the sore throat is described as mild and may result from postnasal drainage in the setting of an upper respiratory infection or allergic rhinitis.

Table 17-1 **Differential Diagnosis of Sore Throat**

| | Infants and Young Children (0–3 Years) | Older Children and Adolescents (3–18 Years) |
|---|---|---|
| Most common | Same as for older children and adolescents, but group A β-hemolytic strep and Epstein-Barr virus are uncommon in this age group | Infections<br>✓ Viral pharyngitis<br>  ✓ Influenza<br>  ✓ Parainfluenza<br>  ✓ Rhinoviruses<br>  ✓ Coronavirus<br>  ✓ Respiratory syncytial virus<br>  ✓ Adenovirus<br>  ✓ Herpes simplex virus<br>  ✓ Enteroviruses (Coxsackie and echoviruses)<br>  ✓ Epstein-Barr virus<br>✓ Bacterial pharyngitis<br>  ✓ Group A β-hemolytic streptococcus (Streptococcus pyogenes) |
| Less common | Other infectious pharyngitis<br>✓ Bacterial<br>  ✓ Groups C and G streptococcus<br>  ✓ *Haemophilus influenzae* type b<br>  ✓ *Neisseria gonorrhoeae*<br>  ✓ *Corynebacterium diphtheriae*<br>  ✓ *Arcanobacterium haemolyticum*<br>  ✓ *Chlamydia trachomatis* and *C. pneumoniae*<br>  ✓ *Yersinia enterocolitica*<br>  ✓ *Coxiella burnetii*<br>  ✓ *Francisella tularensis*<br>✓ Parasitic pharyngitis (*Toxoplasma gondii*)<br>✓ Candidal pharyngitis<br>✓ Mycoplasma pharyngitis (*Mycoplasma pneumoniae* and *M. hominis*) | Other infectious pharyngitis<br>✓ Bacterial<br>  ✓ Groups C and G streptococcus<br>  ✓ *Neiserria gonorrhoeae*<br>  ✓ *Corynebacterium diphtheriae*<br>  ✓ *Arcanobacterium haemolyticum*<br>  ✓ *Chlamydia trachomatis* and *C. pneumoniae*<br>  ✓ *Yersinia enterocolitica*<br>  ✓ *Coxiella burnetii*<br>  ✓ *Francisella tularensis*<br>✓ Parasitic pharyngitis (*Toxoplasma gondii*)<br>✓ Candidal pharyngitis<br>✓ Mycoplasma pharyngitis (*Mycoplasma pneumoniae* and *M. hominis*) |

*(continued)*

*Table 17-1* **Differential Diagnosis of Sore Throat (continued)**

| | Infants and Young Children (0–3 Years) | Older Children and Adolescents (3–18 Years) |
|---|---|---|
| Less common | Other bacterial infections <br> ✓ Epiglottitis <br> ✓ Peritonsillar or retropharyngeal abscess | Other bacterial infections <br> ✓ Epiglottitis <br> ✓ Peritonsillar or retropharyngeal abscess |
| | Anatomic/ingestion <br> ✓ Caustic ingestion | Anatomic/ingestion <br> ✓ Caustic ingestion |
| | Kawasaki disease | Kawasaki disease |

## HISTORY

Although history alone is not sufficient to differentiate group A streptococcal pharyngitis from other etiologies, the history and physical examination are helpful in determining patients at higher risk for streptococcus pharyngitis in whom a throat swab should be obtained. It also can help identify patients who are more likely to have influenza, as they may benefit from treatment in the early days of the illness.

Clinicians should start by obtaining a description of the sore throat. What is the duration? Sore throat lasting more than 14 days is unlikely to be group A streptococcal pharyngitis, which is a self-limited process. Next, focus the history on information that will "rule in" or "rule out" strep. Historical data that support the diagnosis of group A streptococcal pharyngitis include an abrupt onset of the sore throat and fever. The presence of hoarseness, cough and rhinorrhea, conjunctivitis, anterior stomatitis, discrete ulcerative lesions, viral exanthem, and/or diarrhea points to a viral etiology. Younger children with streptococcal pharyngitis frequently have headache, abdominal discomfort, and nausea and/or vomiting. The triad of sore throat, headache, and cough should alert the clinician to the possibility of influenza.

There are several symptoms as well as signs that parents may report that suggest more serious diagnoses. Stridor, respiratory distress, and/or drooling suggest the possibility of epiglottitis. The incidence of epiglottitis has been much reduced since *Haemophilus* type B (HIB) vaccine was introduced in the early 1990s. Trismus or limited neck movement (inability to extend the neck fully or look upward) should raise the possibility of retropharyngeal or peritonsillar abscess.

*Table 17-2* **Microbial Etiologies of Acute Pharyngitis and Their Associated Symptoms**

| Type of Pharyngitis, Pathogen | Associated Disorder(s) or Symptom(s) |
|---|---|
| Bacterial | |
| Streptococci | |
| Group A | Tonsillitis and scarlet fever |
| Group C and G | Tonsillitis and scarlatiniform rash |
| Mixed anaerobes | Vincent angina |
| *Neisseria gonorrhoeae* | Tonsillitis |
| *Corynebacterium diphtheriae* | Diphtheria |
| *Arcanobacterium haemolyticum* | Scarlatiniform rash |
| *Yersinia enterocolitica* | Enterocolitis |
| *Yersinia pestis* | Plague |
| *Francisella tularensis* | Tularemia (oropharyngeal form) |
| Viral | |
| Rhinovirus | Common cold |
| Coronavirus | Common cold |
| Adenovirus | Pharyngoconjunctival fever and acute respiratory disease |
| Herpes simplex virus types 1 and 2 | Gingivostomatitis |
| Parainfluenza virus | Cold and croup |
| Coxsackievirus A | Herpangina and hand-foot-and-mouth disease |
| Epstein-Barr virus | Infectious mononucleosis |
| Cytomegalovirus | Cytomegalovirus mononucleosis |
| Human immunodeficiency virus | Primary HIV infection |
| Influenza A and B viruses | Influenza |
| Mycoplasmal | Pneumonia |
| *Mycoplasma pneumoniae* | |
| Chlamydial | |
| *Chlamydia psittaci* | Acute respiratory disease and pneumonia |
| *Chlamydia pneumoniae* | Pneumonia |

A history should be obtained to aid in management; in pediatric patients; this means ensuring that the child or adolescent is not dehydrated. Is oral intake of fluids diminished? Is there decreased urine output? Significant vomiting (and/or diarrhea) increases the risk for dehydration. Despite the diagnosis, a dehydrated child may require hospital admission if he or she is unable to maintain adequate hydration with oral fluids alone. A child who has a significantly altered level of activity (e.g., is not intermittently playful or is not interacting normally with parents) may alert the clinician to a more serious illness or dehydration.

A past medical history should be obtained even briefly to identify children and adolescents who may be at increased risk for infection. Is the child potentially immunosuppressed? This includes children on immunosuppressive therapy (solid-organ transplant patients, children with malignancy), diabetics, and human immunodeficiency virus (HIV)-positive pediatric patients or children with primary immunodeficiencies.

## PHYSICAL EXAMINATION

There are no physical examination findings that are specific for group A β-hemolytic streptococcal (GAS) pharyngitis. Always start with the child's general appearance, as observation alone may yield significant information. Is the child interacting with family members and with the examiner? Does he or she have a normal level of alertness? Is there any evidence of respiratory distress? A child who is sitting in a "tripod" position (hands outstretched on a flat surface) who is in respiratory distress and is drooling should be presumed to have epiglottitis until proven otherwise. A verbal child or adolescent with a "hot potato" or muffled voice should raise suspicion for a retropharyngeal or peritonsillar abscess.

Fever with or without tachycardia may be seen in children with sore throat; the lack of fever, however, does not rule out the possibility of GAS pharyngitis. Tachycardia may occur either because of fever or from dehydration. Conjunctivitis (inflammation of the conjunctiva) is seen frequently with adenovirus (pharyngoconjunctival fever). Nasal drainage is seen frequently with rhinoviruses and coronaviruses but is much less common in GAS pharyngitis.

Patients with GAS pharyngitis have tonsillopharyngeal erythema with or without exudates, and viral pathogens may cause a similar picture. Palatal petechiae are seen commonly in but are not specific for GAS. Anterior stomatitis (typically vesicular lesions), gingivitis, and discrete ulcerative lesions suggest viral etiologies for pharyngitis. Trismus and asymmetry of the pharynx (unilateral posterior bulging of the pharynx) suggest a peritonsillar abscess. Tender and enlarged bilateral anterior cervical lymphadenopathy is also common for GAS; enlarged posterior cervical lymphadenopathy suggests infectious mononucleosis or cytomegalovirus (CMV). Limitation of neck extension or torticollis should raise suspicion for retropharyngeal abscess

Rashes also can help differentiate GAS pharyngitis from viral etiologies. The classic rash in scarlet fever (caused by GAS) is a fine, erythematous papular rash that is generalized and feels much like sandpaper. These fine papules tend to be clustered in creases such as the antecubital fossae and are called Pastia's lines. Coxsackie A virus can cause papulovesicular lesions on the palmar and plantar surfaces as part of hand-foot-and-mouth disease. Epstein-Barr virus and other viruses can cause viral exanthems.

## LABORATORY AND RADIOGRAPHIC EVALUATION

It is important to remember that viruses account for the large majority of cases of pharyngitis, and throat swabs should be avoided in children without evidence of acute pharyngitis on examination. The diagnosis of acute GAS pharyngitis should be suspected on clinical grounds and then supported by the performance of a laboratory test. Because the incidence of GAS pharyngitis and that of first attacks of acute rheumatic fever are higher in children than in adults, and because there is no specific scoring scale (with history and physical examination) that can predict GAS infection accurately, swabs should be sent and pediatric patients treated when a study is positive. A throat swab should be obtained by touching both tonsillar pillars and the posterior pharynx (in a figure-eight motion). Care should be taken to avoid touching other surfaces, such as the uvula and soft palate, as this dilutes the inoculum.

In most clinical settings, both rapid streptococcus testing and standard throat cultures are available. The sensitivity and specificity of the rapid antigen streptococcus tests vary. A positive rapid streptococcus test or throat culture provides adequate confirmation of GAS pharyngitis, but a negative rapid antigen test requires confirmation by throat culture. In some areas, GAS polymerase chain reaction (PCR) is now available. Retropharyngeal and peritonsillar abscesses are diagnosed on clinical examination, and a computed tomography (CT) scan is helpful to distinguish retropharyngeal cellulitis from retropharyngeal abscess.

## MANAGEMENT

The parents of children with viral pharyngitis should be encouraged to comfort patients with supportive measures and to monitor for signs of dehydration. Antimicrobial therapy should not be given to a child with pharyngitis in the absence of diagnosed GAS or other bacterial infection. Penicillin remains the drug of choice for streptococcal pharyngitis because it is effective at treating pharyngitis and preventing rheumatic fever, has a relatively narrow spectrum, and is safe and inexpensive. Treatment within 9 days of onset is effective in preventing acute rheumatic fever. Treatment may prevent suppurative complications, shorten the length of symptoms, and prevent the spread of infection. The only currently recommended antimicrobial therapy that has been shown in controlled studies to prevent initial attacks of rheumatic fever is intramuscular penicillin (a form now supplanted by

*Table 17-3* ***"Don't Miss" Diagnoses of Sore Throat***

| |
|---|
| Epiglottitis |
| Retropharyngeal/peritonsillar abscess |
| Gonococcal pharyngitis |
| Caustic ingestion |
| Kawasaki disease |

benzathine penicillin G). Patients are contagious until they have received 24 h of effective treatment.

Amoxicillin is a reasonable alternative if there are concerns about compliance with liquid penicillin because of palatability, but amoxicillin has a broader spectrum and thus increases the risk of developing antimicrobial resistance. To date, no group A streptococci resistance to β-lactam antimicrobials have been identified. Erythromycin or other macrolides (e.g., azithromycin) are recommended for penicillin-allergic patients.

If influenza is suspected, rapid testing is available, economic resources permit, and treatment can begin within 36 h of the start of illness, antiviral therapy may be considered. Oseltamivir has been shown to shorten the duration of symptoms, hasten return to normal activities, and reduce the incidence of secondary complications (primarily otitis media), and it can be used in children 1 to 12 years of age. Neuraminidase inhibitors such as oseltamivir and zanamivir have not been shown to benefit at-risk children such as asthmatic patients.

Although the incidence has dropped significantly, epiglottitis is a true emergency and requires immediate evaluation by a team of specialists (typically an otolaryngologist and an anesthesiologist). Children suspected of having epiglottitis should undergo endotracheal intubation in a controlled environment such as the operating room and should never be sent for radiographs, as these children may have acute respiratory failure and arrest (Table 17-3).

## BIBLIOGRAPHY

Bisno AL, Gerber MA, Gwaltney JM, et al. Practice guidelines for the diagnosis and management of group A streptococcal pharyngitis. Infectious Diseases Society of America. *Clin Infect Dis* 35(2):113–225, 2002.

Craig FW, Schunk JE. Retropharyngeal abscess in children: Clinical presentation, utility of imaging, and current management. *Pediatrics* 111(6 Pt 1):1394–1398, 2003.

Friedman MJ, Attia MW. Clinical predictors of influenza in children. *Arch Pediatr Adolesc Med* 158(4):391–394, 2004.

Matheson NJ, Symmonds-Abrahams M, Sheikh A, et al. Neuraminidase inhibitors for preventing and treating influenza in children. *Cochrane Database Syst Rev* 3:CD002744, 2003.

Schwartz B, Marcy SM, Phillips WR, et al. Pharyngitis—principles of judicious use of antimicrobial agents. *Pediatrics* 101(1):171–174, 1998.

Thuma PE. Pharyngitis and tonsillitis. In Hoekelman RAMD, ed., *Primary Pediatric Care*. St. Louis: Mosby, 2001: 1744–1747.

Tsevat J, Kotagal UR. Management of sore throats in children: A cost-effectiveness analysis [see comment]. *Arch Pediatr Adolesc Med* 153(7):681–688, 1999.

# EAR PAIN

*Stephanie Starr*

● LEARNING OBJECTIVES

1. Summarize general differences in approaching ear pain in children as opposed to adults.
2. Describe the pathophysiology of ear pain.
3. List the differential diagnosis for ear pain in children.
4. List the pertinent historical and physical examination information in caring for children with ear pain and explain how it helps narrow the differential diagnosis.
5. Describe options for treating ear pain in children.
6. State the most common diagnoses as well as the diagnoses not to miss for ear pain in children.

## INTRODUCTION

Otalgia, or ear pain, is a common chief complaint of children when they present to the pediatrician's office. In addition, many parents bring preverbal children in for fussiness, ear pulling, or ear rubbing with a suspicion of ear pain. Although ear pain is a very common complaint, the differential diagnosis is not exhaustive, and ear pain rarely indicates a serious disease. Otitis media is the most common reason for ear pain in children; 65 to 95 percent of children have at least one episode of acute otitis media by age 7 years. Otitis media is usually the primary concern for parents who seek care for children with otalgia or perceived otalgia. Children are more likely to present with ear pain because the occurrence of acute otitis media is much higher in infants and young children than it is in adults.

## PATHOPHYSIOLOGY AND ANATOMY

It is worthwhile to review the nerves that serve the ear and its surrounding structures before discussing the differential diagnosis of ear pain in children. The periauricular region includes the auricle, external auditory canal, tympanic membrane, middle-ear space, mastoid air cells, and overlying skin. These regional structures are innervated by the mandibular division of the trigeminal nerve (cranial nerve V), the facial nerve (cranial nerve VII), the glossopharyngeal nerve (cranial nerve IX), the vagus nerve (cranial nerve X), and the C2 and C3 roots of the cervical plexus. Referred pain can arise from any structure in the head and neck that has a common neural pathway with the temporal bone and the periauricular region. Because of this, pathology in the oropharynx, hypopharynx, larynx, tonsils, tongue base, trachea, esophagus, or thyroid gland potentially can cause referred pain to the ear.

## DIFFERENTIAL DIAGNOSIS

Categorizing the differential diagnosis of ear pain on the basis of mechanism and anatomic location can be very helpful, particularly if the diagnosis is not straightforward. Middle-ear pain can result from inflammation of the tympanic membrane, pressure and inflammation from fluid in the middle-ear space (pus, serous fluid, or blood), and unequal pressure between the middle-ear space and the surrounding environment (seen in eustachian tube dysfunction). Pain can originate from the external auditory canal as seen in otitis externa (also known as swimmer's ear), from cerumen impaction, and from foreign bodies lodged in the canal. Inflammation (caused by trauma or cold injury) as well as infection (resulting from cellulitis) can cause auricular pain. In cases in which the diagnosis cannot be made after these periauricular structures are evaluated, etiologies for referred otalgia must be sought. Eustachian tube dysfunction is common and can be exacerbated in environments where the ambient pressure differs significantly from the middle-ear pressure (e.g., flying on aircraft and scuba diving).

The differential diagnosis of ear pain, as with the differential diagnosis of other chief complaints, can be categorized by identifying diseases that are common and diseases that are uncommon but must not be missed because of the potential for significant morbidity and mortality. Acute otitis media is certainly the most common etiology of acute ear pain in children. Mastoiditis, which typically presents in association with otitis media, is much less common but must be identified and treated promptly when present. A summary of the differential diagnosis of ear pain based on the mechanism of pain is presented in Table 18-1; see Table 18-2 for etiologies of ear pain that should not be missed.

## HISTORY

The history of present illness should start by determining the frequency, duration, and character of the ear pain. Is it bilateral or unilateral? Next, associated symptoms should be elicited. Otorrhea in a child without a his-

*Table 18-1* **Differential Diagnosis of Ear Pain (Otalgia)**

|  | Children 0–3 Years | Children and Adolescents 3+ Years |
|---|---|---|
| Most common | Inflammation, infection, and/or pressure from fluid in middle-ear space<br>✓ Acute otitis media<br>✓ Otitis media with effusion<br>✓ Tympanitis | Inflammation, infection, and/or pressure from fluid in middle-ear space<br>✓ Acute otitis media<br>✓ Otitis media with effusion<br>✓ Tympanitis |
|  | Referred pain<br>✓ Tooth eruption<br>✓ Tonsillopharyngitis<br>✓ Periauricular lymphadeno-pathy | Referred pain<br>✓ Tonsillopharyngitis<br>✓ Sinusitis<br>✓ Dental abscess<br>✓ Peritonsillar abscess<br>✓ Temporomandibular joint dysfunction<br>✓ Periauricular lymphadeno-pathy |
|  | Mass<br>✓ Foreign body | |
|  | Inability to equalize pressure between middle ear and surrounding spaces<br>✓ Eustachian tube dysfunction<br>✓ Flying at altitude | Mass<br>✓ Cerumen impaction |
|  | | Inflammation and/or infection of the external auditory canal<br>✓ Otitis externa<br>Inability to equalize pressure between middle ear and surrounding spaces<br>✓ Eustachian tube dysfunction |

*(continued)*

Table 18-1 **Differential Diagnosis of Ear Pain (Otalgia) (continued)**

|  | Children 0–3 Years | Children and Adolescents 3+ Years |
|---|---|---|
| Less common | Inflammation, infection, and/or pressure from fluid in middle-ear space<br>✓ Hemotympanum<br><br>Referred pain<br>✓ Mastoiditis<br>✓ Peritonsillar abscess<br>✓ Temporal bone pain (e.g., histiocytosis X)<br><br>Mass<br>✓ Cerumen impaction<br>Inflammation and/or infection of external auditory canal<br>✓ Otitis externa<br>Auricle inflammation with or without infection<br>✓ Cellulitis<br>✓ Cold injury<br>✓ Trauma | Inflammation, infection, and/or pressure from fluid in middle-ear space<br>✓ Hemotympanum<br><br>Referred pain<br>✓ Mastoiditis<br>✓ Thyroiditis<br><br>Auricle inflammation with or without infection<br>✓ Cellulitis<br>✓ Cartilaginous infection<br>✓ Cold injury<br>✓ Trauma |

tory of pressure equalization (PE) tubes suggests acute otitis media with rupture of the tympanic membrane. Is there fever and/or associated respiratory symptoms such as rhinorrhea, cough, or nasal congestion? A recent history of swimming in an older child increases clinical suspicion for otitis externa. Traumatic ear injuries are an uncommon reason for ear pain, but any history of trauma should be sought, particularly if the diagnosis is not straightfor-

Table 18-2 **"Don't Miss" Diagnoses for Ear Pain**

| |
|---|
| Foreign body<br>Mastoiditis<br>Peritonsillar abscess<br>Dental abscess<br>Hemotympanum |

ward on physical examination. Children with otitis media with effusion (previously called serous otitis media) commonly describe a "popping" sensation, a sense of ear fullness, or decreased hearing in the affected ear.

A brief past medical history also may shed some diagnostic light on a child with ear pain. A child with recurrent acute otitis media may lower the suspicion for otitis media, and this certainly may affect decisions regarding antibiotic therapy if acute otitis media is diagnosed. In addition, children with PE tubes and chronic otorrhea with new pain and drainage, as well as immunodeficient children are at higher risk for unusual organisms. Children with craniofacial abnormalities such as a history of cleft lip and/or palate as well as genetic disorders such as Down, Apert, Crouzon, or Pfeiffer syndromes have a higher frequency of otitis media because of anatomic changes that affect eustachian tube function. Native Americans and Alaskan natives also have a higher incidence of acute otitis media. Children with hearing aids are more likely to present with irritation of the external auditory canal.

## PHYSICAL EXAMINATION

The child's general appearance should be the examiner's first focus, although the large majority of pediatric patients who present with ear pain appear relatively well. Fever increases suspicion for acute otitis media but has poor negative predictive value. Fever is uncommon in otitis externa. Vital signs are otherwise typically normal.

Although the ear examination is most relevant in evaluating children with otalgia, it is one of the most invasive parts of the physical examination for infants and young children. Therefore, it is best to examine the ear at the end of the examination in infants and young children. School-age children typically feel comfortable and will tolerate being examined from head to toe as is done traditionally in examining adult patients. First, the examiner should observe the ear to see if there is any evidence of color change, swelling, or bruising. Symmetry of the ears is also important, as mastoiditis commonly causes the ipsilateral ear to protrude relative to the contralateral ear. Tenderness on palpation of the tragus suggests otitis externa.

Stabilizing the child's ear is the first step toward successfully examining the external auditory canal and tympanic membrane, and this can be done in a number of positions. Infants may be placed comfortably in the supine position, with a parent leaning gently on the baby's arms and legs. The examiner can stabilize the infant's head and adjust the ear with one hand and then introduce the speculum with the other hand. Two-year-olds who appear comfortable are typically at ease sitting on the examination table. As with other parts of the physical examination in this age group, pretending to examine a parent's ear or stuffed animal's ear first can make the experience less frightening for a toddler. Commonly, children 12 to 24 months of age are likely to have stranger anxiety, and attempts to examine the ear are usually more successful when performed on a parent's lap.

After the child's head is stabilized comfortably, the pinna should be pulled gently and simultaneously in a superior, posterior, and lateral vector to straighten the external auditory canal and allow for maximal visualization of the tympanic membrane. Next, the largest speculum tip that will fit comfortably in the child's ear should be used. It is common at this point for a novice examiner to have difficulty visualizing the tympanic membrane (especially the bony landmarks); frequently, visibility is improved by gently advancing the speculum until resistance is met and also by aiming the speculum tip anteriorly (toward the nose). If significant cerumen is present, removal can be accomplished with a cerumen spoon or loop. An erythematous external auditory canal with or without exudate suggests otitis externa.

Many students identify the ear examination as the part of the pediatric physical examination they would like to master during their clerkships. As most seasoned pediatricians will explain, the ear examination takes years of practice to master. It is important to start by having a systematic way to evaluate tympanic membranes:

1. *Color.* This is usually where novice examiners begin. Is the tympanic membrane erythematous? Is it gray (normal)? Does the membrane have a yellow color suggestive of either pus or serous fluid behind the membrane?
2. *Translucency.* Are the bony landmarks visible? How dull is the membrane? Sometimes an air-fluid level can be observed.
3. *Mobility.* Mobility must be determined to document the presence or absence of middle-ear effusion. This is usually most easily performed with pneumatic otoscopy but also can be assessed by using tympanometry.
4. *Position.* This is perhaps the most subtle portion of the examination and the most difficult to ascertain. Bulging tympanic membranes are identified easily and often appear as a "doughnut" as the umbo of the malleolus is tethered to the tympanic membrane and keeps the membrane from fully bulging. The membrane also may be in a neutral position or retracted.

An erythematous, dull, immobile, and bulging tympanic membrane associated with an acute onset of symptoms makes the diagnosis of acute otitis media. An erythematous membrane with good bony landmarks and mobility suggests a viral myringitis. Sometimes prominent vessels can be seen as well. A dull, immobile, nonerythematous, and neutral membrane suggests otitis media with effusion, as does a translucent and colorless membrane with a visible air-fluid level.

If the ear examination appears normal, have the patient point to the area of greatest pain to aid in the diagnosis. In addition, the remainder of the head and neck should be examined. The presence of conjunctivitis with acute otitis media suggests infection with *Haemophilus influenzae*. Because ear pain may be referred in nature, and because upper respiratory tract infections and otitis media with effusion may be associated with pharyngitis and lower respiratory tract symptoms, a thorough examination of the oropharynx, chest, and lungs is important. The neck examination may reveal periauricular lymphadenopathy that may be causing referred ear pain. A chronic history in association with pain near the temporomandibular joint is suggestive of temporomandibular joint dysfunction that is causing masticator muscle spasms. If the ear is normal, a close examination for a dental or peritonsillar abscess also should be performed.

## LABORATORY AND RADIOGRAPHIC EVALUATION

Diagnostic studies are rarely necessary in diagnosing and appropriately treating children with ear pain. The majority of cases of ear pain in children are either acute otitis media or otitis media with effusion. To diagnose acute otitis media, there must be an acute onset of signs and symptoms (such as ear pain, irritability, fussiness, and fever), middle-ear effusion, and signs or symptoms of middle-ear inflammation (distinct otalgia in a verbal child or distinct erythema of the membrane). Otitis media with effusion is diagnosed when middle-ear effusion is present but the criteria for acute otitis media are not met. Eustachian tube dysfunction is suspected when the membrane is retracted.

In selected situations, it may be necessary to document the organism responsible for acute otitis media. Tympanocentesis or carbon dioxide laser–assisted myringotomy should be considered when a child with acute otitis media fails on oral antibiotics and in immunocompromised children. Sending otorrhea for culture may be helpful in identifying and appropriately treating the responsible organism in chronic otitis media when PE tubes (a source of bacterial colonization) are present.

## MANAGEMENT

Because otitis media with effusion and the majority of uncomplicated cases of acute otitis media resolve spontaneously, symptomatic treatment is usually all that is necessary. Many analgesics, such as acetaminophen and ibuprofen, have been used. Topical agents such as benzocaine preparations and naturopathic agents also are used. Home remedies are used by some parents. None of these therapies have been studied systematically for use in ear pain.

A detailed discussion of the treatment of each potential diagnosis for ear pain is beyond the scope of this chapter. There is increasing evidence that uncertain cases of uncomplicated acute otitis media in children 6 months to 2 years of age (as well as certain cases in children more than 2 years of age)

SECTION III / CHIEF COMPLAINTS/COMMON ACUTE ILLNESSES

who appear well can be treated initially with observation alone. It bears mentioning, however, that the first-line drug for acute uncomplicated otitis media is high-dose amoxicillin (80 to 90 mg/kg per day in two doses). If the patient is allergic to amoxicillin and the allergic reaction was not a type I hypersensitivity reaction (urticaria or anaphylaxis), cefdinir (14 mg/kg per day in one or two doses), cefpodoxime (10 mg/kg per day once daily), or cefuroxime (30 mg/kg per day in two divided doses) can be used. In cases of type I reactions, azithromycin (10 mg/kg per day on day 1 followed by 5 mg/kg per day for 4 days as a single daily dose) or clarithromycin (15 mg/kg per day in two doses) can be used in an effort to select an antibacterial agent of an entirely different class. Alternative therapy in a penicillin-allergic patient who is being treated for infection that is known or presumed to be caused by penicillin-resistant *Streptococcus pneumoniae* is clindamycin at 30 to 40 mg/kg per day in three divided doses. In a patient who is vomiting or cannot otherwise tolerate oral medication, a single dose of parenteral ceftriaxone (50 mg/kg) has been shown to be effective for the initial treatment of acute otitis media. Children with otitis media with effusion that persists for at least 3 months and is associated with hearing loss (equal to or worse than 20 decibels hearing threshold in the better ear) should be referred to an otolaryngologist for evaluation and possible PE tube placement.

Children with mastoiditis, chronic otitis media, and peritonsillar abscess may require surgical intervention and parenteral antibiotics.

Acute visits for ear pain provide an opportunity to educate parents about the prevention and benign natural history of acute otitis media. Environmental factors that have been observed to decrease the risk for acute otitis media include breast-feeding for at least the first 6 months and, if possible, minimizing attendance at large day-care settings. Tobacco smoke exposure, pacifier use, and bottle propping have been postulated as risk factors for acute otitis media in infancy, but this has not been proved conclusively.

## BIBLIOGRAPHY

American Academy of Pediatrics, Otitis Media Guideline Panel. Managing otitis media in young children. *Pediatrics* 94(5):766–773, 1994.

Andrews JS. Otitis media and otitis externa. In Hoekelman RAMD, ed., *Primary Pediatric Care*. St. Louis: Mosby, 2001: 1702–1706.

Bauer CAAJ, Herman A. Otologic symptoms and syndromes. In Cummings CW, Fredrickson JM, Harker LA, et al, eds., *Otolaryngology: Head and Neck Surgery*. St. Louis: Mosby–Year Book, 1998: 2551–2552.

Subcommittee on Management of Acute Otitis Media. Diagnosis and management of acute otitis media. *Pediatrics* 113(5):1451–1465, 2004.

# UPPER RESPIRATORY

# TRACT INFECTION

### *Stephanie Starr*

## ● LEARNING OBJECTIVES

1.  Summarize general differences in approaching upper respiratory tract infections in children as opposed to adults.

2.  Describe the pathophysiology of upper respiratory tract infections.

3.  List possible causative organisms for upper respiratory tract infections in children.

4.  Describe the differential diagnosis for upper respiratory tract infection in children, paying particular attention to differences based on age.

5.  List the pertinent historical and physical examination information in caring for children with suspected upper respiratory tract infection and explain how it helps narrow the differential diagnosis.

6.  State the indications for antibiotic treatment for rhinorrhea in childhood.

7.  State the most common diagnoses as well as the diagnoses not to miss for upper respiratory tract infection in children.

## INTRODUCTION

Viral upper respiratory tract infections are the most common infections in children. It is difficult to estimate accurately the cost nationwide associated with provider visits for these infections. Most children have 3 to 8 colds per year, but 10 to 15 percent of children have at least 12 per year, particularly children in group day-care settings. Viral upper respiratory tract infections are 20 to 200 times more common than bacterial sinusitis in children.

The magnitude of viral upper respiratory tract infections has more than financial implications. Authors have estimated that 50 percent of children with upper respiratory tract infections are treated with antibiotics in some settings. It is critical for medical providers to have clear criteria for using antimicrobials to treat respiratory infections in children to minimize the risk of antibiotic resistance.

Viral upper respiratory tract infections traditionally have occurred more frequently in cooler months, leading to the term *cold* and the misconception that exposure to cold temperatures is the cause of these infections. In the northern hemisphere, viral upper respiratory tract infections tend to peak in early autumn, in January, and again in April. There is good evidence that exposure to cold temperatures does not cause a viral upper respiratory tract infection directly or lead to decreased immunity.

## PATHOPHYSIOLOGY AND ANATOMY

Viruses that cause viral upper respiratory tract infections are spread by fomites (fingers and hands, surfaces, and clothing) that contain secretions loaded with virus from the infected individual to other individuals. When viruses come into contact with mucous membranes of the nose, sinuses, nasopharynx, eustachian tube, middle ear, and/or conjunctiva, a viral upper respiratory tract infection ensues. From an anatomic perspective, viral upper respiratory tract infections also can be termed viral rhinosinusitis, as the nasal and sinus mucosa are contiguous. This term is used in the remainder of this chapter and is distinguished from bacterial rhinosinusitis (commonly called "sinusitis").

Viral rhinosinusitis begins with infection of the local respiratory epithelium. It is at this point that affected individuals begin to notice nasal stuffiness and throat irritation. Next, cellular damage occurs and inflammation (thought to be due in part to host production of interleukin 8 and other vasoactive peptides) causes increased vascular permeability and significant mucous secretion manifested by sneezing and watery rhinorrhea. Other symptoms may include malaise, headache, myalgias, and fever. Cough occurs in 60 to 80 percent of these children.

On approximately day 4 of the infection, nasal secretions begin to be thicker because of desquamated epithelial cells, neutrophils, and bacteria that are colonized in the nose. Some providers differentiate mucopurulent rhinitis as a separate disease requiring antibiotics, but it is clear that this change to thicker secretions is part of the natural progression of viral rhinosinusitis and as such does not require antimicrobial therapy. The majority of cases of viral rhinosinusitis last 2 to 7 days and frequently persist as long as 14 days. Cough, rhinorrhea, and nasal congestion can persist for more than 2 weeks in approximately 30 percent of pediatric patients. In addition, children frequently present with sequential episodes of viral rhinosinusitis, making differentiation between viral rhinosinusitis and bacterial rhinosinusitis difficult for clinicians. Historically, families and some providers presumed that children with green rhinorrhea should be treated with antibiotics; the color of the rhinorrhea, however, is not predictive of bacterial rhinosinusitis and is not helpful in making a diagnosis in these patients.

Many viruses can cause viral rhinosinusitis in children. Rhinoviruses and coronaviruses are estimated to cause up to 60 percent of these illnesses in children. In temperate geographic regions, there are frequent episodic outbreaks of some viruses, including respiratory syncytial virus (RSV), influenza A and B, coronaviruses, rhinoviruses, and parainfluenza viruses 1, 2, and 3. Parainfluenza 1 commonly causes croup in very young children but may manifest as a simple viral rhinosinusitis in older children and adults. Parainfluenza virus, influenza virus, and RSV also can cause bronchiolitis in infants. Adenovirus commonly causes an accompanying conjunctivitis and pharyngitis.

## DIFFERENTIAL DIAGNOSIS

Upper respiratory tract infections are the most common reason for rhinorrhea in infants and children. When children present with rhinorrhea (with or without associated symptoms), the examiner still should consider a number of other diagnoses. The differential diagnosis for cough and sore throat is covered in Chaps. 15 and 17, respectively; this chapter focuses more specifically on the differential diagnosis of nasal discharge in children (see Table 19-1). Because infants and young children often have frequent episodes of viral rhinosinusitis, it is important to consider the possibility of sequential episodes of viral rhinosinusitis in the differential diagnosis of prolonged respiratory symptoms. Providers caring for children with chronic lung disease (chronic tracheobronchitis secondary to tracheostomy, bronchopulmonary dysplasia, restrictive lung disease) or immunodeficiency should evaluate these children thoroughly and consider a broader differential diagnosis. It is also important to remember that not all cases of rhinorrhea and nasal congestion are viral rhinosinusitis, bacterial rhinosinusitis, or even allergic rhinitis. Cerebrospinal fluid leak (in a child with head trauma) and congenital syphilis (with classic "snuffles" or nasal drainage) are uncommon but serious etiologies of rhinorrhea.

## HISTORY

It is helpful to begin the history of the present illness by reconstructing a timeline of symptoms. When did the initial symptoms of the illness (nasal discharge, congestion, fever, cough, etc.) begin? Which symptom occurred next?

Table 19-1  **Differential Diagnosis of Nasal Discharge**

|  | Children 0–36 Months | Children 3–18 Years |
|---|---|---|
| Most common | Viral<br>✓ Nonspecific upper respiratory tract infection<br>✓ Influenza<br>✓ Croup<br>✓ Bronchiolitis<br>✓ Acute otitis media<br><br>Bacterial<br>✓ Acute otitis media<br>✓ Pneumonia | Viral<br>✓ Nonspecific upper respiratory tract infection<br>✓ Influenza<br>✓ Acute otitis media<br><br>Bacterial<br>✓ Acute otitis media<br>✓ Pneumonia<br>✓ Rhinosinusitis<br><br>Atypical<br>✓ Pneumonia<br><br>Allergic rhinitis |
| Less common | Allergic rhinitis<br>Bacterial rhinosinusitis<br>Nasal foreign body<br>Cerebrospinal fluid leak<br>Congenital syphilis | Croup<br>Nasal foreign body<br>Cerebrospinal fluid leak<br>Inhaled drugs<br>✓ Cocaine<br>✓ Decongestant nasal sprays |

The duration of the rhinorrhea is important, but the color does not differentiate bacterial from viral rhinosinusitis. Frequently parents are concerned that their child has had rhinorrhea for weeks on end, but careful questioning may reveal that the initial rhinorrhea was heralded by a fever and that the rhinorrhea was nearly resolved but then restarted with a new fever. This should alert the clinician to the possibility of sequential episodes of viral rhinosinusitis. Persistent thick rhinorrhea for more than 14 days raises suspicion for bacterial rhinosinusitis (see Table 19-2). Prolonged rhinitis with new fever and/or irritability or discomfort also raise suspicion for acute otitis media.

Cough is present in 60 to 80 percent of episodes of viral rhinosinusitis. A barky or seal-like cough suggesting croup should raise the possibility of parainfluenza 1 infection. Cough that is worsening may suggest asthma exacerbation, pertussis syndrome, or pneumonia. The triad of fever, headache, and cough is strongly suggestive of influenza infection, particularly during the winter season in temperate climates. Children and adolescents with influenza typically present with significant malaise and myalgias. A history of rash, vomiting, and/or diarrhea points toward a viral etiology.

*Table 19-2* **Clinical Criteria for Diagnosis of Common Bacterial Respiratory Infections in Children**

| | |
|---|---|
| Acute otitis media | ✓ Acute onset of signs and symptoms (ear pain, irritability, fussiness, fever) *and*<br>✓ Presence of middle-ear effusion *and*<br>✓ Signs/symptoms of middle-ear inflammation (distinct ear pain or erythema of the tympanic membrane) |
| Acute bacterial rhinosinusitis | ✓ Persistent thick rhinorrhea without improvement for 10–14 days *or*<br>✓ More severe upper respiratory tract symptoms and signs [temperature greater than or equal to 39°C (102.2°F), facial swelling, facial pain] |
| Community-acquired pneumonia (bacterial or atypical) | ✓ Tachypnea; abnormal adventitial lung sounds (rales) or evidence of consolidation on lung examination<br>✓ Consider confirmation by chest radiograph |

Allergic rhinitis is much less common in children under 3 years old than in older children and adolescents. A history of long-standing clear rhinorrhea, particularly when it is associated with sneezing, an itchy nose, or symptoms of allergic conjunctivitis (itchy, red, and/or watery eyes), helps make the diagnosis of allergic rhinitis. Although uncommon, a history of head trauma and an abrupt onset of clear rhinorrhea always should raise suspicion for a fracture of the cribriform plate and a cerebrospinal fluid leak. As with all acute pediatric illnesses, it is important to determine whether the child is tolerating oral liquids well and has been having a good urine output.

A brief past medical history should be obtained to identify children with a history of asthma and children with a higher risk of infection and pulmonary compromise (such as chronic lung disease or immunodeficiency). It is typical to test pregnant women routinely for syphilis with a nontreponemal test; a positive prenatal test suggestive of syphilis should prompt a thorough examination of the infant in the newborn period. Although congenital syphilis is quite uncommon, an infant with a history of chronic rhinorrhea as well as intrauterine growth concerns, hepatosplenomegaly, hyperbilirubinemia, and/or chronic rash (a maculopapular rash that becomes brown with desquamation or a vesicular bullous eruption) should prompt evaluation for this disease.

## PHYSICAL EXAMINATION

The physical examination should narrow the differential diagnosis further or confirm the diagnosis suspected at the end of the history. The examination always begins with observation. Is the child alert and playful? Is she or he tired but interactive? Is he or she listless or irritable? Is there evidence of increased work of breathing (chest retractions, nasal flaring, grunting)? Is the child cyanotic? Vital signs are essentially normal in children with viral rhinosinusitis, but tachycardia can be seen in those with fever and dehydration. Tachypnea in the presence of respiratory symptoms should alert the examiner to a lower respiratory tract illness such as pneumonia or bronchiolitis. The best individual finding for ruling out pneumonia in infants and young children is the absence of tachypnea.

The HEENT (head, ears, eyes, nose, and throat) examination starts with observation of the conjunctiva. Injection or conjunctivitis can be seen with adenovirus infection as well as in conjunction with otitis media (*Haemophilus influenzae* is the classic culprit). An exudative conjunctivitis suggests a bacterial source. The appearance of the rhinorrhea does not differentiate between a bacterial rhinosinusitis and a viral rhinosinusitis. Unilateral nasal discharge, especially in the absence of other symptoms, raises suspicion for a foreign body, and the nasal cavity should be inspected. Unfortunately, the physical examination generally does not assist in differentiating viral rhinosinusitis from bacterial rhinosinusitis. Facial pain is unusual in children; facial tenderness is rare in young children and may be unreliable in older children and adolescents. Significant unilateral pain over the body of a frontal or maxillary sinus may increase the probability of bacterial rhinosinusitis. Periorbital swelling is suggestive of ethmoid sinusitis. Pharyngitis or evidence of inflammation and erythema of the pharynx on examination is nonspecific but frequently is seen in adenovirus infection. The tympanic membranes and middle-ear spaces should be examined closely to rule out the possibility of acute otitis media.

In addition to the ear examination, the lung examination is the other critical portion of the physical examination in children with prolonged respiratory symptoms, as acute otitis media and pneumonia should be eliminated as possible diagnoses. Bacterial and atypical pneumonias typically manifest with focal rales on auscultation of the lungs. Bronchiolitis usually presents with a combination of bilateral rales and coarse expiratory breath sounds that resemble wheezes. Rashes such as urticaria, fleeting maculopapular eruptions, or papulovesicular lesions on the palms and soles (characteristic of hand-foot-and-mouth disease) suggest viral etiologies.

## LABORATORY AND RADIOGRAPHIC EVALUATION

Viral rhinosinusitis is a clinical diagnosis, and no diagnostic studies are required. One exception is in the case of suspected influenza infection when a child meets the criteria for antiviral therapy and rapid antigen testing is feasible. Viral rhinosinusitis is differentiated from common bacterial respiratory infections (rhinosinusitis, acute otitis media, and pneumonia) by specific clinical criteria (see Table 19-2).

There is no role for imaging (plain films or computed tomography) in differentiating viral rhinosinusitis from acute bacterial rhinosinusitis, as sinus membrane thickening and fluid levels may be seen in both conditions. Again, the best individual finding for ruling out pneumonia in infants and young children is the absence of tachypnea.

## MANAGEMENT

Infants and children with viral rhinosinusitis generally require only supportive measures. Parents of infants and young children may use a bulb syringe with or without nasal saline drops to aid the removal of nasal secretions and improve comfort. Many providers also suggest humidifier use to facilitate secretion removal. As with other acute infections, antipyretics should be considered if a child appears significantly uncomfortable while febrile, but otherwise the fever accompanying these and other illnesses do not require routine treatment. Fluid intake and rest should be encouraged. Family members should be encouraged to practice careful handwashing to prevent the spread of this infection and future viral infections.

Over-the-counter cold medications are plentiful but have not been shown conclusively to improve symptoms in pediatric patients, and can cause side effects, particularly in infants. Most of these preparations include an antihistamine, a decongestant, or a combination of the two. Other preparations may include analgesics (such as acetaminophen) and/or cough suppressants. Although there is some evidence that antihistamine therapy (clemastine fumarate specifically) in adults with viral rhinosinusitis leads to a marginal decrease in sneezing and nasal secretions, those effects have not been demonstrated in young children. Patients and their parents should be advised to avoid nasal decongestant sprays because of the rebound effects that typically occur after 2 to 3 days of use. Zinc has been used increasingly to treat symptoms of viral rhinosinusitis, but adult studies have shown conflicting results; therefore, it cannot be recommended in the routine treatment of children with these infections. There is also no conclusive evidence that ascorbic acid therapy taken during an episode of viral rhinosinusitis is effective in alleviating the associated symptoms.

Antiviral therapy is currently available for the treatment of influenza infection. Oseltamivir is U.S. Food and Drug Administration (FDA)-approved for patients 1 year of age and older, and zanamivir may be used in patients 7 years of age and older. These medications are effective if started within 36 to 48 h of the onset of symptoms. A recent Cochrane Database review recommends oseltamivir over zanamivir because it has been shown to decrease the incidence of acute otitis media in this setting and is effective in younger children. Vomiting is a common side effect. Neither drug is recommended in children with chronic medical conditions (such as asthma) because benefit has not been shown with either drug in pediatric patients with chronic disease. There is also a theoretical risk for bronchospasm with zanamivir. Potential antirhinoviral drugs are being studied, but to date there has been no conclusive evidence of benefit for viral rhinosinusitis.

Children with respiratory infections should be treated with antibiotics only if a specific bacterial or atypical infection has been diagnosed in accordance with the criteria listed above. *It cannot be overemphasized that mucopurulent rhinorrhea (with or without color change) does not signify bacterial infection and does not require antibiotic therapy if the criteria for bacterial rhinosinusitis are not met.* This can present a significant challenge for providers when they are pressured by parents to prescribe antibiotics. Parent and patient education about the natural history of viral rhinosinusitis should be a routine part of all visits for viral rhinosinusitis; this education can be quite effective in clarifying misunderstandings and providing parental reassurance. Judicious use of antibiotics is critical to minimize antimicrobial resistance, unnecessary health-care costs, and side effects from unnecessary antibiotics. Children with chronic lung disease (e.g., children with tracheomalacia or chronic tracheobronchitis from tracheostomy) and/or immunodeficiency may benefit from antibiotic therapy in selected circumstances. Parents of children diagnosed with viral rhinosinusitis should be instructed to return for evaluation if the child has prolonged symptoms (past the natural history of the disease) or if symptoms suggestive of acute otitis media or pneumonia develop.

Other etiologies of nasal discharge should be treated directly. Nasal foreign bodies should be removed. Children with specific illnesses such as croup or viral infection with asthma exacerbation should be treated accordingly.

---

### *"Don't Miss"* Diagnoses for Nasal Discharge

Bacterial pneumonia
Atypical pneumonia
Nasal foreign body
Viral upper respiratory tract infection with asthma exacerbation
Cerebrospinal fluid leak
Congenital syphilis

---

## BIBLIOGRAPHY

Fahey TN, Stocks N, Thomas T. Systematic review of the treatment of upper respiratory tract infection. *Arch Dis Child* 79(3):225–230, 1998.

Friedman MJ, Attia MW. Clinical predictors of influenza in children. *Arch Pediatr Adolesc Med* 158(4):391–394, 2004.

Margolis P, Gadomski A. The national clinical examination. Does this infant have pneumonia? [see comment]. *JAMA* 279(4):308–313, 1998.

Matheson NJ, Symmonds-Abrahams M, Sheikh A, et al. Neuraminidase inhibitors for preventing and treating influenza in children. *Cochrane Database Syst Rev* 3:CD002744, 2003.

O'Brien KL, Dowell SF, Schwartz B, et al. Acute sinusitis—principles of judicious use of antimicrobial agents. *Pediatrics* 101(1):174–177, 1998.

Rosenstein N, Phillips WR, Gerber MA, et al. The common cold—principles of judicious use of antimicrobial agents. *Pediatrics* 101(1):181–184, 1998.

Subcommittee on Management of Acute Otitis Media. Diagnosis and management of acute otitis media. *Pediatrics* 113(5):1451–1465, 2004.

Subcommittee on Management of Sinusitis and Committee on Quality Improvement. Clinical practice guideline: Management of sinusitis. *Pediatrics* 108(3):798–808, 2001.

Thuma PE. Common cold. In Hoekelman RAMD, ed., *Primary Pediatric Care*. St. Louis: Mosby, 2001: 1399–1401.

# ABDOMINAL PAIN

## M. Robin English

1. Know the components of a thorough history and physical examination for a pediatric patient with abdominal pain and understand the importance of the history and examination in developing a differential diagnosis.

2. Know the presenting signs and symptoms of the common causes of abdominal pain.

3. Understand the underlying etiology and/or pathophysiology for each of the common causes of abdominal pain.

4. Identify the appropriate initial workup and management for each of the common causes of abdominal pain.

## INTRODUCTION

Abdominal pain is one of the most common presenting symptoms a pediatrician encounters. It also can prove to be one of the most challenging complaints to approach, as children and adolescents are often unable to describe the timing and character of their pain. Young infants and toddlers can experience abdominal pain without localizing it, presenting with fussiness or inconsolability. Older children often describe a "tummy ache," with little else to offer in terms of characterization. Adolescents often are able to describe their pain, but the differential diagnosis becomes so much broader in this age group that a new set of challenges arises. In addition, abdominal pain is a common somatic complaint in pediatrics, and this means that the pain is not due to an underlying physiologic process but rather to stress or another nonorganic etiology.

The pediatrician's role in evaluating pediatric or adolescent abdominal pain is to take a complete history and perform a complete physical examination to decide whether the pain requires immediate surgical or medical attention. Many diseases that cause abdominal pain in these age groups are nonemergent, but the severity of the few surgical etiologies and the potentially serious consequences of missing these diagnoses make a high index of suspicion important. Many children ultimately are diagnosed with functional abdominal pain, but it is important to rule out more serious illnesses before assigning this diagnosis. This chapter discusses the features of the history and physical examination that are crucial in determining the etiology of the pain.

As a complete history and physical examination are performed, the examiner begins to develop a differential diagnosis. This differential diagnosis may change several times during the course of the history and examination as new information comes to light. There are several ways to approach the differential diagnosis of abdominal pain. Some clinicians prefer to think about the problem in terms of the organs that may be involved, such as stomach problems or kidney problems. Others choose to look at the chronicity or timing of the pain to help them develop the differential diagnosis. This chapter is arranged primarily by organ system, but it also highlights the importance of considering the time course of abdominal pain in formulating a differential diagnosis. Diagnostic tests and management options for many common pediatric diseases causing abdominal pain are discussed.

## HISTORY

The history is of the upmost importance when one is seeing a pediatric patient with abdominal pain, and an extensive history of the present illness is crucial. As with any other history obtained when one sees a patient with pain, the location, quality and severity, timing, relieving and aggravating factors, and associated symptoms all should be explored. The location of pain in children usually is identified by them as periumbilical, and if the pain is consistently in a different location, the suspicion for an underlying pathology should increase. Older children should be asked if the pain is sharp or achy in nature and probably will be able to quantify the pain on a pain scale. Children or parents should be asked whether the pain interferes with regular activity, such as play, sleep, and school activities. The timing of the pain, including onset, duration, and course (i.e., recurrent, constant, intermittent), is also important, because the differential diagnosis differs from acute pain to chronic or recurrent pain (Table 20-1).

*Table 20-1* **Etiologies of Abdominal Pain by Time Course**

|  | Acute | Recurrent or Chronic |
|---|---|---|
| Stomach | Gastritis | Peptic ulcer disease<br>Chronic gastritis |
| Liver | Viral hepatitis | |
| Biliary system | Cholelithiasis<br>Cholecystitis | |
| Pancreas | Pancreatitis | |
| Intestine (surgical) | Appendicitis<br>Intussusception<br>Incarcerated inguinal<br>hernia | |
| Intestine (nonsurgical) | Gastroenteritis | Constipation<br>Inflammatory bowel disease |
| Kidney | Nephrolithiasis<br>Urinary tract infection | |
| Genital system | Ovarian or testicular<br>torsion<br>Pelvic inflammatory<br>disease<br>Ectopic pregnancy | |
| Other | Henoch-Schönlein<br>purpura | Malignancy<br>Functional |

Some causes of chronic pain, such as peptic ulcer disease and constipation, can present with acute exacerbations. Relieving and aggravating factors such as food intake, medications, and position may offer a clue as to the etiology as well. Associated symptoms such as vomiting, diarrhea, rashes, fever, joint pain, constipation, activity, and appetite may be important in determining whether the etiology is localized to one organ or is more systemic in nature. Adolescents should be questioned independently, as an accurate sexual history is important. Finally, a complete review of systems should be performed to uncover pertinent history that was not obtained previously.

Information obtained in the history of the present illness is used by the examiner to help focus his or her approach. If this history is very suggestive of an acute surgical problem, the examiner may forgo less pertinent history, such as the developmental, social, or family history, to pursue the examination and subsequent treatment quickly. If the initial history is suggestive of a more chronic etiology, the examiner should take the time to gather all aspects of the history, as more information about the differential diagnosis may be uncovered. Historic clues to the etiology of abdominal pain will be discussed with each specific disease entity later in this chapter.

## PHYSICAL EXAMINATION

A complete physical examination of the patient should be performed, including attention to hydration and vital signs. A child's general demeanor may provide valuable clues to the etiology of the pain. A child with an acute or surgical abdomen often will remain very still and resist movement or ambulation, whereas a child who is talkative or smiling or who moves around the examination table with little difficulty probably will not have a surgical etiology for her or his pain.

The first aspect of the abdominal examination is inspection, looking for distended veins, discoloration, or distention. Next, the abdomen should be auscultated, listening carefully for bowel sounds in all four quadrants. This should be done before palpation, as palpation by itself can evoke bowel sounds. Gentle palpation over all aspects of the abdomen should be done with care, and the examiner may elicit a more accurate examination by leaving his or her hand on the abdomen for a few seconds before performing deep palpation, especially in infants and younger children. Both upper quadrants should be palpated for the presence of hepatomegaly or splenomegaly. Maneuvers that evaluate for peritoneal irritation, such as rebound tenderness, heel tap, and obturator signs, should be performed, especially if a surgical problem is suspected. Percussion is helpful in determining rebound tenderness, gaseous distention, and organomegaly. An external anal and genital examination generally is indicated. A rectal examination may be indicated, although this is often very uncomfortable for young children. A pelvic examination usually is indicated for adolescent females.

The site of abdominal tenderness or pain can be an important clue to the organ system involved. Epigastric pain usually represents pathology in the stomach, hepatobiliary system, or pancreas. Distal small bowel, appendix, and proximal colon pathology often causes periumbilical pain, although as was noted above, many children point to the umbilicus first as the site of their pain regardless of etiology. Distal colon, urinary system, and pelvic organ diseases often present with suprapubic or back pain. Specific physical examination findings suggestive of the etiology for a child's abdominal pain will be discussed below with each specific disease entity.

## DIFFERENTIAL DIAGNOSIS OF ABDOMINAL PAIN

### STOMACH

#### GASTRITIS

Gastritis generally is defined as inflammation of the stomach lining that may be acute or chronic. Acute gastritis may be caused by a number of influences, including viral illnesses and stress, both psychological and physiologic. Medications that commonly cause gastritis in children are nonsteroidal anti-inflammatory drugs and steroids. Chronic gastritis may be caused by the factors noted above. Also implicated in chronic gastritis is *Helicobacter pylori* infection. However, most children found to have *H. pylori* infection are actually asymptomatic.

A history of nausea without diarrhea, aggravation with food ingestion, or medication use may be obtained. These children are generally well-appearing and have mild midepigastric tenderness. Usually, no laboratory or radiologic evaluation is necessary. Specifically, it is not recommended to perform tests for *H. pylori* in these children. Children may be treated with a course of an H2 receptor antagonist, and a proton pump inhibitor can be prescribed if there is no improvement.

#### PEPTIC ULCER DISEASE

Peptic ulcer disease occurs as a result of increased acid production and decreased local protective factors, such as secretion of bicarbonate and mucus. It may be idiopathic or may be caused by medications or infection with *H. pylori*. Children with peptic ulcer disease may complain of recurrent epigastric abdominal pain, which may awaken them at night; heartburn; nausea; or hematemesis. Midepigastric tenderness is generally present on physical examination. These findings are typically more severe in peptic ulcer disease than in simple gastritis without ulcer.

Children with signs and symptoms of peptic ulcer disease without evidence of bleeding can undergo a trial of H2 receptor antagonists. If there is no improvement or if there is gastrointestinal bleeding, a referral to a pediatric gastroenterologist for an endoscopy is appropriate. Endoscopy is useful to obtain biopsies for *H. pylori* and to evaluate for other causes of dyspepsia. In fact, a biopsy is the diagnostic method of choice for diagnosing *H. pylori*; serologies and urea breath tests are not recommended because of unreliability.

The treatment of peptic ulcer disease involves H2 receptor antagonists, proton pump inhibitors, and cytoprotective agents such as sucralfate. If a biopsy shows evidence of *H. pylori* infection and there is evidence of gastric or duodenal ulcers on endoscopy, treatment should consist of 2 weeks of double antibiotic therapy (using a combination of amoxicillin, clarithromycin, and/or metronidazole) and 1 month of a proton pump inhibitor.

Compliance with this drug regimen is important for complete eradication of the organism.

## LIVER/BILIARY SYSTEM/PANCREAS

### CHOLELITHIASIS/CHOLECYSTITIS

Cholelithiasis, or gallstones, is uncommon in healthy children. Predisposing factors in pediatric patients include hemolytic disease, cystic fibrosis, prolonged parenteral nutrition, and obesity. Most gallstones in children are pigmented rather than cholesterol stones. The history may reveal recurrent, colicky right upper quadrant pain that is often worse after eating fatty foods. The pain may radiate to the scapula or shoulder. If cholelithiasis is suspected, the examiner should look for evidence of an underlying disease such as failure to thrive, obesity, or jaundice. Often, the examination will reveal right only upper quadrant tenderness to palpation. Ultrasound of the gallbladder is the diagnostic method of choice. Cholecystectomy is the surgical procedure required for treatment, and it can be done laparoscopically.

Cholelithiasis often can lead to cholecystitis. Cholecystitis also can develop without the presence of stones (acalculous cholecystitis); this may be due to bacterial infection of the gallbladder or trauma. Patients may complain of vomiting, epigastric or right upper quadrant pain, and fever. The physical examination typically reveals significant right upper quadrant tenderness and guarding, and a Murphy sign (abrupt cessation of inspiration on deep palpation of the right upper quadrant) may be present. Ultrasound of the gallbladder probably will show enlargement and thickening of the wall. A complete blood count may show leukocytosis but is not required for the diagnosis. The treatment of choice is cholecystectomy and possibly antibiotics.

### HEPATITIS

Most cases of hepatitis in children and adolescents are viral in etiology, and hepatitis A and Epstein-Barr viruses are two primary etiologies for abdominal pain. Children with hepatitis A present with fever, vomiting, anorexia, and dull abdominal pain in the right upper quadrant. Physical examination shows right upper quadrant tenderness and possibly dehydration. Jaundice is seen more commonly in infected older children but is rare in infected infants. Laboratory evaluation typically shows elevation of liver enzymes and bilirubin, and a prothrombin time may be prolonged. Elevation of hepatitis A virus–immunoglobulin M (HAV-IgM) confirms the diagnosis of hepatitis A; this is typically part of a routine hepatitis panel. Children with hepatitis A have a good prognosis, with symptoms resolving in less than a month, but fulminant hepatitis progressing to end-stage liver disease has been reported rarely. Contacts of children with hepatitis A should receive hepatitis A immune globulin.

Hepatitis that occurs with Epstein-Barr infection usually is seen as part of the infectious mononucleosis syndrome, and so hepatosplenomegaly, lymphadenopathy, and tonsillar exudates may be present. Epstein-Barr virus (EBV) can be confirmed either by a positive Monospot or by elevation of EBV-IgM. Nonspecific viral hepatitis and Epstein-Barr hepatitis typically resolve without treatment and have excellent prognoses.

## PANCREATITIS

Pancreatitis is caused by autodigestion by proteolytic and lipolytic enzymes after an initial insult. Common causes in pediatric patients include viral illnesses, medications (e.g., steroids, valproic acid, some antibiotics), trauma, cystic fibrosis, and Kawasaki disease, although the complete list of etiologies is quite extensive. The history should include any medications and recent illnesses. Most children present with vomiting and midepigastric pain that radiates to the back. Many prefer to sit forward or lie on the side. The physical examination usually reveals a very uncomfortable and ill-appearing child. In acute hemorrhagic pancreatitis, which is rare in children, bluish discoloration of the periumbilical area (Cullen sign) or flanks (Grey Turner sign) may be evident.

The diagnosis of pancreatitis can be made by obtaining amylase and lipase levels, which will be elevated. Elevated lipase is more specific for pancreatitis than is elevated amylase. Radiologic findings may include evidence of pancreatic enlargement or peripancreatic fluid collections as seen on computed tomography or ultrasound. Management includes aggressive pain control, intravenous fluids, and taking nothing by mouth. Most patients recover in 1 to 3 weeks, although a few have a more prolonged course.

## INTESTINE (SURGICAL)

### APPENDICITIS

Appendicitis should be high in the differential diagnosis of acute abdominal pain in all children as it requires prompt surgical attention. It usually is caused by luminal obstruction followed by increased pressure and subsequent vascular thrombosis of the appendiceal wall. These patients often present with the acute onset of nausea, vomiting, and anorexia. The pain of appendicitis usually starts in the periumbilical area and then moves to the right lower quadrant after a few hours. Pain that is very severe and then improves suddenly should raise the examiner's suspicion of perforation. The physical examination usually reveals a child who is ill-appearing and unwilling to walk or move without caution. Pain in the right lower quadrant is usual, and rebound tenderness may be elicited by percussion. A rectal examination may be painful and usually is not required for the diagnosis.

Laboratory findings are variable. These children may have leukocytosis or a high erythrocyte sedimentation rate, but these findings should not be used to make or rule out the diagnosis. Children and adolescents suspected of having appendicitis should be seen by a surgeon immediately. Many surgeons proceed with surgery without further radiologic testing if the clinical picture is very suspicious for appendicitis. If the diagnosis is in question, a computed tomography scan of the abdomen may be helpful.

The treatment consists of surgical removal, with the addition of broad-spectrum antibiotics if perforation has occurred. The prognosis is generally good.

## INCARCERATED INGUINAL HERNIA

Incarcerated hernia occurs when the contents of a hernia sac (usually the small intestine) cannot be reduced into the abdominal cavity. It is seen most commonly in the first year of life. The history may reveal fussiness, vomiting, and the acute onset of generalized abdominal pain and/or inguinal pain. Incarcerated hernia is one of the diagnoses that highlight the importance of performing a genital examination in children with abdominal pain because the abdominal pain may be more pronounced than inguinal or scrotal pain and therefore lead the examiner to another diagnosis. The physical examination will reveal generalized abdominal tenderness and a firm, tender, and often discolorated mass in the inguinal region.

Management of an incarcerated hernia involves attempting to reduce the contents of the hernia sac manually, which usually can be done without surgical intervention with the use of sedation. Strangulation, which develops when the blood supply becomes compromised, can occur if the hernia is not reduced in a timely manner. Strangulation and an unreducible hernia are indications for immediate surgical intervention. If the hernia can be reduced manually, a herniorrhaphy should be scheduled after the edema and pain have resolved. It is important to remember that some boys with an incarcerated hernia also have infarction of the ipsilateral testis.

## INTUSSUSCEPTION

Intussusception is another important diagnosis to recognize in pediatrics. It occurs most commonly in children between 6 months and 3 years of age, and it is the most common cause of intestinal obstruction in this age group. It occurs when a loop of the intestine telescopes into a portion of the intestine immediately distal to it and is seen most commonly in the ileocecal area. Common lead points include Meckel diverticulum and enlarged Peyer patches. Older children with intussusception should be evaluated for lymphoma, as this can act as a lead point in this age group. The history may reveal bilious or nonbilious vomiting, lethargy, and irritability. Many mothers note that the child seems to be in pain, but they cannot identify the source of the pain. Affected children often pull up their legs and cry intermittently but may act normally between episodes of pain. Lethargy is common and may be the predominant feature. The characteristic "currant jelly" stool is often a late finding, and so the presence of normal stools should not rule out the diagnosis. A sausage-shaped mass may be palpable, and abdominal distention may be noted.

Intussusception is considered an emergency, and so diagnosis and treatment should be sought as soon as the diagnosis is suspected. An abdominal radiograph may show evidence of obstruction, but the test of choice for diagnosis is an air-contrast or barium enema. Many centers favor air-contrast enemas because of a slightly decreased risk of perforation compared with barium enemas. These enemas are usually therapeutic as well as diagnostic, as the pressure from the air or barium reduces the intussusception. However, a surgeon should be aware that the enema is being performed, because failure to reduce the obstruction is an indication for immediate surgical reduction. Most children have very rapid improvement in their irritability, lethargy, and vomiting after reduction.

## INTESTINE (NONSURGICAL)

### CONSTIPATION/ENCOPRESIS

Constipation is one of the most common causes of abdominal pain in the pediatric and adolescent population. Usually it is due to a nonorganic cause such as lack of dietary fiber, but occasionally organic causes such as spinal cord tumors or Hirschsprung disease are identified. The history usually reveals recurrent, vague, generalized abdominal pain. Questions regarding toilet habits and diet are important. Frequently, a history of withholding stool and irregular voiding patterns is elicited, and affected children tend to have poor fiber intake. The physical examination usually reveals a well-appearing child. Stool may be palpated through the abdominal wall, and generalized mild tenderness may be elicited on palpation. An anorectal examination to look for anal fissures or tags and to assess rectal tone should be performed. If the constipation is new in onset, a thorough neurologic examination is indicated to evaluate for a spinal cord lesion.

Encopresis is defined as involuntary stool leakage and may be misinterpreted by the parent or child as diarrhea. Encopresis results from severe constipation. A large stool partially obstructs the colon, and more proximal liquid stool leaks around the blockage. This, combined with decreased rectal tone, causes leakage of the stool into the child's underwear. Understandably, this becomes a social problem for the child.

The diagnosis of constipation can be confirmed with an abdominal radiograph. Management consists of dietary counseling and stool softeners, often in combination with enemas. In cases of fecal impaction, the first step is to disimpact the rectum. This is best accomplished by administering polyethylene glycol either orally or through a nasogastric tube until the stools become clear. This may take several days. After disimpaction, therapy should focus on keeping the stools soft and getting the child to have regular bowel movements. This can be a complicated problem to address, and many children have chronic difficulties with recurrent impaction.

### GASTROENTERITIS

Gastroenteritis, either viral or bacterial, can cause significant abdominal pain in children. The history usually includes diarrhea and vomiting of fairly acute onset, and other family members may be ill as well. The physical examination may show vague abdominal tenderness and increased bowel sounds, but focal or severe tenderness is unusual. Some bacterial pathogens, specifically *Yersinia enterocolitica* and *Campylobacter jejuni*, can cause an appendicitis-like clinical picture known as pseudoappendicitis. A stool culture or rapid antigen test can help identify the responsible bacterial or viral pathogens. Most of these illnesses resolve with fluid therapy and time.

### INFLAMMATORY BOWEL DISEASE

Both ulcerative colitis and Crohn disease can cause abdominal pain, but usually other symptoms, such as diarrhea, are present. These diseases should be considered in children and adolescents with chronic abdominal pain. The history also may reveal tenesmus, crampy abdominal pain with bowel movements, and bloody or nonbloody diarrhea. Questions about weight loss, anorexia, and other constitutional symptoms also should be explored. The physical examination often shows vague, generalized abdominal tenderness. A careful search for extraintestinal manifestations of these diseases (arthritis, growth failure, skin lesions) should be performed as well. The diagnosis and management of ulcerative colitis and Crohn disease are covered in Chap. 30.

## KIDNEY

### NEPHROLITHIASIS

Children and adolescents with nephrolithiasis can present with intense abdominal pain. The history often reveals hematuria, although this is variable. The pain produced by stones is generally episodic or colicky in nature. There may be a family history of kidney stones. Pain typically begins in the flank and is referred to the inguinal region. The physical examination is often normal, although vague tenderness may be present.

Laboratory evaluation may reveal microscopic hematuria or high urinary calcium, although neither is required for the diagnosis. A spiral computed tomography scan or ultrasound often can confirm the presence of stones. As kidney stones often are composed of calcium, they frequently can be seen on plain abdominal radiographs as well. Most children with small stones improve with hydration and do not require surgical intervention or lithotripsy; larger stones may need to be removed surgically.

## URINARY TRACT INFECTION/PYELONEPHRITIS

It is not unusual for abdominal pain to be the primary symptom of a urinary tract infection (UTI). Children with simple cystitis often present with acute suprapubic pain, and a history of dysuria, frequency, or urgency may be obtained. The pain associated with pyelonephritis tends to be unilateral flank pain that may be sharp or dull. Fever is often present. On physical examination, costovertebral angle tenderness can be elicited by gently tapping on the flank region.

Laboratory evaluation should include a urinalysis and urine culture obtained by the cleanest means possible. Infants and toddlers should be catheterized for the specimen if a strong suspicion for UTI is present. Older children and adolescents usually can provide a clean specimen via clean-catch collection. Ultrasound may show evidence of pyelonephritis but is not required for the diagnosis. The abdominal pain typically resolves after the infection is treated with antibiotics.

# GENITAL SYSTEM

## OVARIAN/TESTICULAR TORSION

Torsion of the ovary or testicle constitutes a surgical emergency and should be identified and treated quickly to improve the outcome. Ovarian torsion usually is seen in school-age children and adolescents, but bilateral ovarian torsion also can occur in infancy. It may occur spontaneously or in conjunction with an ovarian cyst or another mass. The pain is acute in onset and may be intermittent and sharp. Vomiting may be a prominent associated feature. The physical examination shows lower abdominal tenderness and often a lower abdominal mass. The diagnosis often can be confirmed with pelvic ultrasound with Doppler flow; at other times, complete visualization of the adnexa may be difficult. Surgical intervention should occur promptly, and oophoropexy of the contralateral ovary is recommended by some sources.

Testicular torsion occurs when a testis that is not normally fixed in the scrotum twists within the tunica vaginalis. The torsion may be preceded by minor trauma. These patients present with acute, severe testicular pain, but abdominal pain may be more prominent than the testicular pain, again demonstrating the importance of a genital examination when there is a complaint of abdominal pain. A cremasteric reflex (elevation of the testicle with gentle upward stroking of the inner thigh) is absent in most cases, and so this is an important sign to try to elicit. The affected testicle will be tender, edematous, and often erythematous, with a horizontal position. The diagnosis can be confirmed with testicular ultrasound with Doppler flow, but if the history and physical examination are very suggestive of testicular torsion, surgical intervention should not be delayed while one waits to do the ultrasound. The chance of salvaging the testicle increases the sooner the torsion can be relieved. Bilateral orchiopexy is indicated after detorsion.

## PELVIC INFLAMMATORY DISEASE

Pelvic inflammatory disease (PID) is an infection of the female genital tract. It is commonly caused by *Neisseria gonorrhoeae* or *Chlamydia trachomatis* as well as other bacteria. This disease should be suspected strongly in adolescent females with lower abdominal pain. Affected adolescents often present with vomiting and fever as well. As with all adolescents, a social history, including sexual activity, should be obtained from the adolescent. Lower abdominal tenderness is typical, although right upper quadrant pain can occur if perihepatitis (Fitz-Hugh-Curtis syndrome) is present. The abdomen should be palpated carefully for masses, as tuboovarian abscess is a common complication. A full pelvic examination should be performed. Findings on pelvic examination that are suggestive of PID are vaginal or cervical discharge, adnexal tenderness, and cervical motion tenderness.

Laboratory evaluation should include cervical cultures and a wet prep for *Trichomonas*. Screening for other sexually transmitted diseases, such as syphilis and human immunodeficiency virus (HIV), and a urine pregnancy test also should be done. Treatment should not be withheld until culture results are known but should be initiated immediately. Indications for hospitalization include inability to tolerate oral medications or feedings, tuboovarian abscess, fear of noncompliance, pregnancy, and failure to improve or comply with outpatient therapy. Many practitioners feel that all adolescents with PID should be hospitalized. Several regimens for PID treatment have been developed, and all require at least two antibiotics. A frequently used combination is cefoxitin plus doxycycline. Long-term complications include infertility and chronic pelvic pain. All adolescents with PID should be counseled on the importance of safe sex practices.

## PREGNANCY/ECTOPIC PREGNANCY

It is important to screen for pregnancy in all adolescent females who present with abdominal pain, especially if another cause is not immediately evident. This screening should be done before any radiologic studies, even if pregnancy is not strongly suspected. Intrauterine pregnancy can present with abdominal pain, but acute, severe pain may be indicative of an ectopic pregnancy. The abdominal pain seen in patients with ectopic pregnancy can be variable, including lower abdominal pain and back pain.

Ectopic pregnancy can be diagnosed with a urine pregnancy test and pelvic ultrasound. Gynecologic consultation should be obtained when the diagnosis is confirmed.

## OTHER

### HENOCH-SCHÖNLEIN PURPURA

Abdominal pain may be the initial presenting symptom of Henoch-Schönlein purpura, with the rash and other symptoms presenting within a day or two. The abdominal pain can be quite severe and colicky in nature. Vomiting and diarrhea, which can be bloody, also may be present. A particular consideration in a child with Henoch-Schönlein purpura and abdominal pain is the risk of intussusception, in which an area of vasculitis serves as the lead point. The pain from intussusception can be difficult to distinguish from the pain of the disease itself, and so it is important to maintain a high index of suspicion. Henoch-Schönlein disease is covered in greater depth in Chap. 38.

### MALIGNANCY

Malignancies such as leukemia and abdominal lymphomas can present with abdominal pain in children and adolescents, but it is unusual for abdominal pain to be the only symptom. In addition, the physical examination should reveal other abnormalities, such as an abdominal mass, hepatosplenomegaly, pallor, bruising, or lymphadenopathy.

### FUNCTIONAL ABDOMINAL PAIN

Functional disorders are those in which symptoms are not caused by an organic disease. Functional abdominal pain is very common in the pediatric and adolescent populations. Parents, patients, and pediatricians can become frustrated when abdominal pain persists but no underlying cause can be found. The Rome II criteria were developed to assist with the management of functional gastrointestinal disorders.

Irritable bowel syndrome is characterized by 12 or more weeks of abdominal pain in a year. Other features include bowel changes, which may consist of diarrhea, constipation, or a combination of the two, and abdominal distention. Abdominal pain often is relieved with defecation. Another functional disorder is known as functional recurrent abdominal pain (FRAP). This is characterized by 12 or more weeks of persistent abdominal pain, usually without bowel changes or a relationship to defecation. Most children with FRAP miss school and experience loss of other regular daily functioning.

The goal of the pediatrician evaluating a child with recurrent abdominal pain is to get a thorough history that excludes organic diseases. Clues that recurrent abdominal pain actually may be due to an organic cause include weight loss, recurrent vomiting, chronic diarrhea, fever, and consistent pain that is localized to one area of the abdomen. A normal physical examination is typical with functional pain, but it does not rule out an organic cause.

Treatment of functional gastrointestinal disorders can be complicated and challenging. Psychosocial triggers should be identified and addressed. The pediatrician should emphasize the absence of serious disease and the importance of maintaining daily functioning. Giving the child a diagnosis of "functional abdominal pain" and then educating the parents about the diagnosis probably is more effective in reassuring them than is telling them that there is nothing wrong with their child. Several therapies have been studied with varied success, including cognitive-behavior therapy and diet therapy. There is no consistent placebo-controlled evidence that medication is helpful in the management of functional abdominal pain.

---

### "Don't Miss" Diagnoses for Abdominal Pain

Appendicitis
Incarcerated inguinal hernia
Intussusception
Ovarian/testicular torsion
Pelvic inflammatory disease
Pregnancy/ectopic pregnancy
Urinary tract infection

---

## CONCLUSION

Many of the etiologies of abdominal pain in pediatrics and adolescence are self-limited and benign in nature. However, the few emergent or serious diseases that can present with abdominal pain necessitate a high index of suspicion at all times when this complaint is encountered. Keeping both the time course and the characteristics of the pain in mind can help the examiner take an organized and focused approach to developing a differential diagnosis and subsequent plan of management for the patient.

## BIBLIOGRAPHY

Ashcraft K. Acute abdominal pain. *Pediatr Rev* 21:363–366, 2000.

Chelimsky G, Czinn S. Peptic ulcer disease in children. *Pediatr Rev* 22:349–354, 2001.

Gold BD, Colletti RB, Abbott M, et al. Helicobacter pylori infection in children: Recommendations for diagnosis and treatment. *J Pediatr Gastroenterol Nutr* 31:490–497, 2000.

Hyman PE, Rasquin-Weber A, Fleisher DR, et al. ROME II: Childhood functional gastrointestinal disorders. In Drossman DA, ed., *The Functional Gastrointestinal Disorders*, 2d ed. Lawrence, KS: Allen Press, 2000: 533–575.

Kohli R, Li B. Differential diagnosis of recurrent abdominal pain: New considerations. *Pediatr Ann* 33:113–122, 2004.

# VOMITING

*Michael A. Barone*

1. Describe the evaluation of a vomiting child.
2. Using knowledge of the differential diagnosis, understand the necessary components of the medical history and physical examination in a vomiting child.
3. Understand the basic principles of the pathophysiology of vomiting and be able to relate them to the actions of pharmacotherapy for vomiting.

## INTRODUCTION

Like many conditions in pediatrics, vomiting can be considered both a symptom and an illness. Although many of its causes are benign and self-limited, an astute pediatrician always takes vomiting seriously as its potential causes and complications can be quite severe. Parents understandably are concerned about vomiting in a child of any age because it causes distress and threatens the child's nutritional status, an aspect of the child's health to which they devote great time and energy. In light of the fact that the causes of vomiting range from simple dietary indiscretion to serious intracranial pathology, a careful history focusing on the onset, progression, and pattern of symptoms is crucial. The physical examination must include not only the abdomen but the entire patient. This chapter focuses on the workup of a vomiting child, possible diagnoses, and the necessary steps in the management of vomiting.

## PATHOPHYSIOLOGY

Care should be taken in the history to differentiate a child who is truly vomiting from one who is regurgitating or exhibiting other signs of gastroesophageal reflux, a common condition in young infants in which gastric contents are passively refluxed up the esophagus. Vomiting should be considered the forceful expulsion of gastric contents from the mouth. The contents may be digested or undigested food, gastric or intestinal fluids (with or without bile), or blood. The coordinated vomiting reflex is thought to be governed by the "vomiting center" in the medulla. That center receives input via vestibular stimulation, visceral afferent stimulation, and chemoreceptors in an area of the brain at the floor of the fourth ventricle known as the chemoreceptor trigger zone (CTZ). Acetylcholine, histamine, and dopamine have been implicated as neurotransmitters in the stimulation of vomiting. In recent years, serotonin also has been cited for its role in this reflex, leading to the introduction of antiemetic agents, which antagonize serotonin receptors (see "Management," below).

In addition to the distress and discomfort that vomiting may cause a child, the risk of dehydration should not be underestimated. If vomiting (emesis) is persistent and prohibits the intake of fluids and nutrition, free-water deficits, ketosis, and electrolyte abnormalities will ensue. Throughout this period, one may observe progressively diminished urine output, decreased saliva and tear production, tachycardia, decreased peripheral profusion, and eventually changes in mental status, often leading to further nausea and emesis.

## DIFFERENTIAL DIAGNOSIS

In light of the vast nature of the differential diagnosis of vomiting, it is useful to categorize etiologies by the age of the patient. Table 21-1 lists possible causes of vomiting in children. As the differentiation between vomiting and gastroesophageal reflux is based primarily on clinical grounds, the table focuses on vomiting alone.

## HISTORY

A careful history will focus on the onset of vomiting, noting a gradual or abrupt start to the symptoms. Frequency, characteristics (e.g., blood, bile) of the emesis, differential tolerance of foods, and whether the symptoms are abating, static, or progressive are extremely helpful historic clues. Has the child had access to new surroundings (e.g., lead poisoning) or been with contacts who are also ill, and if so, what is the temporal nature of the child's

*Table 21-1* **Differential Diagnosis of Vomiting**

NEWBORNS
  Intestinal Obstruction
    Esophageal atresia
    Gastrointestinal duplications
    Hypertrophic pyloric stenosis
    Intestinal web, atresia, stenosis
    Malrotation of gastrointestinal tract (with or without midgut volvulus)
    Hirschsprung disease
    Imperforate anus
    Meconium ileus/meconium plug
    Incarcerated hernia
  Various Gastrointestinal Causes
    Necrotizing enterocolitis
    Protein allergy/eosinophilic gastroenteritis
  Infectious Causes
    Urinary tract infection
    Gastroenteritis (viral, bacterial, parasitic)
    Posttussive emesis (pertussis, respiratory syncytial virus)
    Sepsis/meningitis
  Neurologic Causes
    Hydrocephalus
    Intracranial hemorrhage
    Kernicterus
  Metabolic and Endocrine Causes
    Inborn errors of metabolism
    Adrenal insufficiency (e.g., congenital adrenal hyperplasia)
    Hypoglycemia
  Renal Causes
    Obstructive uropathy (e.g., posterior urethral valves)
    Uremia
    Renal tubular acidosis

OLDER INFANTS/EARLY TODDLERS
  Intestinal Obstruction
    Foreign body/bezoar
    Hypertrophic pyloric stenosis
    Malrotation (with or without midgut volvulus)
    Intussusception
    Incarcerated hernia
    Hirschsprung disease

*(continued)*

*Table 21-1* **Differential Diagnosis of Vomiting (continued)**

Various Gastrointestinal Causes
    Protein allergy eosinophilic gastroenteritis
    Celiac disease
    Appendicitis
Infectious Causes
Infectious gastroenteritis (viral, bacterial, parasitic)
Otitis media
Hepatitis
Sepsis/meningitis
Posttussive emesis (pertussis/respiratory syncytial virus)
Pneumonia
Upper respiratory infection
Sinusitis
Urinary tract infection
Neurologic Causes
    Intracranial mass lesions
    Intracranial hemorrhage
    Cerebral edema
    Hydrocephalus
Metabolic and Endocrine Causes
    Inborn errors of metabolism
    Adrenal insufficiency
Renal Causes
    Renal tubular acidosis
    Uremia
    Obstructive uropathy
Toxicities
    Lead or other heavy metal
    Medication overdose (e.g., aspirin)
    Alcohol
    Food poisoning (e.g., staphylococcal enterotoxin)

OLDER CHILDREN
    Intestinal Obstruction
        Adhesions
        Malrotation (with or without midgut volvulus)
        Superior mesenteric artery syndrome
        Incarcerated hernia
        Meconium ileus equivalent (cystic fibrosis)

*(continued)*

*Table 21-1*  **Differential Diagnosis of Vomiting (continued)**

Various Gastrointestinal Causes
    Trauma (e.g., hematoma)
    Inflammatory bowel disease (e.g., Crohn disease)
    Peptic ulcer disease
    Pancreatitis
    Cholelithiasis
    Appendicitis
    Celiac disease
    Paralytic ileus
Infectious Causes
    Gastroenteritis (viral, bacterial, parasitic)
    Urinary tract infection
    Hepatitis
    Ménétrier gastritis
    Streptococcal pharyngitis
Neurologic Causes
    Migraine, cyclic vomiting
    Brain mass lesion
    Intracranial hemorrhage
    Cerebral edema
    Pseudotumor cerebri
Renal Causes
    Uremia
Metabolic and Endocrine Causes
    Diabetic ketoacidosis
    Acute intermittent porphyria
    Inborn errors of metabolism
Toxicities
    Alcohol
    Medication overdose/poisoning (e.g., acetaminophen)
    Food poisoning (e.g., staphylococcal enterotoxin)
Various Causes
    Pregnancy
    Ovarian or testicular torsion

illness compared with that of the contacts? Did it occur before or after (infection) or simultaneously with (possible food poisoning) the contacts? Other constitutional symptoms, such as headache, fever, diarrhea, presence of pain, respiratory symptoms, dysuria, irritability, and changes in mental status, are important to elicit.

In consideration of the etiologies listed above, open-ended histories with some targeted, directed questions often lead to the ultimate diagnosis before any other studies have to be performed. For example, infants with esophageal atresia exhibit postprandial emesis of formula and breast milk, most often with respiratory distress, as salivary secretions pool in the proximal esophageal pouch. The presence or absence of bile in vomitus in the case of suspected gastrointestinal obstruction can differentiate the location of the blockage. Pyloric stenosis, for example, is associated with nonbilious vomiting as the gastric outlet obstruction is proximal to the ampulla of Vater, the second portion of the duodenum. Vomiting symptoms are progressive in pyloric stenosis because of continued elongation, hypertrophy, and pylorospasm. Often vomiting is described as "projectile," but this finding is neither universally sensitive nor specific. Infants are hungry; they tend to feed well in the period before dehydration and electrolyte abnormalities ensue, but vomiting becomes a postprandial rule over time. Infants with imperforate anus, Hirschsprung disease, or meconium ileus develop distention with a paucity or absence of stools. Protein allergy and eosinophilic gastroenteritis may be associated with other allergic diatheses, such as atopic dermatitis. Infectious gastroenteritis often is associated with fever, and by virtue of its name, diarrhea should be present at some point in the illness. Children with evolving hydrocephalus may have a history of prematurity and intracranial hemorrhage (e.g., posthemorrhagic hydrocephalus). They may exhibit a fixed downward gaze known as "sunsetting," along with a growth velocity in head circumference that is abnormal for age. Questions investigating possible maltreatment (child abuse) should be explored in any infant with an intracranial hemorrhage.

Inborn errors of metabolism such as urea cycle defects (e.g., ornithine transcarbamylase deficiency) can lead to lethargy, coma, hypoglycemia, and hyperammonemia. Similarly, disorders of organic acid metabolism can cause lethargy and protracted emesis. In these cases, a history of failure to thrive, chronic emesis, or an unusual odor of the child should be taken. A family history of children needing specialized nutrition or early unexplained infant deaths also may be suggestive of inborn errors of metabolism. Infants with adrenal insufficiency caused by congenital adrenal hyperplasia may be virilized, whereas older children with adrenal insufficiency caused by Addison disease may exhibit vomiting with hyperpigmentation [as a result of increased adrenocorticotropic hormone (ACTH) secretion].

Children with intussusception classically exhibit colicky pain, which often leads them to draw up their legs and cry. Discrete episodes of irritability with somnolence or lethargy in between may be seen. Stools may be loose early in the process but can have a reddish mucoid quality (currant jelly) as the bowel mucosa becomes compromised from ischemia. Children with celiac disease may exhibit vomiting along with diarrhea, growth delay, and abdominal distention. The onset of the symptoms is worth noting as one would not expect symptoms to become manifest until gluten is introduced into the diet.

In older patients, certain diagnoses also can be gleaned through a careful history. The superior mesenteric artery (SMA) syndrome, though rare, is associated with vomiting and feeding intolerance as the SMA obstructs the duodenum proximal to the ligament of Treitz. Symptoms occur in the supine position in thin children in whom low weight has caused reduction of fat in the mesentery. In this condition, the duodenum becomes extrinsically compressed between the aorta and the SMA vessel. The presentation of inflammatory bowel disease (e.g., Crohn disease, ulcerative colitis) may be associated with vomiting, with other features of note being weight loss, passage of blood in stools, oral ulcerations, rash, and arthritis/arthralgia.

Causes of vomiting resulting from central nervous system abnormalities also can be elicited from a careful history. Early morning emesis that is due to elevation in intracranial pressure from lying supine is concerning for a brain tumor or another cause of increased intracranial pressure, such as pseudotumor cerebri. Although migraine headache typically is associated with throbbing pain, many patients have vomiting as well. In younger children, vomiting may be the presenting feature of migraine because it causes greater distress than does the headache or because of the complete absence of a headache complaint. As an example, the cyclic vomiting syndrome is considered a migraine variant.

Patients presenting with vomiting, ill appearance, rapid breathing, and polyuria/polydipsia should be considered to have diabetic ketoacidosis until proven otherwise. Ingestions are also important considerations in vomiting patients, particularly adolescents. Alcohol intoxication or acetaminophen overdose (often as part of a suicide attempt) can lead to substantial emesis. Careful questions about medications, ingestions, and any over-the-counter herbal or performance-enhancing preparations should be asked.

## PHYSICAL EXAMINATION

Since so many causes of vomiting do not have their origins in abdominal factors, a thorough physical examination is paramount. Beginning with vital signs and growth parameters, numerous clues to the etiology exist. Although tachycardia typically is a sign of dehydration, bradycardia with hypertension should be concerning for a central nervous system (CNS) etiology (part of

Cushing's triad along with irregular respiration). Fever is often a hallmark of infectious diseases, but absence of fever or hypothermia, particularly in a neonate, should not be used to rule out infection. Elevated respiratory rate can be seen as a result of the metabolic acidosis caused by dehydration or an inborn error of metabolism. Alternatively, tachypnea may be due to pneumonia, which can lead to vomiting via referred pain to the abdomen and the creation of a paralytic ileus. Assessment of growth parameters is crucial. Although one may expect some acute weight loss as a result of dehydration, the clinical features of failure to thrive should lead one to consider diagnoses such as uremia, renal tubular acidosis, diabetes, and inborn errors of metabolism along with gastrointestinal causes such as malabsorptive disorders (cystic fibrosis, celiac disease), protein allergy, and pyloric stenosis.

Obviously, a thorough abdominal examination is essential in a vomiting patient. Beginning with observation, distention or gray discoloration of the abdomen may herald a catastrophe such as a midgut volvulus or necrotizing enterocolitis (NEC). Hirschsprung disease typically leads to distention with constipation.

Hyperactivity of bowel sounds often suggests infectious gastroenteritis, whereas quiet or absent bowel sounds may be noted in a patient with generalized ileus or peritonitis (e.g., perforated appendix). Palpation of the abdomen should be able to detect pain, voluntary or involuntary guarding, rebound tenderness, or organomegaly. A palpable mass may be detected in conditions such as pyloric stenosis (e.g., an "olive," a small pyloric mass palpable in the epigastrium to the right of the midline) and intussusception (often a right upper quadrant mass). Subtle physical findings also abound, such as the possible association of pyloric stenosis with an absent mandibular frenulum in infants. Thorough examination of the groin and umbilicus to evaluate for incarcerated hernias is needed. Examination of the scrotum will detect testicular trauma or torsion in males.

If vomiting continues, children begin to show signs of dehydration such as tachycardia, dry mucous membranes, poor capillary refill in the peripheral vascular beds (normal is less than 2 s), and eventually mental status changes. Regardless of the etiology, the fluid loss resulting from vomiting should be considered an abnormal loss to the body's typical fluid balance. As a result, the presence or absence of the signs of fluid deficit listed above must be noted as they play a substantial role in the further management of the patient.

## LABORATORY AND RADIOLOGIC EVALUATION

Often clinical grounds alone can determine an adequate etiology for vomiting. Laboratory and radiologic studies should be used for the monitoring of complications (e.g., dehydration, malnutrition) and establishing an additional need for diagnostic certainty.

A number of clinical scenarios require immediate directed testing. One is bilious vomiting in a neonate. In light of the high likelihood of a congenital gastrointestinal tract (GI) tract abnormality, an abdominal x-ray should be followed by an upper gastrointestinal contrast study. The findings may demonstrate the "double-bubble" appearance of duodenal atresia, or duodenal obstruction with right-sided bowel in malrotation with volvulus. Ultrasound can be useful to examine the pyloric channel in suspected hypertrophic pyloric stenosis, but many prefer the upper GI series as it also can provide information about the position of the ligament of Treitz, which is misplaced in malrotation. Although ultrasound also can be useful to diagnose intussusception, an air- or barium-contrast enema offers both diagnostic and therapeutic benefit because of its ability to reduce the intussusception back into the proximal bowel. In addition to the history and physical, computed tomography (CT) has gained popularity in the diagnosis of appendicitis. Endoscopy may be considered in cases of possible peptic ulcer disease or inflammatory bowel disease.

If the history supports it, expanded chemistry panels examining pancreatic enzymes such as lipase (pancreatitis) and liver enzymes (cholelithiasis, hepatitis) can be useful. Bacterial cultures of stool, throat, and urine obtained in the most sterile fashion possible can help differentiate infectious causes of vomiting. Patients with worrisome CNS symptoms (headache, diplopia) or signs (visual field deficits, cranial nerve deficits) should undergo neuroimaging. Magnetic resonance imaging (MRI) is more sensitive for posterior fossa masses, but CT may be more immediately useful as it is widely available and can detect hemorrhage with accuracy.

Monitoring of the patient's electrolytes is often useful in conjunction with the parameters of urine output and weight. Dehydration may lead to prerenal azotemia, acidosis, and serum electrolyte abnormalities. Certain classic electrolyte profiles exist. Pyloric stenosis often is associated with hypochloremic, hypokalemic metabolic alkalosis. Diabetic ketoacidosis will present with hyperglycemia, hyponatremia (because of elevated serum glucose), and metabolic acidosis. Inborn errors of metabolism should be expected when an elevated anion gap acidosis and hypoglycemia are present.

## MANAGEMENT

In general, therapy for vomiting revolves around the prevention and correction of dehydration and electrolyte abnormalities. Although not widely used in pediatrics, antiemetic agents may be helpful in certain situations. Although fluid and electrolyte therapy may be the *primary* treatment needed in some patients (e.g., viral gastroenteritis), the importance of such therapy may be considered secondary in a patient with, for example, a bowel obstruction caused by a midgut volvulus. In this case, management must focus on the etiology and the patient must be prepared for definitive surgery. Other examples of ameliorating vomiting by correcting the primary etiology include administering insulin to patients in diabetic ketoacidosis, providing a sustaining carbohydrate infusion (typically 10% dextrose at twice the maintenance rates) to reverse catabolism in children with inherited metabolic disorders, and instituting a gluten-free diet in a patient with celiac sprue.

Conservative therapy for vomiting consists of offering small amounts of liquid by mouth as soon as the child tolerates them. Many children exhibit a tendency to drink as much as possible because of thirst or the need for comfort. This is ill advised and generally leads to further episodes of vomiting. No defined period of bowel rest is mandated for a vomiting child. Parents should be encouraged to observe for the signs of dehydration and try to prevent their appearance. Oral electrolyte solutions (e.g., Pedialyte) are useful in infants, but older children only occasionally accept them because of their salty taste. These solutions provide a particular concentration of sodium and carbohydrate to facilitate cotransport and optimal water absorption across the intestinal brush border. In older children, a more practical fluid choice, although not perfect, may be diluted fruit juices or sports drinks. Fluids with high osmolalities may exacerbate diarrhea if it is concurrent.

If vomiting continues and the child becomes notably dehydrated, a more formal approach to oral rehydration or in some cases parenteral rehydration is necessary. Guidelines for oral rehydration are available through the Centers for Disease Control and Prevention. They consist of deficit replacement with 50 to 100 mL/kg of oral rehydration solution by mouth (given in small aliquots) over 3 to 4 h and an additional 2 to 4 oz (60 to 120 mL) by mouth per vomiting episode for children < 10 kg, with 4 to 8 oz (120 to 240 mL) by mouth administered to children ≥ 10 kg. Water must not be used, particularly for infants and young children, because of the risk of hyponatremia and seizures. Children may be placed back on a regular diet when they can tolerate it. The time to do this varies with the individual child, but most children will achieve this within 1 to 2 days after the vomiting has subsided.

Pharmacologic therapy for vomiting might include appropriate antibiotics for specific bacterial infections (e.g., streptococcal pharyngitis or urinary tract infection) or therapy for migraine. Multiple classes of antiemetic medications exist, and although they should be used with care because of the side effects, a brief description is in order.

As was mentioned above, vomiting is thought to be mediated via three pathways, each of which leads to stimulation of the vomiting center in the medulla. Given the specific neurotransmitters involved, drugs with antihistaminic, anticholinergic, or antiserotoninergic properties may aid in stopping vomiting. Antihistamines such as diphenhydramine (Benadryl) and hydroxyzine (Atarax) can be used in children. Dopamine antagonists such as prochlorperazine (Compazine) and promethazine (Phenergan) are also effective and are available in suppository form for children with complete intolerance to oral intake. Side effects include sedation and dystonia. Newer agents such as ondansetron (Zofran) and dolasetron (Anzemet) antagonize the action of serotonin at the 5HT3 receptor. These agents are costly but can be very effective in postoperative vomiting, vomiting induced by chemotherapy, and vomiting caused by severe gastrointestinal infections.

---

### "Don't Miss" Diagnoses of Vomiting

Newborn
  - Hypertrophic pyloric stenosis
  - Malrotation of the gastrointestinal tract (with midgut volvulus)
  - Incarcerated hernia
  - Hydrocephalus
  - Inborn errors of metabolism
  - Adrenal insufficiency
Older infants and toddlers
  - Intussusception
  - Appendicitis
  - Intracranial mass lesion
  - Inborn errors of metabolism
  - Poisoning
Older children
  - Streptococcal pharyngitis
  - Pancreatitis
  - Diabetic ketoacidosis
  - Acetaminophen poisoning
  - Testicular torsion and ovarian torsion
  - Pregnancy

---

## BIBLIOGRAPHY

Flake ZA, Scalley RD, Bailey AG. Practical selection of antiemetics. *Am Fam Phys* 69:1169, 2004.

*For Healthcare Providers: Guidelines for the Management of Acute Diarrhea.* Available at http://www.bt.cdc.gov/disasters/hurricanes/dguidelines.asp.

Stevens MW, Henretig FM. Vomiting. In Fleisher GR, Ludwig S, eds., *Textbook of Pediatric Emergency Medicine*, 4th ed. Philadelphia: Lippincott Williams & Wilkins, 2000: 625–633.

Tunnessen WW. *Signs and Symptoms in Pediatrics*. Philadelphia: Lippincott Williams & Wilkins, 1999.

Ulshen MH. Vomiting. In Hoekelman RA, ed., *Primary Pediatric Care*, 4th ed. St. Louis: Mosby, 2001: 1298.

# DIARRHEA

*Michael A. Barone*

## LEARNING OBJECTIVES

1. Describe the evaluation of children with diarrhea.
2. Using knowledge of the differential diagnosis, understand the necessary components of the medical history and physical examination in children with acute diarrhea or chronic diarrhea.
3. Understand the basic principles of the pathophysiology of diarrhea and be able to use them to guide any necessary diagnostic tests or use of therapies.

## INTRODUCTION

It is well known that diarrhea remains a leading cause of childhood morbidity and mortality throughout the world. This is due to the high burden of disease in developing countries, where diarrhea causes 3 million to 4 million deaths per year. In developed countries, the consequences of diarrhea are less severe, but nevertheless, the average child has two to three episodes of diarrhea per year, and in the United States and Canada, approximately 350 to 400 children per year die from diarrhea. The evaluation of acute and chronic diarrhea is common practice for any pediatrician. Therefore, an understanding of the specific types of diarrhea, their causes, and potential therapies is critical for those administering medical care to children.

Before considering the causes and potential treatments for diarrhea, one should consider whether the child in question has diarrhea at all. As the diet of children varies, so does the consistency and frequency of a normal stooling pattern. Parents are reassured when stools are well formed, come on schedule, and are easy to pass. This is unlikely to be the case on each day of a child's life. Changes of stool consistency to liquid generally cause greater concern to parents than do increases in the frequency of stooling. By definition, however, diarrhea refers to an abnormal daily stool volume, typically more than 10 mL/kg per day. Therefore, a single low-volume liquid stool per day cannot be considered diarrhea. However, a child may be considered to have diarrhea, despite stools being semiformed, if she or he is having numerous stools per day with significant fluid loss. From a practical perspective, most children with diarrhea have an increase in stool number and a decrease in stool consistency. Other characteristics of abnormal stool include the presence of blood or mucus.

This chapter considers the classification of different types of diarrhea, as well as the evaluation of various causes of acute and chronic diarrhea. In addition, although most cases of diarrhea in children are self-limited, the management of specific diarrheal syndromes is discussed.

## PATHOPHYSIOLOGY

An understanding of the pathophysiology of diarrhea requires knowledge about the role of the gastrointestinal (GI) tract in normal fluid homeostasis. Normal stool volume is approximately 5 mL/kg per day (5 g/kg per day). The fact that diarrhea is apparent when stool volumes exceed 10 mL/kg per day highlights the important role of the bowel in fluid absorption. The small bowel generally absorbs 90 percent of fluid intake, and although less fluid typically is absorbed in the large bowel, the colon maintains a reserve capacity for absorption that must be overcome for diarrhea to develop. Consider a normal infant ingesting 180 mL/kg per day, for example, a 4-kg infant drinking 90 mL of infant formula every 3 h (3 oz every 3 h). Assuming normal stools, the GI tract will absorb more than 170 mL/kg per day in this child, given its own intestinal secretion. Absorption of fluid occurs through water following osmotic gradients maintained across the GI tract. If the gradients are disturbed as a result of increased osmolality in the lumen, net water loss will occur. Such a perturbation may occur with the persistence of osmotically active substances in the lumen of the GI tract (e.g., malabsorption) or the active secretion of osmotically active substances into the lumen, as may occur in infection. This provides the basis for the most common types of diarrhea clinically seen: *osmotic diarrhea* and *secretory diarrhea*. Other types of diarrhea include that caused by *motility disorders* and that resulting from *inflammatory disease*.

Osmotic diarrhea is the most common type in children, and it generally is due to an infectious disease (e.g., rotavirus) that damages the villous absorption surface. Malabsorption of nutrients such as carbohydrates can present an osmotic load to the distal bowel, resulting in fluid efflux into the lumen. Osmotic diarrhea also may occur when hyperosmolar fluids (e.g., high-sugar-containing juices) are ingested in excess amounts, overwhelming the maximum carbohydrate absorption capacity of the child's GI tract.

The process of fluid loss through the active secretion of water and electrolytes into the intestinal lumen is the basis for secretory diarrhea. Secretory diarrhea should be suspected when diarrhea continues in a child *despite the interruption of feeding*. Diarrhea in cholera is classically of the secretory form. The effect of the enterotoxin on enterocytes leads to increased chloride secretion and impaired ability to reabsorb sodium. As a result, water is drawn into the GI tract, leading to stool fluid losses. Another example of secretory diarrhea is the rare but well-characterized congenital chloride diarrhea, in which there is a defect in $Cl^-/HCO_3^-$ exchange, thus impairing active chloride reabsorption from the lumen. Abnormal motility of the GI tract, as is seen in irritable bowel syndrome, also can cause diarrhea. Motility of the GI tract also may be increased in certain secretory and osmotic diarrheas. Finally, inflammatory disorders, either acute (infectious) or chronic (inflammatory bowel disease), may cause diarrhea as a result of water following the mucus, blood, and protein that are sloughed into the intestinal lumen.

## DIFFERENTIAL DIAGNOSIS

By definition, the term *chronic diarrhea* is used to describe diarrhea lasting more than 14 days. Among all patient populations, chronic diarrhea is most common in infants, the population most vulnerable to malnutrition if the ongoing diarrhea impairs the absorption of nutrients. The causes are numerous and include primary diseases of the bowel but also many systemic conditions. Table 22-1 lists common and uncommon causes of both acute diarrhea and chronic diarrhea. Although certain forms of diarrhea generally affect certain age groups, there is some overlap for neonates, infants, and toddlers.

## HISTORY

As with most illnesses in pediatrics, significant progress toward diagnosis can be made through a detailed medical history. First, it is useful to ask about the duration of the symptoms to help with the assessment of acute versus chronic diarrhea. Next, questions about the frequency and consistency of stool are important, noting any unusual features, such as blood or mucus. Recall that a child with one to two loose stools per day without other symptoms is unlikely to be losing enough fluid to be classified as having diarrhea. Noting the characteristics of onset is also helpful as chronic cases of diarrhea generally begin in a more indolent manner than do, for example, cases of acute infectious diarrhea. The presence of systemic features such as

*Table 22-1* **Differential Diagnosis of Diarrhea**

ACUTE DIARRHEA
  Infectious Causes
    Viral enteritis
      Rotaviruses, Norwalk agent, caliciviruses, enteric adenoviruses, astro-
      viruses, *Cytomegalovirus* (immunocompromised hosts), *Clostridium*
      *difficile*
    Bacterial enteritis
      *Salmonella, Shigella, Yersinia, Vibrio* spp., *Campylobacter, Escherichia coli,*
      *Staphylococcus aureus, Aeromonas*
    Parasitic enteritis
      *Cryptosporidium, Cyclospora, Entamoeba, Giardia, Isospora*
    Other bacterial infections: Urinary tract infection

  Gastrointestinal Causes
    Food allergy
    Overfeeding
    Starvation diarrhea
    Intussusception
    Malrotation with volvulus
    Appendicitis
    Constipation with overflow
    Lactose intolerance
    Necrotizing enterocolitis in neonates

  Miscellaneous Causes
    Antibiotic-associated diarrhea
    Laxative abuse

CHRONIC DIARRHEA
  See causes for acute diarrhea
  Gastrointestinal Causes
    Food allergy (e.g., cow's milk allergy)
    Toddler's diarrhea
    Disaccharidase deficiency (e.g., lactose intolerance)
    Short bowel syndrome (e.g., necrotizing enterocolitis)
    Microvillus syndrome
    Pancreatic insufficiency
      Cystic fibrosis
      Shwachman syndrome
    Celiac disease

*(continued)*

*Table 22-1* **Differential Diagnosis of Diarrhea (continued)**

Inflammatory bowel disease
   Crohn disease
   Ulcerative colitis
Overfeeding/dietary indiscretion
Congenital chloride diarrhea
Autoimmune enteropathy
Irritable bowel syndrome
Immunologic Causes
   Acquired immune deficiency syndrome
   Combined immunodeficiency (severe combined immunodeficiency)
   Ataxia telangiectasia
Endocrine Causes
   Hyperthyroidism
   Adrenal insufficiency (e.g., Addison disease)
Neoplastic Causes
   Neuroblastoma
   Pheochromocytoma
   Vasoactive intestinal peptide–secreting tumor
Various Causes
   Laxative abuse
   Chronic antibiotic use (e.g., *Clostridium difficile* toxin)
   Dysautonomia syndromes (e.g., Riley-Day syndrome)

fever suggests infection; therefore, it is useful to know if the patient's illness is isolated or simultaneous with illness in playmates and family members. In this regard, a dietary record or history is also important to assess possible ingestion of contaminated foods (e.g., undercooked meat, raw eggs).

Since a child's nutritional status hinges on the absorption of nutrients, questions about recent weight loss or frank failure to thrive are important for both acute (e.g., rehydration need) and chronic (e.g., evaluation and treatment of malabsorption syndrome) purposes. Other systemic illnesses also should be discussed. For example, has there also been recurrent pulmonary disease or wheezing (e.g., cystic fibrosis)? Has there been a history of reported infections (e.g., immunodeficiency state or Shwachman syndrome)? Have there been common rashes such as eczema (food allergy) or uncommon rashes such as pyoderma gangrenosum (inflammatory bowel disease)? Other useful lines of questioning include the following:

- Dietary history, including intolerances (lactose) and allergic manifestations (such as hives) to certain foods.

- Is there excessive intake of hyperosmolar fluids such as soda or fruit juice?
- Does the diarrhea subside when the child's diet is interrupted? (secretory versus osmotic diarrhea)?
- Does the child attend a day-care center where epidemics of infectious gastroenteritis are common?
- Has there been recent antibiotic use for an unrelated reason (e.g., otitis media)?
- Has there been recent travel to areas with a potentially contaminated water supply?
- Are there "pets" living in the home? Some domestic animals may transmit bacteria such as *Campylobacter*; reptiles are a well-known reservoir for *Salmonella*.

Children with viral enteritis often have fever and preceding or concurrent vomiting (viral gastroenteritis). The presence of blood in the stool should suggest invasive bacterial or parasitic infection, but the absence of visible blood in the stool does not exclude such infections. Children with cow's milk allergy may pass occult or frank blood in the stool. Typically, these children represent a small percentage (5 percent) of infants fed cow's milk protein–based formula, but this also may occur in a nursing infant as a result of the transmission of antigenic proteins through breast milk. Whereas the former case would respond to a change in the infant formula protein (e.g., from cow's milk protein to soy protein or an elemental formula), the latter case may respond to a more restricted maternal diet with the mother removing the suspected offending protein.

The entity of "toddler's diarrhea" is worthy of special mention. This condition, which may be referred to as chronic nonspecific diarrhea of childhood or irritable colon syndrome, demonstrates a typical pattern of a thriving infant or toddler passing numerous foul-smelling, nonbloody stools while awake. The stools are watery and may contain undigested food particles, particularly vegetables. This should be distinguished from diarrhea simply resulting from increased GI lumen osmolality in a child with excessive ingestion of sugary juices or sodas, although there may be some overlap clinically. Clearly, removing any offending dietary habits would be the first step in management. Children with true chronic nonspecific diarrhea of childhood seem to have increased GI motility, and this may be the primary source of the problem. Many experts agree that this disorder is a variant of irritable bowel syndrome in adults.

Severe constipation also may present as diarrhea. In children with fecal retention, stool impaction may develop with the presence of liquid feces proximal to the impaction. Leakage of stool into the pants or diapers may be the presenting symptom that is interpreted as diarrhea by the parents. Here a careful history is paramount, noting that the problems began with constipation. The physical examination of the abdomen and rectum also can be diagnostic.

Immunodeficiencies should not be overlooked as a cause of diarrhea. Acquired immunodeficiencies such as human immunodeficiency virus (HIV) infection should be a concern in any child with prolonged diarrhea. As a result, questions about maternal HIV risk factors or questions investigating possible postnatal HIV exposure in the child (breast-feeding) should be asked. The many disorders that constitute severe combined immunodeficiency may cause diarrhea as a result of chronic viral infection. Questions regarding a history of chronic thrush, a rash that is not resolving, jaundice, or pulmonary disease should be considered.

## PHYSICAL EXAMINATION

As in the examination of a child with vomiting, a careful, thorough examination is a must in a child with diarrhea. Many of the conditions listed above have primary or secondary findings that may not be appreciated on an abdominal examination alone. A general assessment is important as it can help differentiate a well child (toddler's diarrhea) from an ill child (malabsorption or dehydration). Abnormal vital signs may suggest dehydration (tachycardia) or infection (fever). Tachypnea may be seen in a child compensating for the metabolic acidosis that results from dehydration and ketosis. Although low blood pressure is not a sensitive sign of dehydration in a child, the presence of hypertension may be suggestive of hyperthyroidism, pheochromocytoma, or dysautonomia.

The assessment of growth parameters is critical. Acute weight loss may be expected because of dehydration, but a decrease in growth velocity over time or growth parameters that suggest malnutrition should lead one to consider malabsorption syndromes or other serious systemic diseases. As was mentioned above, rashes may be a clue to food allergy, inflammatory bowel disease, or immunodeficiency. They also may be seen, however, in ubiquitous GI viral infections.

In the consideration of infectious causes of diarrhea, a few syndromes merit mention. Many types of *Escherichia coli* can cause diarrhea; they include Shiga toxin–producing *E. coli* (STEC), enterotoxigenic *E. coli* (ETEC), enterononinvasive *E. coli* (EIEC), and enteropathogenic *E. coli* (EPEC). Clinical infection with STEC (the most common serotype is O157:H7) may cause bloody diarrhea with progression to the hemolytic-uremic syndrome (HUS) in about 5 to 10 percent of patients. Therefore, features of uremia (edema, hypertension), hemolytic anemia (tachycardia, jaundice), and thrombocytopenia (bruising, bleeding) should be assessed carefully in the physical examination.

Infections with *Salmonella* organisms are also capable of manifesting in many ways. These infections include gastroenteritis, septicemia with or without suppurative sequelae, and fever syndromes such as enteric fever/typhoid fever. Typhoid fever is characterized by unrelenting fever, hepatosplenomegaly, abdominal pain, headache, and the presence of either diarrhea or constipation. Two other features, although uncommon, are worthy of a careful look in the physical examination: (1) the presence of relative bradycardia despite fever and dehydration and (2) a discrete salmon-red rash (rose spots) over the trunk.

Gastrointestinal or systemic causes of chronic diarrhea also may have notable features on physical examination. For example, patients with cystic fibrosis may have evidence of pulmonary disease (chronic cough, wheezing). Patients with inflammatory disease may present with arthritis or growth failure. In Crohn disease, the presence of mouth ulcers or perirectal skin tags can often provide insights into the diagnosis.

## LABORATORY AND RADIOLOGIC EVALUATION

Most children with acute infectious gastroenteritis require no laboratory tests unless there is concern about complications such as dehydration. Among the many potential viral etiologies for infectious diarrhea, few specific tests exist outside research laboratories. Furthermore, one must consider their utility in a particular patient's case. Would knowing that a 15-month-old child's diarrhea was due to rotavirus change the management? In some cases, the answer may be yes if one is concerned about community epidemiology or hospital infection control. Alas, in many cases, the answer is no. Nevertheless, commercially available rapid diagnostic tests exist for rotaviruses, enteric adenoviruses, and astroviruses. These tests typically use enzyme immunoassay or direct fluorescent antibody techniques.

Diagnostic evaluation for bacterial pathogens consists of specific and nonspecific testing. Nonspecific testing includes examination of the stool for red blood cells and/or white blood cells. Examination for white blood cells, done either by microscopy or by stool lactoferrin assay, can help assess the presence of an invasive or toxin-producing organism. Beyond these two rapid tests, stool cultures generally are performed if indicated. Because of the burden of normal, nonpathogenic bacteria in stool samples, the detection of stool pathogens is a time-consuming and labor-intensive process. The clinician should not expect full results in 24 h. As each laboratory is different, one should be aware of which organisms may be isolated in his or her laboratory's "routine" culture. If there is a clinical concern for a less common organism such as *Vibrio* ssp., *Yersinia,* or *E. coli* O157:H7, a call should be placed to the laboratory to alert the personnel, and special media can be used.

Studies for parasitic infection of the GI tract include microscopic examination for ova and parasites as well as antigen studies such as those available for *Giardia lamblia* and *Cryptosporidium parvum*. Although antigen detection is more sensitive, it should be noted that when parasitic infection is suspected, more than a single stool specimen is warranted. For example, it is recommended that at least three stool specimens be submitted for microscopic examination (ova and parasite examination) when there is clinical suspicion for *Giardia*.

There are various other tests to discover the etiology of chronic diarrhea, including antibody tests in the case of celiac disease (antitissue transglutaminase) or acquired immune deficiency syndrome (HIV-1/HIV-2 antibody). Other disorders may require the involvement of a gastroenterologist to allow for a tissue diagnosis. Endoscopy is done in virtually every case for the diagnosis of inflammatory bowel disease, microvillus syndromes, and autoimmune enteropathies.

## MANAGEMENT

As the causes of acute and chronic diarrhea are so vast, definitive management of the other disorders mentioned above is beyond the scope of this chapter. Most children, however, recover spontaneously from diarrhea and require only simple supportive measures for care.

With increased fluid losses from the stool, the concern for dehydration looms. In a child who is not vomiting, the parents should be encouraged to increase the child's intake to keep pace with the losses. Ample urine output throughout the day is a good measure of success. With avoidance of fatty foods and high concentrations of sugars (juices), a regular diet should be offered. This would include infant formula or breast milk in an infant and an age-appropriate diet for an older child. There is often a concern about transient lactose intolerance resulting from diarrhea. These concerns are overstated, as most infants and children digest lactose sufficiently after diarrheal illness. Obviously, one should consider lactose intolerance if stools increase in frequency and volume when lactose is ingested.

For children whose vomiting impairs oral intake or for children becoming dehydrated from diarrhea alone, one should consider the use of an oral electrolyte solution. The goal of such therapy is to enhance fluid absorption by utilizing glucose-sodium cotransport. It should be noted that there is no reason for children to be on clear fluids alone or bowel rest if they are able to maintain their hydration status during diarrhea. Well-designed oral rehydration solutions (ORSs) such as Pedialyte (formulated for maintenance water and electrolyte needs), Rehydralyte, and World Health Organization (WHO) solution (both formulated for rehydration water and electrolyte needs) will serve to treat a child with diarrhea better than will fruit juices, fruit drinks, or commercially available sports drinks (e.g., Gatorade). Sports drinks tend to have higher sugar contents than ORSs, leading to increased osmolality in the lumen and subsequent GI losses. If a child refuses an ORS, he or she may not be substantially dehydrated. However, from a practical perspective, it is better to have the child ingest a sports drink than a juice drink loaded with high-fructose corn syrup.

A summary of recommendations for ORS in the dehydrated patient is as follows:

| | |
|---|---|
| No dehydration | 4–8 oz (120–240 mL) of ORS per watery stool. Continue regular diet. |
| Mild dehydration (3–5 percent) | 40–60 mL/kg of ORS over 4 h along with stool replacement (120–240 mL ORS/stool) and regular diet. |
| Moderate dehydration (6–9 percent) | 80–100 mL/kg of ORS over 4 h along with stool replacement (120–240 mL ORS/stool) and regular diet. |
| Severe dehydration (≥10 percent) | Child should be considered candidate for parenteral rehydration. |

Although it might seem logical that all bacterial infections of the GI tract require antibiotic treatment, that is not the case. Infections with *Campylobacter* and *Salmonella* frequently resolve without antibiotics, and their treatment typically is not recommended in normal hosts. Some *Salmonella* infections, such as those in neonates, infants, immunocompromised patients, and those with sickle cell disease, do require treatment. Although infections with *Shigella* can be self-limited as well, patients with gastroenteritis caused by this organism generally should be treated with antibiotics; trimethoprim-sulfamethoxazole is the drug of choice, but local resistance patterns should be considered. There is ongoing debate and investigation about whether treating diarrhea caused by *E. coli* O157:H7 increases the risk of the hemolytic-uremic syndrome.

Antidiarrheal medications should be avoided in general. Anticholinergics and opiates that slow down GI motility can lead to overgrowth of organisms and prolonged presence of toxins in the gut. This may have detrimental consequences for the child. Other medications that absorb water or have antisecretory effects (Kaopectate, Pepto Bismol) may give the impression that diarrhea is resolving and hence lead to less judicious fluid replacement by caregivers.

Dietary adjuncts to diarrhea treatment include a regular diet as discussed above. Dietary substrates have been shown to enhance the regeneration of enterocytes. Diets higher in fiber, low in total daily fluid, and void of fruit juices can be helpful in cases of chronic nonspecific diarrhea. Increasing fat content in the diet also may be helpful in this case. Finally, the use of probiotics deserves special mention. *Lactobacillus* species and other probiotics, which are available in cultured foods or as a single agent, have wide acceptance in the practicing pediatric community for the treatment of both acute and chronic diarrhea. The recommendation occurs most often in the setting of acute gastroenteritis or antibiotic-associated diarrhea. Recent data show small but significant benefits in these settings in terms of reduced frequency of stooling and reduced duration of illness.

As with many pediatric illnesses, the best therapy is prevention. The promotion of breast-feeding and instruction of all patients and families in good hygiene practices could reduce the burden of diarrhea significantly. Day-care centers should strictly follow policies to prevent transmission of stool pathogens. Currently, no vaccines routinely aimed at diarrheal illness are given in the United States. In 1998 and 1999, a rotavirus vaccine was recommended as part of the routine U.S. immunization schedule. Because of an increased number of cases of intussusception in vaccine recipients, that recommendation was retracted. Ongoing investigation continues in rotavirus vaccinology as the potential for decreased morbidity and mortality is enormous considering the burden of disease in the developing world.

---

### *"Don't Miss" Diagnoses of Diarrhea*

Acute Diarrhea
- Shiga toxin producing *Escherichia coli* diarrhea (e.g., O157:H7)
- *Shigella* enteritis
- Giardiasis
- *Clostridium difficile* toxin pseudomembranous colitis
- Urinary tract infection
- Intussusception
- Constipation with overflow

Chronic Diarrhea
- Cystic fibrosis (pancreatic insufficiency)
- Celiac disease
- Inflammatory bowel disease
- Immunodeficiency states (AIDS, severe combined immunodeficiency)
- Laxative abuse
- Pheochromocytoma or vasoactive intestinal peptide–secreting tumor

---

## BIBLIOGRAPHY

Berman J. Heading off the dangers of acute gastroenteritis. *Contemp Pediatr* 20(7):57–76, 2003.

Fleisher GR. Diarrhea. In Fleisher GR, Ludwig S, eds., *Textbook of Pediatric Emergency Medicine,* 4th ed. Philadelphia: Lippincott Williams & Wilkins, 2000: 203–207.

*For Healthcare Providers: Guidelines for the Management of Acute Diarrhea.* Available at http://www.bt.cdc.gov/disasters/hurricanes/dguidelines.asp.

Ghishan FK. Chronic diarrhea. In Behrman RE, Kliegman RM, Jenson HB, eds., *Nelson Textbook of Pediatrics,* 17th ed. Philadelphia: Saunders, 2004: 1276–1281.

Lasche J, Duggan C. Managing acute diarrhea: What every pediatrician needs to know. *Contemp Pediatr* 16(2):74–83, 1999.

Pickering LK, Snyder JD. Gastroenteritis. In Behrman RE, Kliegman RM, Jenson HB, eds., *Nelson Textbook of Pediatrics,* 17th ed. Philadelphia: Saunders, 2004: 1272–1276.

Ulshen MH. Diarrhea and steatorrhea. In Hoekelman RA, Adam HM, Nelson NM, et al, eds., *Primary Pediatric Care,* 4th ed. St. Louis: Mosby, 2001: 1020–1033.

Vanderhoof JA. Chronic diarrhea. *Pediatr Rev* 19(12):418–422, 1998.

# RASH

## M. Robin English

⚬ LEARNING OBJECTIVES

1. Understand the importance of identifying rashes on the basis of the type of skin lesion and the time course.

2. Understand the underlying etiology and/or pathophysiology for rashes caused by infectious diseases, inflammatory conditions, and hypersensitivity reactions.

3. Know the appropriate initial workup and management for rashes caused by infectious diseases, inflammatory conditions, and hypersensitivity reactions.

## INTRODUCTION

Identifying rashes in the pediatric and adolescent population can be a challenging task. Rash is a feature of many different types of pediatric diseases, from infection to allergy, and so it is one of the most common chief complaints a pediatrician encounters. Many rashes seen in children are relatively benign in nature and do not herald a serious underlying disease. However, a few rashes are important to recognize immediately, as they represent the visible evidence of a severe infection or inflammatory condition.

It often seems that experienced pediatricians or dermatologists can merely look at a rash and make an immediate diagnosis on the basis of a "gestalt" impression: "I've seen this before." However, these clinicians actually take a focused history and recognize patterns and types of lesions; this enables them to make the diagnosis quickly and accurately. This chapter discusses the importance of the history and physical examination in helping an examiner take this systematic approach. It is beyond the scope of the chapter to include all diseases or entities that may present with a rash, but several common pediatric dermatologic conditions, including their diagnosis and management, are reviewed.

## HISTORY

As with all complaints, the history one obtains from a patient with a rash is instrumental in developing a differential diagnosis. One of the most important aspects is the timing of the rash. Rashes of acute onset often have either infectious or allergic etiologies. Chronic rashes may be due to inflammatory or allergic causes. Patients or parents should be asked when the rash started and whether it has maintained the same appearance or changed in any way. The location of the rash at its onset and the manner in which it has spread to other parts of the body may provide important clues to the etiology. If the parents have given medications for the rash, such as topical creams or antihistamines, the improvement or worsening of the rash with such therapy should be noted. The quality and severity of the rash, including pruritus and pain, are important. Associated symptoms such as upper respiratory symptoms, fever, joint pain, vomiting, abdominal pain, and general activity should be explored as well.

The history for a patient with rash also should include any administration of medications in the last few weeks. Some rashes, such as erythema multiforme, may occur in response to medication taken weeks earlier, whereas others may be caused by an acute allergic reaction to a drug taken recently. Other exposures the child may have had, including new foods, new detergents, and plant contact such as poison ivy, should be elicited. Adolescents should be asked to give a sexual history independently from their parents, as disseminated gonorrhea, syphilis, and human immunodeficiency virus infections all can present with rashes. Chronic or frequent illnesses are important, and a family history of dermatologic or rheumatologic conditions should be obtained. As usual, a thorough review of systems may help identify additional signs and symptoms.

## PHYSICAL EXAMINATION

The most effective way to use physical examination findings to develop a differential diagnosis for rash is to characterize the types and patterns of the skin lesions seen. Lesions can be differentiated into primary lesions, which usually are seen first and are often most representative of the rash, and secondary lesions, which occur later and represent changes to the primary lesions (Tables 23-1 and 23-2).

Dermatologic diseases often contain more than one type of lesion and can be classified accordingly. For example, the papulosquamous disorders are

*Table 23-1* **Descriptions and Examples of Primary Skin Lesions**

| Lesion | Description | Conditions |
| --- | --- | --- |
| Macule | Flat, circumscribed, any size, blanching | Viral exanthem, tinea versicolor, drug reaction |
| Papule | Raised, < 1 cm, solid, circumscribed | Viral exanthem, scarlet fever, drug reaction, molluscum contagiosum |
| Nodule | Raised, 0.5–2 cm, solid, may be deep | Erythema nodosum, rheumatic fever |
| Plaque | Raised, flat-topped, > 1 cm | Atopic dermatitis, pityriasis rosea, tinea corporis |
| Vesicle | Raised, fluid-filled, < 0.5 cm, circumscribed | Herpes infection, varicella, contact dermatitis |
| Bulla | Raised, fluid-filled, > 0.5 cm, circumscribed, tense or flaccid | Bullous impetigo, epidermolysis bullosa |
| Wheal | Raised, circumscribed edema, evanescent, pink | Urticaria, insect bites, erythema multiforme |
| Pustule | Raised, pus-filled (bacterial or sterile), yellowish | Impetigo, psoriasis, pustular acne |
| Petechia | Flat, nonblanching, < 2 mm, red to purple | Meningococcemia, viral exanthem, bleeding disorder |
| Purpura | Flat, nonblanching, 2 mm–1 cm, red to purple | Meningococcemia, bleeding disorder, Henoch-Schönlein purpura |

those which present with raised, scaling lesions (e.g., pityriasis rosea, psoriasis). Vesiculopustular disorders include scabies, herpes infections, and impetigo. Maculopapular eruptions, which contain both macules (flat lesions) and papules (raised lesions), are typical of viral exanthems. The pattern of the skin lesions is also important. Lesions may be confluent or discrete, linear or annular (ring-shaped), monomorphic or polymorphic. The color of the lesions should be noted. The distribution of the lesions on the child's body gives a clue to the etiology as well. Some diseases have a predilection for certain areas, for example, the flexural surfaces or the palms and soles. Gloves always should be worn when examining a rash.

A thorough general examination is as important in determining the etiology of a rash as is the description of the rash itself. The child's general appearance can provide a good deal of information. An ill-appearing febrile child should alert the clinician to the possibility of a serious infection or severe hypersensitivity reaction as a cause for the rash. A child who is play-

Table 23-2 *Descriptions and Examples of Secondary Skin Lesions*

| Lesion | Description | Conditions |
|---|---|---|
| Excoriation | Abraded loss of skin, usually secondary to self-induced trauma | Atopic dermatitis, scabies, contact dermatitis, varicella |
| Crusting | Dried secretions, overlying primary lesions, e.g., pus, serum | Impetigo, varicella, atopic dermatitis, contact dermatitis |
| Scaling | Accumulated desquamation; may be flaky or greasy or thick | Pityriasis rosea, tinea corporis, seborrheic dermatitis, psoriasis |
| Fissure | Linear crack in skin | Atopic dermatitis |

ful and well-appearing probably does not have a serious infectious etiology regardless of the severity of the rash. Many infectious and rheumatologic conditions present with rashes and joint findings, and so a complete joint examination is indicated. In addition, signs such as edema, abdominal tenderness, heart murmur, or eye abnormalities may signal an underlying rheumatologic condition. Rheumatologic conditions that present with rash are discussed in Chap. 38.

## DIFFERENTIAL DIAGNOSIS

### INFECTIONS
### Viral

#### Generalized Viral Exanthem

Rashes are seen commonly in many viral infections. In many cases, the identification of the virus is not possible, but the appearance and course of the rash, in association with other disease features, make the diagnosis of nonspecific viral exanthem the most likely. The history often reveals fever, upper respiratory symptoms, vomiting, diarrhea, or cough. These children are typically well-appearing on examination. The rash is generalized and may be represented by any primary lesion, including maculopapules, petechiae, urticaria, or purpura. The differential diagnosis for these children should include the etiologies mentioned below because the rashes can be similar. No specific diagnostic test is required, and no treatment is needed. The prognosis is excellent, with most exanthems resolving within a few days. Some rash-causing viruses, such as measles and rubella, are seen rarely in the United States today because of widespread immunization practices.

### Roseola Infantum

One virus that produces a fairly specific set of symptoms is roseola, which is caused by human herpesvirus 6. The illness begins with 3 or 4 days of high, spiking fevers that may be accompanied by febrile seizures. The rash typically is not present during this time. Once the febrile period is over, the rash, which is characterized by generalized erythematous macu-lopapules, develops. This is different from many viral exanthems in which the fever and rash are present simultaneously. Most of these children are well-appearing with an otherwise normal examination. Roseola requires no test for diagnosis and no treatment.

### Erythema Infectiosum

Erythema infectiosum, or fifth disease, is another viral exanthem that can present with distinct features. The virus implicated in this disease is par-vovirus B19. As with roseola, an illness characterized by fever, myalgia, and malaise often precedes the rash by approximately 7 days. These children are generally well-appearing on examination. The initial cutaneous mani-festation is known as the "slapped cheek" appearance, in which the child's cheeks become intensely erythematous. Later cutaneous manifesta-tions include generalized erythema and a lacy, reticular rash over the extremities. If the diagnosis is in question, an elevated parvovirus B19-specific immunoglobulin M (IgM) antibody can confirm it, but this test requires several days and is usually unnecessary. No treatment is required, although care should be taken to decrease exposure to pregnant women and children with hemolytic disease, because of the risk of fetal hydrops and aplastic crisis in those groups, respectively. However, children are conta-gious before the onset of the rash, during which time the disease may not be suspected because of its similarity to other nonspecific viral illnesses.

### Herpes Simplex Virus

There are many manifestations of herpes simplex infections in children, but the most common is gingivostomatitis. These children usually present with fever, irritability, and decreased ability to take oral fluids. On physical examination, they may be ill-appearing and dehydrated. The typical enan-them (mucous membrane eruption) is vesicles or ulcers on erythematous bases on the lips, gingiva, and tongue. Treatment includes hydration and pain management. In healthy children, a few studies have shown more rapid improvement of symptoms with systemic acyclovir therapy. Herpesvirus can affect other parts of the skin as well, such as the genital area and areas affected by atopic dermatitis. Typical lesions are vesicles and ulcers on ery-thematous bases. Treatment with acyclovir should be initiated early in these cases to achieve the best results.

### Varicella Zoster Virus

Varicella zoster virus is the etiologic agent for chickenpox, a disease not commonly seen by pediatricians today because of a safe and effective vaccine that became available in 1995. However, it is important to keep the disease in mind and be able to recognize it. Affected children typically present with a prodromal phase, as in many other viruses, of fever, malaise, and headache. They may appear ill on examination. The rash is characterized by many types of lesions, including macules, papules, and vesicles. The presence of all lesions is pathognomonic of the disease (Fig. 23-1). Usually a clinical diagnosis can be made without laboratory testing. Treatment is supportive, including hydration, antipyretics, and antipruritus medications. Older children, immunocompromised children, and those with serious internal complications should be treated with acyclovir.

## BACTERIAL

### Cellulitis

Cellulitis is defined as an acute bacterial infection of the skin and soft tissue. The organisms most commonly responsible are *Streptococcus pyogenes* (group A streptococci) and *Staphylococcus aureus*, but *Strep. pneumoniae* and

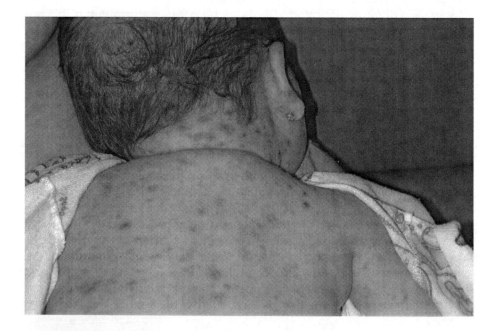

*Figure 23-1* **Varicella.**

*Haemophilus influenzae* also can be causes. In cases of facial cellulitis, infection with anaerobes must be considered strongly.

Affected patients typically present with the acute onset of redness, pain, and swelling of the skin, often after an insect bite or other trauma to the skin. Fever may be present, especially if the organism has spread to the blood or underlying tissues. If systemic infection is present, the child may appear ill on examination; otherwise the child is generally well-appearing. The affected area is tender, warm, edematous, and very erythematous. The quality of the edema may help distinguish cellulitis from an allergic reaction: Cellulitis causes firmness and induration, whereas allergic reactions cause boggy edema. When cellulitis is diagnosed, it is helpful to measure the size of the erythema to help determine improvement or worsening with treatment.

To make an accurate bacteriologic diagnosis, one may aspirate the leading edge of the erythema for a culture. However, many physicians advocate starting antibiotics against group A streptococci and *S. aureus* without getting a culture unless no clinical improvement is noted. If methicillin-resistant *S. aureus* (MRSA) is prevalent in the community, this should be taken into consideration in prescribing antistaphylococcal coverage. Many cases improve within 1 to 2 days after starting appropriate antibiotics, but some infections become more suppurative and form an abscess under the skin. This occurs commonly and must be treated with incision and drainage, at which time a culture of the material can be obtained to identify the pathogen.

### Impetigo

Impetigo (known to some as "Indian fire") is a superficial bacterial infection of the skin. It is caused most commonly by *Strep. pyogenes* and *S. aureus*. The onset is acute, and lesions may be found anywhere on the body; it is common to see them around the mouth and nose. The lesions start as small erythematous macules that become pustules, vesicles, or bullae within several days. These lesions rupture easily, causing the oozing of yellow fluid, which crusts (commonly honey-colored crusts). Pustules and vesicles are caused more commonly by *Streptococcus* species, and bullae are seen more commonly with *S. aureus* infections (Fig. 23-2). Children with impetigo are generally well-appearing.

The treatment of impetigo can be oral or topical. Topical mupirocin has been shown to be as effective for resolution of lesions as oral antibiotics. As with cellulitis, if MRSA is a common pathogen in the community, oral antibiotics against this organism should be initiated. It is important to remember that some strains of streptococci are nephritogenic and cause poststreptococcal glomerulonephritis after the infection has resolved, regardless of antibiotic use.

### Scarlet Fever

Scarlet fever is seen most commonly in school-age children. It is caused by infection with *Strep. pyogenes*. Patients usually present with the acute

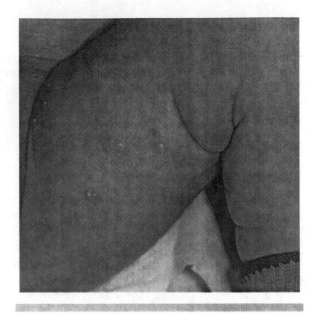

*Figure 23-2* **Bullous impetigo.**

onset of sore throat, vomiting, headache, fever, and rash. Infected children may be ill-appearing on examination. Examination of the mouth reveals a strawberry tongue, palatal petechiae, and erythematous tonsils. Circumoral pallor is a common finding. The rash is maculopapular and typically begins on the torso, spreading later to involve the entire body. The rash has a few distinct characteristics: a rough, sandpaper quality and an accentuation in the body creases, which are known as Pastia's lines.

The diagnosis can be confirmed with a throat culture, which usually shows growth of the organism. Treatment of scarlet fever is similar to treatment of streptococcal pharyngitis without rash and includes an oral course of antibiotics (penicillin or erythromycin) or intramuscular penicillin. Rheumatic fever, which occurs as a poststreptococcal sequela, can be prevented with an adequate course of antibiotics. Children with scarlet fever generally have an excellent prognosis.

### Meningococcemia

Meningococcemia occurs as a result of invasive infection with *Neisseria meningitidis*. The rash often is preceded by a flulike illness characterized by fever, malaise, and chills. Once the initial lesions of the rash are present, they can disseminate quite rapidly. Affected children may be ill-appearing at presentation or may look relatively well initially, deteriorating over the course of the evaluation. Shock is common. Macules may be present initially, but the classic lesions of meningococcemia are petechiae, purpura, and ecchymoses.

The diagnosis is confirmed by blood culture or by Gram stain of a skin lesion, which reveals gram-negative diplococci. Ideally, cerebrospinal fluid also should be evaluated for culture of the organism, but many children with meningococcemia are too unstable to undergo an invasive procedure such as lumbar puncture. Treatment with intravenous fluids and intravenous antibiotics should be initiated as soon as the diagnosis is suspected. Appropriate antibiotics include penicillin and ceftriaxone; 7 days is usually an adequate course. Survivors of meningococcemia often show sequelae of the disease, which include gangrene and subsequent amputation of digits or limbs.

## Fungal

### Monilial Infections

The two most common manifestations of moniliasis, or candidiasis, in the pediatric population are oral thrush and candidal diaper dermatitis. *Candida albicans* is the most common species to cause these two entities. Oral thrush is seen frequently in neonates and infants, but its presence after 1 year of age in the absence of antibiotic administration should raise the suspicion of an underlying immunodeficiency. The history is usually unremarkable, although some parents report decreased feeding. The physical examination reveals a well-appearing infant with whitish gray plaques on the tongue, buccal mucosa, and gingiva. These plaques are not easily removed by gentle scraping with a tongue blade, distinguishing them from residual milk. The diagnosis can be confirmed by performing a potassium hydroxide stain on a scraping, but most pediatricians prefer to initiate therapy on the basis of their clinical suspicion. The therapy used most is oral nystatin solution, which should be applied four times a day, and treatment should be continued for several days after the disappearance of the lesions.

Candidal diaper dermatitis occurs when irritant diaper dermatitis becomes secondarily infected with *C. albicans*. The physical examination reveals very erythematous patches with scaling and surrounding erythematous papules known as satellite lesions. This eruption does not spare the inguinal folds, and this helps distinguish it from simple irritant diaper dermatitis. A potassium hydroxide preparation confirms the diagnosis. Treatment involves application of topical antifungal ointment: Nystatin is used commonly. Treatment should be continued for a week after the rash has resolved, and parents should be counseled to continue their usual regimen of frequent diaper changes and barrier creams.

### Tineal Infections

The two most common dermatophytoses seen in pediatrics are tinea capitis and tinea corporis. Tinea capitis is a superficial fungal infection of the scalp, and it is caused most commonly by *Trichophyton tonsurans*. Less common causes include *Microsporum* spp. and other *Trichophyton* spp. The history may reveal exposure to another child with tinea capitis. There may be hair loss in the affected area, which also may be pruritic. The physical examination reveals a discrete area of alopecia with broken-off hairs, the so-called black dot sign. Scaling usually is noted as well. Occasionally, a local inflammatory response known as a kerion occurs, causing a boggy mass either surrounding or underneath the alopecia. Occipital or posterior cervical lymphadenopathy is common. The diagnosis can be confirmed with a potassium hydroxide stain or a culture. Treatment is an 8-week course of oral griseofulvin, which should be given with fatty foods to increase absorption. Topical antifungal creams are ineffective. Steroids can be used if a kerion is present, although some kerions resolve with griseofulvin alone.

Tinea corporis is a superficial fungal infection of the skin and is known commonly as ringworm. *Trichophyton* spp. are most commonly implicated. The lesion is generally circular and raised, with a scaly or pustular border. Erythema of the lesion may be present. As with tinea capitis, the diagnosis is made with a potassium hydroxide preparation of the scraping or with a fungal culture. Treatment involves administration of an antifungal cream. Corticosteroid creams should be avoided.

### Scabies

Scabies is caused by infection with the mite *Sarcoptes scabiei*, which is transmitted through close personal contact. The history includes intense pruritus and often reveals other family members with similar symptoms. Infants, who may be unable to communicate pruritus, frequently present with irritability. The rash in older children is seen most commonly in the folds of the skin, between fingers and toes, and along the waistline. Infants often have lesions on the hands, feet, and head. Typical lesions are pustules, papules, and sometimes vesicles. A very specific lesion that is seen is a serpiginous burrow, which represents the track of the adult female mite, but this is not always seen in children. To diagnose scabies, a scraping of a lesion collected with mineral oil should be examined microscopically. The mite can be seen easily in most cases. The treatment of choice in children and adolescents is permethrin cream, which should be applied neck to toe in older children and head to toe in infants. The cream is left on overnight and rinsed off 8 to 14 h later. All family members should be treated simultaneously. Bedding, clothing, and towels should be washed in hot water.

## INFLAMMATORY CONDITIONS

### ATOPIC DERMATITIS

Atopic dermatitis is a chronic inflammatory skin condition that affects up to 15 percent of the pediatric and adolescent population. Much research is being conducted to elucidate fully the immunopathogenesis of this disease. Essentially, the introduction of antigen to the skin evokes a complicated inflammatory cascade that involves interleukins and leukocytes. Atopic dermatitis can present as early as 3 months of age, and many children outgrow the condition by preschool age. The majority of affected children have a positive history of another allergic disease, such as asthma or allergic rhinitis, and a family history of atopy is very common. Other features of the history may include chronic itching or discomfort and exacerbations with weather changes or periods of stress. Food allergies have been implicated as a trigger, but actually only a minority of cases are truly exacerbated by foods. Children or parents should be asked about chronic rhinitis, cough, or wheezing.

The physical examination of children with atopic dermatitis differs by age. Infantile atopic dermatitis is seen more commonly on the face and neck, and the lesions include erythematous papules and vesicles, often with crust formation. The diaper area usually is spared, possibly because of chronic moisture. The extensor surfaces of the arms and legs often are involved. In older children and adolescents, the distribution changes to include the flexural surfaces, especially the popliteal and antecubital fossae. Lichenification with erythematous plaque formation is typical as a result of the chronic drying of the skin. Keratosis pilaris—cornified plugs in the hair follicles—is seen commonly in older children with severe atopic dermatitis as well. The physical examination also should include a thorough lung examination and evaluation for other atopic stigmata, such as allergic facies.

The treatment of atopic dermatitis is complicated, and parental education is extremely important. The keys to successful management are moisture and controlling inflammation and pruritus. Many physicians differ on how often to bathe the child, with some recommending every other day and others recommending twice a day. All agree on the minimal use of soap, gently patting the child dry to retain maximal moisture, and applying topical therapy (either lubricants alone or steroids followed by lubricants) immediately after bathing. Emollient ointments are generally better at retaining moisture than lotions and should be applied liberally to the entire body. Topical steroids usually are required, except in very mild cases. The lowest-potency steroids that are effective should be used; more potent steroids can be used in pulse fashion for 1 to 2 weeks for severe flares. Very low potency steroids should be used on the face. Short courses of oral steroids sometimes are used for severe exacerbations.

Two topical immunomodulators are available and have been approved for children over 2 years of age: tacrolimus and pimecrolimus. They have been shown to be effective in the treatment of atopic dermatitis, and they may allow physicians to avoid long-term use of topical steroids in children with mild to moderate eczema. They are safe for use on the face, which is another advantage. Oral antihistamines can be used to help control itching.

Another important aspect of management is the avoidance of triggers, which differ from one child to another.

Children with atopic dermatitis are at risk for secondary infection. Most of them are colonized with *S. aureus,* and so a vigilant watch for impetigo and cellulitis is important. Many atopic dermatitis exacerbations are associated with this secondary infection. Infections should be treated promptly with antistaphylococcal antibiotics.

Herpes simplex virus is another common agent that secondarily infects eczematous lesions; this is known as eczema herpeticum and should be treated with acyclovir.

## CONTACT DERMATITIS

Contact dermatitis is inflammation of the skin in response to either an irritant or an allergen. Irritant contact dermatitis is due to a local toxic effect of an irritant; examples include diaper dermatitis (in which fecal enzymes act as the irritant) and phytophotodermatitis (in which a substance in some plants, such as citric acid or leaves, acts locally to affect the skin). Allergic contact dermatitis is caused by an immunologic response to an antigen such as poison ivy or nickel and other metals. The history should focus on exposures to these or any other substances. The physical examination often reveals erythematous vesicles or unroofed blisters in a pattern consistent with the exposure. Irritant diaper dermatitis tends to spare the intertriginous folds.

The diagnosis can be confirmed by patch testing after the dermatitis has resolved, but often the configuration of the rash and the history of exposure allow an accurate diagnosis without testing. The treatment for contact dermatitis is topical steroids. Infants with irritant diaper dermatitis respond to frequent diaper changes and barrier creams. However, in instances in which the rash persists despite frequent diaper changes and barrier creams or if the dermatitis is moderate to severe, a low-potency topical steroid such as 1% hydrocortisone cream may be used.

## SEBORRHEIC DERMATITIS

Seborrhea is an inflammatory response that is seen in the areas of the body with high sebaceous gland activity. Fungal infection with *Pityrosporum* sp. may play a role in the pathogenesis of the disorder. Seborrhea is seen most commonly in infants, but adolescents can be affected as well. Affected infants are well-appearing and usually otherwise healthy, although severe seborrhea can indicate an underlying immunodeficiency. Two clinical manifestations of seborrheic dermatitis can be seen in infants. Dermatitis of the scalp, known as cradle cap, presents with yellowish, greasy scales on the scalp, with occasional spread to the face and neck. Seborrheic diaper dermatitis is characterized by greasy, often erythematous scaly lesions over the perineum and in the intertriginous folds. Adolescents often present with greasy yellowish scales in the intertriginous areas and scalp. The diagnosis usually can be made on the basis of the clinical presentation. Treatment includes the use of an antiseborrheic shampoo such as selenium sulfide and topical steroids for severe inflammation; however, many cases of cradle cap resolve without treatment.

## HYPERSENSITIVITY REACTIONS

### URTICARIA

Urticaria is a common hypersensitivity reaction in pediatrics. It can be caused by several mechanisms, including immunoglobulin E (IgE)-mediated histamine release and complement activation. Urticaria may be acute or chronic, and the differential diagnosis changes depending on the time course. Common causes of acute urticaria are insect stings, viral or strepto-coccal infections, and drug reactions. Chronic urticaria may be associated with collagen vascular disease, chronic infection, and chronic environmental exposure. Physical urticarias are reactions to heat, cold, or exercise. Therefore, the history should focus on inciting factors and the duration of the lesions to help determine the etiology. Urticarial lesions usually last less than 24 to 48 h, and it is typical for them to disappear and reappear in other parts of the body. Individual lesions that last longer than 48 h should raise the suspicion of another diagnosis, such as vasculitis. The physical examination in urticaria reveals the presence of wheals, which are raised, circumscribed pinkish areas of edema caused by extravasation of plasma from small capillaries. A complete physical examination should be performed in all cases to look for other signs of infection or inflammatory disease. Management of urticaria consists of removing any potential triggers and giving oral antihistamines. Lack of improvement or a more chronic time course may signal the need for further diagnostic evaluation and treatment.

### ERYTHEMA MULTIFORME

Erythema multiforme (EM) is considered by some to be a spectrum of hypersensitivity syndromes: EM minor, EM major (also known as Stevens-Johnson syndrome), and possibly toxic epidermal necrolysis. It can have many different etiologies, including infection and medication use, but many cases are idiopathic. Common infections include herpes simplex virus (especially for recurrent EM minor) and *Mycoplasma pneumoniae* (particularly in older children and adolescents with EM major), although other infections have been implicated. Antiepileptic medications and antibiotics are frequently implicated medications. The history should focus on these triggers and other associated symptoms, such as fever, mucosal lesions, and decreased appetite. EM minor typically involves only mild constitutional symptoms, whereas EM major can cause more systemic symptoms such as vomiting, diarrhea, malaise, or high fever.

The typical skin lesion in EM is the target lesion, which often begins with a wheal or macule that develops a central clearing. Lesions commonly occur

on the extremities and can be seen on the palms and soles. Mucosal involvement is limited to one area in EM minor, usually the mouth. The presence of
two or more mucosal surfaces and the formation of generalized bullae are
characteristic of EM major (Fig. 23-3). Children with EM minor are well-
appearing, whereas those with EM major are often very ill-appearing and
dehydrated.

The most important aspect of management in EM is the identification of
the inciting medication or infection if possible. All potential medication triggers should be discontinued immediately, and infection should be treated
promptly. Mild cases resolve without any treatment. Treatment of severe
cases is largely supportive. Oral antihistamines and pain medications can be
used to improve itching or pain. Careful vigilance of bullous lesions is
important in identifying secondary infection. Oral mouthwashes and anesthetics may be necessary for severe oral involvement, and some children will
be unable to take liquids or food by mouth for several days, necessitating
nasogastric feeding. The use of systemic steroids is controversial. Some
physicians prescribe intravenous immunoglobulin G to reduce symptoms,
but this has not been proved to improve the outcome in clinical trials.
Morbidity is highest in children with severe involvement. Those with extensive lesions should be treated similarly to patients with burns.

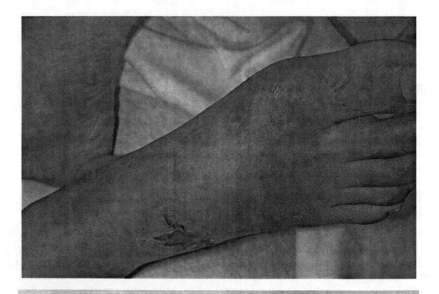

*Figure 23-3* **Stevens-Johnson syndrome.**

---

**"Don't Miss" Diagnoses for Rashes**

---

Cellulitis
Scarlet fever
Meningococcemia
Erythema multiforme

---

## CONCLUSION

Rashes are common in pediatrics, and their etiologies can range from simple, self-limited infections to severe hypersensitivity reactions. It is always important to get a complete history and perform a complete physical examination, paying close attention to the general appearance of the child and the characteristics of the lesions. Categorizing the differential diagnosis on the basis of these findings enables the examiner to take a focused approach to this broad complaint.

## BIBLIOGRAPHY

Andreae M. How to recognize and manage herpes simplex virus type 1 infections. *Contemp Pediatr* 21:41–60, 2004.

Hansen RC. Atopic dermatitis: Taming "the itch that rashes." *Contemp Pediatr* 20:79–97, 2003.

Hurwitz S, ed. *Clinical Pediatric Dermatology*, 2d ed. Philadelphia: Saunders, 1993.

Mancini AJ. Bacterial skin infections in children: The common and the not so common. *Pediatr Ann* 29:29–35, 2000.

Pickering LK, ed. *Red Book: 2003 Report of the Committee on Infectious Diseases*, 26th ed. Elk Grove Village, IL: American Academy of Pediatrics, 2003.

Weston WL, Badgett JT. Urticaria. *Pediatr Rev* 19:240–244, 1998.

# TRAUMA

*Lynn M. Manfred*

## LEARNING OBJECTIVES

1. Be able to evaluate a child with a head injury.
2. Know the treatment of common fractures.
3. Recognize burns secondary to child abuse.
4. Know the management of nursemaid's elbow.

## MAJOR TRAUMA

Trauma is one of the leading causes of morbidity and mortality in children. Major trauma results commonly from automobile accidents, falls from high places, abuse, and recreational activities. At the scene of the accident or injury, the child's neck and back should be immobilized and the airway should be secured. Initial assessment in the emergency room should be airway, breathing, circulation, disability, exposure (in trauma patients) (ABCDE), with follow-up of any abnormalities that are found (see Chap. 39 for a detailed discussion of initial assessment in the emergency room). In younger children, the head is proportionally bigger and heavier than it is in older children and adults. Thus, a child's head is more susceptible to injury.

The mechanism of injury is very important in the evaluation of an injured child. Motor vehicle accidents, especially high-speed ones, require particular attention. Large numbers of children are incorrectly restrained in child safety seats or not restrained at all. Children who have been in high-speed accidents must be checked for intracranial, neck, back, peripheral neurologic, flexion-extension, and abdominal injuries. Stabilizing central nervous system (CNS) injuries while treating other, sometimes more obvious, injuries can be lifesaving for some children.

Any injuries that are out of proportion to the stated mechanism of injury should be referred for evaluation by a child protection worker or the local department of social services. Substance use is a common comorbidity with major trauma in older children and teens. Evaluating the patient for the presence of substances and monitoring for withdrawal symptoms are important.

## HEAD INJURIES

Trauma patients should have a careful evaluation of the CNS. Primary blows to the head can cause significant injury, but the secondary injuries that result from hypotension or increasing intracranial pressure often increase the severity of the injury and subsequent disability. Thus, every effort should be made to assure adequate blood flow carrying adequate oxygen and glucose to the CNS. Blood pressure and perfusion should be kept as normal as possible. If rising intracranial pressure is a concern, early intubation with hyperventilation to a $PCO_2$ of 20 to 25 has been shown to decrease the disability from the injury. Other measures should be taken, such as elevating the head of the bed and direct monitoring of intracranial pressure.

Obvious skull injuries should be scanned to determine their extent. Deep depressed skull fractures should be elevated by neurosurgeons. Linear skull fractures are rarely a problem unless they cross the path of a major vessel such as the middle meningeal artery. In older children and adults, this vessel sits in the groove inside the skull and is easily fractured when there are skull injuries to the area. Younger children do not have this anatomy and are less likely to have traumatic injury to the vessel.

Bleeding into the closed space of the skull can come from arteries, venous sinuses, or veins. A rapid decline in mental status may result from an epidural bleed and constitutes a neurosurgical emergency since herniation can be imminent. Slower-developing disabilities can result from subdural fluid collections or swelling of the brain tissue itself from concussion or an intraparenchymal bleed. These conditions require careful observation and monitoring to prevent rising pressures that cause additional damage to the brain and eventual herniation of the intracranial contents from the skull trapping the brainstem. As the brainstem herniates, the pulse pressure increases, the heart rate slows, and the patient becomes apneic.

More commonly, the clinician sees less severe closed head injuries from a fall or a sports injury. Many of these patients have lost consciousness for a brief period. They should have a complete neurologic evaluation and imaging of the CNS. Children with neurologic abnormalities who have prolonged loss of consciousness or amnesia for the event and the time surrounding it should have a scan to evaluate the extent of the injury. The majority of these patients will have a normal scan or evidence of swelling in only a small section of the brain. These children should be removed from participation in sports until the symptoms of headache and dizziness have resolved. The American Academy of Pediatrics and the American Academy of Sports Medicine have developed joint guidelines for the management of children with concussions.

Children who are fully alert with a normal neurologic examination and who stay that way for a few hours do not need additional evaluation.

## SEAT BELT INJURIES

Children wearing seat belts that fit above the superior iliac crests are prone to injury of the intraabdominal contents, especially the bladder. Urine should be checked for blood, and if blood is found, the integrity of the genitourinary tract should be evaluated.

## OTHER TRAUMA

### FRACTURES

Fractures are a common reason for emergency room visits. Long bone injuries are usually the result of auto accidents, recreational activities (skiing, snowboarding, motorized racing, or bicycle riding), falls, and other high-speed activities. These injuries require careful follow-up as there is a high incidence of disproportionate growth in the injured extremity as it heals. Similarly, any involvement of the growth plate requires special consideration and close follow-up. Elbow injuries put the ulnar nerve at risk of injury, and neck and back injuries can hurt other nerves or the spinal cord.

Falls on outstretched hands can cause wrist fractures, commonly of the Colles type. Some of these falls can result in predominantly growth plate injury that may not be readily apparent in the initial x-rays. Clavicles can easily be fractured with direct trauma. Fingers and toes are vulnerable to fractures and sprains, as children play more games with balls (baseball, basketball, soccer, etc.).

Treatment is focused on creating sufficient alignment and approximation of the fracture sites to allow for good healing. Children remodel fractures, and so the angulation rarely has to be perfect.

Toddlers presenting with refusal to walk may have a "toddler's fracture." This is a spiral fracture of the tibia or femur caused by an immobilized foot and a fall in a rotating or twisting motion. Abuse consisting of shaking the child and holding the ankles can be the etiology of leg fractures in children, especially among those too young to walk.

Spiral fractures, compression fractures, and greenstick fractures generally heal with immobilization and good nutrition.

## SPRAINS

Sprains are ligamentous injuries to joints that cause swelling and pain. They are not structurally unstable, but reinjury can delay healing and even cause permanent swelling and disability. Ankles often are inverted forcibly, causing triangulate ligament injury, and fingers can easily be hyperextended and sprained.

## DISLOCATIONS

By far the most common dislocation in pediatrics is dislocation of the radial head from the elbow joint with traction on the distal extremity, better known as a nursemaid's elbow. Children present with refusal to use the extremity. If the dislocation is of short duration, the swelling may be minimal. The differential includes clavicle, humerus, and forearm fractures, though there is often point tenderness over the fracture. These dislocations frequently are relocated by an experienced pediatrician in the office or in an urgent care facility. Supination of the palm and flexion of the elbow often are successful. Care must be taken to decrease the risk of recurrence.

Shoulders can be dislocated by anterior force from above and posteriorly. Football falls are common causes of anterior shoulder dislocations. Removing the shirt and observing from the front will reveal that the humeral head is inferior and medially displaced into the space below the clavicle. Relocation is achieved by traction on the elbow. Often a muscle relaxant with analgesia is given to facilitate the relocation.

## OVERUSE INJURIES

With increasing frequency, children are presenting with overuse injuries. They are more active in sports and activities and engage in them with more intensity than previous generations. Overuse injuries first were recognized in young pitchers whose elbows became sore. Carpal tunnel injuries are seen in computer mouse users, shin splints in soccer and runners, and extensor tendinitis in tennis players and golfers. These injuries have no clear traumatic event and have a gradual onset of pain, swelling, and disability. Often the pain will be worse after inciting and aggravating activities.

## BURNS

Burns must be taken seriously, and careful consideration must be given to the possibility of nonaccidental burns. Trauma surgeons use the rule of nines to approximate the percentage of a child's body surface that is burned. For older children and adolescents, the head, one arm, the front of one leg, the back of one leg, the anterior trunk to the pelvis, and the posterior trunk each represent about 9 percent of the body surface area. For infants, 18 percent of the body surface area is on the head and the legs have less than 9 percent each. These are general estimates; more detailed charts are available in emergency medicine and surgery textbooks. The depth and location of the burns are very important. Distal burns may make perfusion of the affected area difficult and may slow healing. Circumferential burns also can damage the blood supply to the affected area. Symmetric circumferential burns are particularly concerning for their possibility of abuse, usually by immersion.

Burns to the face are also very serious. Specialized care should be sought, and the patient should be followed carefully. Toddlers can easily burn the palmar surface of the hands as they explore their environment. They also are prone to pulling on dangling objects so that they spill hot beverages over themselves.

Impressive fluid losses can be expected from open burn surfaces. These open areas are also prone to infection, which delays healing and creates more scarring. Caring for burns involves decreasing the open area and covering it with substances that decrease the risk of infection.

## BITES

Small children exploring their environment can frighten or annoy animals, even ones they know well. The surprised animal may bite exposed surfaces. For older children, this is usually the hand or the leg. For infants, it can be the head or upper extremities. Bites are puncture wounds that drive the oral bacteria of the animal deep into the tissue planes of the bitten areas.

Signs and symptoms of infection after animal bites almost always occur 24 to 72 h after the bite. Redness, swelling, and tenderness develop around the site of injury and often are accompanied by purulent or serosanguineous drainage. *Pasteurella* species are the most common isolates from both dog bites (50 percent) and cat bites (75 percent). Although *Pasteurella* species are the most common isolates from animal bites, mixed aerobic and anaerobic infection are present in 56 percent of all animal wounds (48 percent of dog bites and 63 percent of cat bites). Because the risk of a mixed infection, especially with *Staphylococcus aureus* and anaerobes, is high with animal bites, oral amoxicillin-clavulanate is recommended. In addition to treatment with antibiotics, care for animal bites includes careful cleansing of the bite, immobilization and elevation of larger injured areas, the administration of tetanus prophylaxis when required, and evaluation of the need for rabies prophylaxis.

## CLOSED HEAD INJURIES

Many children, particularly toddlers, have falls and other injuries that involve head injuries. The vast majority of these incidents occur without loss of consciousness or extracranial injury. When the mechanism of injury is not high-impact, as when a toddler trips and hits his or her head on a coffee table, the patient can be evaluated and observed in an urgent care setting. If there has been no prolonged loss of consciousness, the neurologic examination is normal, and the child has not vomited more than twice, that child can be observed for 6 h. If there is no progression of symptoms, the risk of significant injury is small and the child may be discharged with instructions to the caregiver to return if any new symptoms develop, such as vomiting, ataxia, or dizziness.

## LACERATIONS

Lacerations are common in pediatric practice. The sites and severity of the lacerations vary with the age of the child. Infants who are starting to cruise and walk are often quite unsteady on their feet. Living room tables are easy targets for their heads, which are proportionately heavier than they will be later in life. The distance these infants fall is short, and so there is rarely a loss of consciousness. These youngsters have not developed the protective reflexes that allow older children and adults to put their hands up. They often have lacerations to the head. The head is a very vascular place, and so any bleeding is usually profuse. Many of these lacerations must be closed in layers, including the galea when it is lacerated. Injuries on the scalp can be closed with staples after irrigation and exploration of the wound. These wounds heal quickly, and sutures and staples can be removed in 5 to 7 days.

Older children and adolescents fall, causing lacerations predominantly to the extremities. Most of these lacerations can be closed simply if they are not over joints or the abdomen. Wounds that may penetrate joint spaces or the abdomen or chest must be explored and closed carefully. Antibiotics are required if penetration is into the joint space or the abdomen.

Lacerations over extremities are also prone to lacerating tendons and other soft tissue structures. Hand lacerations should be evaluated carefully to detect injury to the tendons. The hand should be able to make a fist and resist squeezing pressures.

Hand lacerations acquired in fights should be treated as human bites. The clinician should have a high index of suspicion that metacarpophalangeal (MCP) lacerations on the dorsal surface of the hand in fact were acquired in a fight.

Lacerations over MCP joints also may occur because the patient put his or her hand through a piece of glass. Injuries to the feet often involve glass as well. A careful search for glass fragments should be made, and any that are found should be removed as they delay healing and serve as a locus for infection.

Injuries to the extremities mandate a careful evaluation of the sensation in the area.

---

***"Don't Miss" Diagnoses for Trauma***

---

Increased intracranial pressure after closed head trauma
Nursemaid's elbow
Burns secondary to child abuse

---

## BIBLIOGRAPHY

American Academy of Pediatrics, Committee on Quality Improvement. The management of closed head injury in children. *Pediatrics* 104:1407–1415, 1999.

Reese R, Ludwig S, eds. *Child Abuse: Medical Diagnosis and Management.* Philadelphia: Lippincott Williams & Wilkins, 2001.

# JOINT AND LIMB

# PROBLEMS

*M. Robin English*

## LEARNING OBJECTIVES

1. Understand the importance of the history and physical examination in developing a differential diagnosis for joint pain and gait disturbances.

2. Understand the presenting signs and symptoms for infectious, rheumatologic, hematologic, oncologic, and orthopedic conditions that may cause joint and limb pain.

3. Understand the underlying etiology and/or pathophysiology for infectious, rheumatologic, hematologic, oncologic, and orthopedic conditions that may cause joint and limb pain.

4. Know the appropriate initial workup and management for infectious, rheumatologic, hematologic, oncologic, and orthopedic conditions that may cause joint and limb pain.

## INTRODUCTION

Children and adolescents who have gait disturbances (limp) or joint pain challenge pediatricians to consider an extensive differential diagnosis. The etiologies of such symptoms are varied and include rheumatologic disorders, orthopedic disorders, infections, congenital deformities, and neuromuscular diseases. It is up to the pediatrician to define the cause of the problem, which can be difficult to do initially because many children present with a limp only and are unable to describe the nature or location of the pain. Some childhood illnesses that cause a limp or joint pain are simple general pediatric diseases that can be diagnosed and treated by a pediatrician.

However, others require subspecialty consultation and more complicated therapy and follow-up. A thorough history and physical examination usually help the pediatrician determine whether laboratory or radiologic evaluation and subspecialty involvement are necessary.

A limp, which is merely abnormal ambulation, can be caused by joint pain, bone pain, anatomic anomalies, or neuromuscular weakness. Joint pain can be seen with a number of diseases, and any joint in the body can be involved. Some diseases have a predilection for large weight-bearing joints, whereas some have a propensity to cause problems in small joints. This chapter reviews the important elements of the history in a child who presents with a limp or joint pain, and the critical features of the physical examination are discussed. Many of the diseases that can present with these symptoms are covered elsewhere in this book; this chapter discusses common conditions that pediatricians encounter.

## HISTORY

The history of a child who presents with a limp should start with the timing of the limp. The acute onset of limp may be a symptom of acute trauma or infection, whereas a limp that has been present and possibly worsening over weeks may indicate an underlying orthopedic or rheumatologic disease. It is important to explore a history of antecedent trauma, even seemingly insignificant trauma, keeping in mind that toddlers often fall without their parents' knowledge and that many older children experience minor trauma and do not divulge it to their parents. The effect that the limp has had on the child's daily activity is also important, for example, whether it interferes with the ability to attend school or play sports. The child should be asked, if possible, for the location of any pain, but it is crucial to remember that referred pain is common, especially in the lower extremities. For example, knee pathology often causes hip pain, and hip problems frequently cause knee pain only. A social history, including child-care arrangements and the people who live with the child, is important, especially in toddlers, because small fractures resulting from nonaccidental trauma can cause a limp and the history probably will not reflect the trauma.

When a child presents with joint pain, it is important to ascertain whether a single joint or multiple joints are involved. Some rheumatologic illnesses present with a migratory pattern of joint pain, meaning that one joint will be involved for a few days and then the pain will "move" to another joint. As with limp, the ability of the child to continue with normal daily activities can give the examiner an idea of the severity of the pain.

The total duration of the pain also is important. Morning stiffness is a complaint that should raise suspicion of rheumatoid arthritis. Children or parents should be asked if joint swelling or redness accompanies the pain, which would indicate arthritis. A history of recent illnesses, especially gastroenteritis, should be elicited. Adolescents should be asked about their sexual history independently from their parents, as some sexually transmitted diseases can present with arthritis. Also important is the recent administration of immunizations, especially measles-mumps-rubella (MMR) vaccine, because joint pain is a rare side effect of vaccination against rubella.

Associated symptoms such as fever, malaise, pain in other areas, or rash are important historic features that can help the examiner develop a differential diagnosis for both joint pain and limp because these symptoms often are seen in rheumatologic and malignant diseases. The effect of any over-the-counter medication the child may have taken is helpful as well. All these factors should be included in the history of present illness for either limp or joint pain. Past medical problems and a family history of rheumatologic or other diseases also should be asked about. As usual, a thorough review of systems is indicated to gain further information for a complete differential diagnosis.

## PHYSICAL EXAMINATION

The examination of a child who presents with a limp starts with a thorough general examination. One important task is to observe the child's ambulation to identify features of the limp. Some children simply refuse to walk, insisting on being carried or staying in the parent's lap. This probably indicates pain. Some children with pain agree to walk but demonstrate a pattern of decreased weight-bearing time on the affected side that is called an "antalgic gait." Children with knee swelling may hold the affected leg out straight while walking, but they also may refuse to walk. Children who demonstrate a broad-based gait may actually be ataxic rather than limping from pain, and children with neurologic disturbances such as spasticity and muscle weakness may show a Trendelenburg gait (leaning away from the center of gravity with each step but with equal weight bearing bilaterally) or toe walking. These two gait disturbances are not secondary to joint or limb problems but rather to neurologic diseases and therefore are not discussed in this chapter.

The examination of the joints includes visualization, palpation, and range of motion of all joints. The joints should be evaluated for tenderness and warmth as well as erythema and swelling. Evidence of joint effusion includes palpation of fluid (as in knee effusions) or, more commonly, a decrease in range of motion. At times, it may be difficult to assess whether a decrease in range of motion is due to effusion or pain. Joints that are painful without any evidence of warmth, swelling, effusion, or erythema can be classified as arthralgia, whereas joint pain accompanied by those features is indicative of arthritis. This can be an important distinction to make, because the differential diagnosis changes if arthritis is present. This will be discussed in the context of individual diseases later in this chapter.

Table 25-1  *Typical Time Course and Pattern of Diseases Affecting the Joints*

| | Acute | Chronic | Single Joint | Multiple Joints | Large Joints | Small Joints |
|---|---|---|---|---|---|---|
| Septic arthritis | X | | X | | X | X |
| Gonococcal arthritis | X | | X | X | X | |
| Reactive arthritis | X | | X | | X | |
| Transient synovitis | X | | X | | X | |
| Henoch-Schönlein purpura | X | | | X | X | |
| Polyarticular juvenile rheumatoid arthritis | | X | | X | | X |
| Pauciarticular juvenile rheumatoid arthritis | | X | | X | X | |
| Rheumatic fever | X | | | X | X | |
| Systemic lupus erythematosus | | X | | X | | X |

A complete physical examination is as important as the joint examination. The examiner should look for any rashes or other skin abnormalities. The heart should be evaluated for murmurs, and the abdomen should be examined for evidence of hepatosplenomegaly. Because some malignancies can present with joint pain or limp (secondary to bone pain), it is important to look for evidence of anemia or thrombocytopenia, such as pallor, petechiae, or bruising.

Once the history and physical examination are complete, the differential diagnosis can be refined according to the time course and the pattern of joint involvement (Table 25-1). Specific historic and physical examination findings are discussed in the context of individual diseases later in this chapter.

## DIFFERENTIAL DIAGNOSIS

### INFECTIONS AND POSTINFECTIOUS CONDITIONS

#### OSTEOMYELITIS

Osteomyelitis is defined as a bacterial infection of the bone. It usually occurs as a result of hematogenous spread of bacteria to the bone, but it also may be the result of local infiltration of bacteria, as in complicated wounds or deep soft tissue infections. It may be acute, chronic, or recurrent, and the time course can help determine the most likely bacteria causing the infection. *Staphylococcus aureus* is the most common cause of acute osteomyelitis, but *Streptococcus pyogenes*, *Kingella kingae*, and other organisms are common causes as well. *Salmonella* sp. can cause osteomyelitis in children with sickle cell disease. *Pseudomonas aeruginosa* often is implicated in cases of osteomyelitis that occur after puncture wounds of the foot. Osteomyelitis can occur with or without evidence of joint involvement.

Children with osteomyelitis typically present with bone pain. Younger children who may be unable to communicate pain may present with fussiness or decreased movement of the affected limb (pseudoparalysis). Fever may be present. These children may be ill-appearing if bacteremia is present. The examination is usually normal except for the affected limb, which often shows point tenderness, warmth, erythema, or edema. At times, however, no external sign of infection can be seen, and the only presentation may be a limp or nonspecific limb pain.

The laboratory evaluation for a child with osteomyelitis often shows an increased white blood cell count. Acute-phase reactants, such as the erythrocyte sedimentation rate and C-reactive protein, are likely to be elevated. Plain radiographs typically do not show evidence of the infection until 7 to 10 days after symptoms have been present. A bone scan or magnetic resonance imaging scan is more likely to be positive early in the disease process, and so one of those studies should be done to confirm the diagnosis. A blood culture may be positive for the offending organism, but the most accurate way to confirm the bacterial cause is direct aspiration of the bone.

Treatment consists of intravenous antibiotics aimed against *S. aureus*, keeping in mind the methicillin-resistance patterns in the community, or against other suspected or confirmed organism. Many clinicians advocate intravenous therapy for a few weeks until acute-phase reactants have decreased, at which time oral therapy can be instituted for another few weeks. The total time of therapy is usually 4 to 6 weeks.

A particular infection that merits mention because of its propensity to cause isolated limp or nonspecific pain is diskitis, which can occur in conjunction with vertebral osteomyelitis. Point tenderness over the involved disk or vertebral body may be elicited. The bacteriology, diagnosis, and treatment for diskitis are the same as those for osteomyelitis as outlined above.

## SEPTIC ARTHRITIS

Acute septic arthritis can be isolated or can be associated with osteomyelitis. It is defined as a bacterial infection of the joint. The pathogenesis is similar to that of osteomyelitis, with hematogenous seeding of bacteria to the joint or local spread of the infection from a wound. The bacterial pathogens responsible for septic arthritis are similar to those which cause osteomyelitis, with *S. aureus* being the most common. An organism that can cause arthritis in adolescents is *Neisseria gonorrhoeae*, which occurs with disseminated gonococcal infection. Neonates are at risk for septic arthritis from group B streptococcal infection, which often occurs concurrently with osteomyelitis.

Children with septic arthritis usually present with pain in a single joint, although referred pain to other joints can occur, especially between the hip and the knee. Refusal to walk is very common when lower extremity joints are affected. Children often prefer to hold their limbs in a specific position to relieve the pain: flexed and externally rotated at the hips or flexed partially at the knee. These children may be ill-appearing if systemic infection is present, and fever is usual. Significantly decreased range of motion and swelling of the affected joint are typical. Warmth, erythema, and tenderness are also common. Disseminated gonococcal infection can cause a migratory polyarthralgia of the knees, ankles, and wrists, which may be associated with a rash characterized by macules and hemorrhagic pustules over the joints. Gonococcal arthritis also can cause frank arthritis of a single joint. Adolescents suspected of having gonococcal infection should have a complete pelvic examination.

Laboratory evaluation may reveal elevation of the white blood cell count, erythrocyte sedimentation rate, and C-reactive protein. Plain radiographs may show widening of the joint space or soft tissue swelling. Ultrasound is useful, especially when hip effusion is suspected (hip swelling may be difficult to ascertain on physical examination). Blood culture often reveals the organism, but the most important test is aspiration of joint fluid. Typical findings on the synovial fluid include a very elevated white blood cell count and a positive Gram stain and culture. Immediate orthopedic consultation for the aspiration and for surgical irrigation of the joint is indicated.

Treatment consists of intravenous antibiotics for several weeks. Septic arthritis carries a good prognosis if it is diagnosed and treated early. If the diagnosis is delayed, degenerative joint disease can result.

## REACTIVE ARTHRITIS

Arthritis can occur as a postinfectious reaction in some children. Common preceding infections that cause reactive arthritis include *Salmonella, Shigella, Yersinia*, and *Campylobacter*. The history in these patients should establish the preceding infection, and the joint pain usually occurs within a few weeks after the infection has resolved. Usually only one joint is involved, most often the knee or ankle, but occasionally polyarthritis can occur. The physical examination typically reveals transient swelling and tenderness of the affected joints. These children are usually well-appearing, and the remainder of the examination is usually normal. Laboratory evaluation may reveal a high erythrocyte sedimentation rate but is generally unnecessary for the diagnosis. The prognosis is excellent.

## TRANSIENT/TOXIC SYNOVITIS

Transient synovitis, also known as toxic synovitis, is a fairly common occurrence in pediatrics. It occurs as a postviral syndrome. The history usually reveals an upper respiratory infection 1 to 2 weeks before presentation. Children typically present with the acute onset of hip pain, although referred pain to the leg or knee is also common. Fever is usually not present. On physical examination, these children are generally well-appearing. Some refuse to walk, but most demonstrate an antalgic gait. Examination of the hip may be painful and therefore difficult, but range of motion usually is not extremely limited. Overlying signs of inflammation such as warmth and erythema are not present.

It can be difficult to differentiate transient synovitis from septic arthritis of the hip on physical examination; therefore, laboratory evaluation, including a complete blood count and erythrocyte sedimentation rate, and plain radiographs should be performed. The results of these tests usually are normal in transient synovitis. Treatment includes rest and nonsteroidal anti-inflammatory medications, and the pain usually resolves within a few days.

## RHEUMATOLOGIC CONDITIONS

Joint pain is part of the presentation of most rheumatologic diseases; this demonstrates the importance of taking a thorough history and performing a complete physical examination, because many other features besides joint pain will be present in these diseases. Laboratory evaluation always should be performed for the purpose of making the diagnosis, and so it is important to think carefully about how the results of the tests will be used before ordering them. Initial laboratory tests in suspected rheumatologic diseases include complete blood count, erythrocyte sedimentation rate, and C reactive protein. More specific tests such as rheumatoid factor and antinuclear antibody can be obtained as suspicion warrants. The details of these diseases are discussed in Chap. 38; this chapter describes the joint findings specifically. The joint pain in rheumatologic diseases generally responds very well to anti-inflammatory medications.

## HENOCH-SCHÖNLEIN PURPURA

A majority of children with Henoch-Schönlein purpura (HSP) present with joint pain, which can be present early in the disease. The history often reveals migratory pain, and the knees, ankles, and other large joints typically are involved. The physical examination will reveal swelling, erythema, and tenderness of the affected joints, and many of these children will refuse to walk. Other features of the disease, including abdominal pain and palpable purpura on the lower extremities and buttocks, also will be present. HSP is discussed in more detail in Chap. 38.

## JUVENILE RHEUMATOID ARTHRITIS

Joint pain is a prominent feature in most cases of juvenile rheumatoid arthritis (JRA). Children with systemic JRA may not present with joint pain initially. Pauciarticular JRA includes the involvement of four or fewer joints, typically large joints such as the knee. Polyarticular JRA involves five or more joints, and the small joints of the wrists and fingers are affected commonly. JRA is discussed in more detail in Chap. 38.

## RHEUMATIC FEVER

Rheumatic fever occurs as a sequela of group A streptococcal disease. The joint involvement is migratory in nature, typically affecting large joints such as the knees, elbows, ankles, and wrists. The joints are very painful both to touch and with movement and are usually erythematous and edematous. This polyarthritis is one of the five major Jones criteria; arthralgia is one of the four minor criteria, but it cannot be considered a minor criterion if polyarthritis is present. Rheumatic fever is discussed in more detail in Chap. 38.

## SYSTEMIC LUPUS ERYTHEMATOSUS

Arthritis is one of the 11 criteria required for the diagnosis of systemic lupus erythematosus (SLE). Arthralgia is also a feature that is seen commonly. The joint involvement in SLE is typically polyarticular, with the joints of the hands being affected frequently. The pain may be migratory. SLE is discussed in more detail in Chap. 38.

## HEMATOLOGIC AND ONCOLOGIC CONDITIONS

Several hematologic diseases and cancers in children can cause bone pain, and it is important to keep them in mind. These diseases highlight the importance of asking about constitutional symptoms such as weight loss or fatigue. African-American children should be asked if they have sickle cell disease even if no previous complications, such as vasoocclusive crisis, have occurred. The initial test ordered for children with bone pain should be a plain radiograph of the affected area. This will rule out diagnoses such as fracture and may provide clues that lead toward malignancy as a diagnosis. The bone and joint complaints of three of these diseases are discussed below. Further details about these diseases are discussed in Chap. 31.

## BONE TUMORS

Primary bone tumors, namely, Ewing sarcoma and osteosarcoma, are an important cause of bone and joint pain, especially in the adolescent population. The history typically reveals localized pain and swelling, and patients often give a history of minor trauma to the area. The pain is usually persistent and worsens over time. The physical examination shows point tenderness with localized swelling. If the tumor is close to a joint, decreased range of motion and swelling or arthralgia without effusion can be seen. These tumors can be seen on a plain radiograph, which is the initial test of choice.

## LEUKEMIA

Acute lymphoblastic leukemia commonly presents with bone or joint pain and limp as a chief complaint. The pain is due to leukemic infiltration of the joint or marrow cavity. These children complain of deep bone pain that may or may not be localized. The bone examination in these children is typically normal, without the swelling that is seen in primary bone tumors, but tenderness may be present. Stigmata of cytopenias such as bruising, bleeding, or pallor also may be evident. Plain radiographs may show "leukemia lines," which are radiolucent lines in metaphyseal areas.

## SICKLE CELL PAIN CRISIS

Pain crisis is a common occurrence in children with sickle cell disease. It is caused by vasoocclusion and subsequent ischemia to the tissue. Areas that are affected commonly by this are the arms, legs, and back. The pain can be quite severe. The physical examination, however, is often normal in the affected areas, with no swelling, erythema, or warmth. The diagnosis of osteomyelitis always should be considered in children with sickle cell pain crisis, and so it is important to look for these external signs of infection. A complete blood count and a reticulocyte count are important to obtain to see the degree of anemia and marrow response.

## ORTHOPEDIC CONDITIONS

Children presenting with limp, or bone and joint pain, often have diseases attributable to abnormalities of the bones themselves. These diseases are covered in detail in Chap. 36.

## GROWING PAIN

Growing pain, or idiopathic leg pain, is a common occurrence in children. The etiology is unknown. The history typically reveals deep pain, usually in the legs, that occurs most often at night. The pain often is relieved when a parent massages the legs. The physical examination is completely normal. Laboratory evaluation is generally not necessary, but if there is significant anxiety on the part of the patient or parent, normal laboratory values can be reassuring. Treatment consists of reassurance and time.

## CONCLUSION

Limp and joint pain and/or bone pain sometimes result from benign, self-limited diseases in pediatrics. However, in many cases a serious underlying infection or inflammatory condition is responsible for the pain. It is always important to take a thorough history, including the duration of the pain, and perform a complete examination even if the area of pain is localized and small. This approach will help ensure that serious diagnoses are not overlooked.

---

**"Don't Miss" Diagnoses for Joint and Limb Problems**

Bone tumor
Leukemia
Osteomyelitis
Rheumatic fever
Septic arthritis
Sickle cell pain crisis

---

## BIBLIOGRAPHY

Godler DR. A practical approach to the child who limps. *Contemp Pediatr* 19:56–63, 2002.

Narasimhan N, Marks M. Osteomyelitis and septic arthritis. In Behrman RE, Kliegman RM, Arvin AM, eds., *Nelson Textbook of Pediatrics*, 15th ed. Philadelphia: McGraw-Hill, 1996: 724–733.

Pickering LK, ed. *Red Book: 2003 Report of the Committee on Infectious Diseases*, 26th ed. Elk Grove Village, IL: American Academy of Pediatrics, 2003.

Trueworthy RC, Templeton KJ. Malignant bone tumors presenting as musculoskeletal pain. *Pediatr Ann* 31:355–359, 2002.

# CENTRAL NERVOUS

# SYSTEM PROBLEMS

*Lynn M. Manfred*

● LEARNING OBJECTIVES

1. Recognize the etiologies of the most common and most serious problems of the central nervous system, including infections, seizures, headaches, masses, and bleeds.

2. Describe the differential diagnosis for the most common central nervous system disturbances, including, seizures, headaches, weakness, ataxia, and mental status changes, in pediatric patients.

Central nervous system (CNS) problems are very common in the pediatric population. The head of a small child is disproportionately large compared with the rest of the body, making it particularly vulnerable to trauma (see Chap. 39). The CNS is growing and changing rapidly in young children, and so small disturbances can lead to bleeds, tumors, or seizures. As in adults, metabolic and infectious problems elsewhere in the body affect the brain.

## INFECTIONS

### MENINGITIS AND ENCEPHALITIS

Infection of the CNS should be considered in any child with a fever and no obvious source of infection or mental status changes. Children older than 18 to 24 months with a supple neck probably do not have meningitis; however, a supple neck is not a reliable sign in younger children. Infants may present with a protruding anterior fontanel and either somnolence or irritability. Children also can present with seizures, confusion, or other mental status changes. Whenever meningitis is a consideration, a lumbar puncture should be performed. Table 26-1 shows the most common etiologies of meningitis by age group and typical spinal fluid findings. Empirical therapy for children older than 3 months consists of a third-generation cephalosporin plus vancomycin. Vancomycin is discontinued if the culture demonstrates that the organism is sensitive to the third-generation cephalosporin. Treatment is usually for 7 days for *Neisseria meningitidis* and *Haemophilus influenzae* B but 10 to 14 days for *Streptococcus pneumoniae*.

Mortality from acute bacterial meningitis is 5 to 10 percent, and 50 percent of the long-term survivors have significant morbidity, including hydrocephalus, seizures, developmental delays, learning disabilities, or hearing loss. The most common long-term complication of bacterial meningitis is hearing loss.

In contrast to meningitis, encephalitis is an acute inflammatory infection of the brain, not its coverings. Children and the elderly are the most commonly infected, most with viruses. Thirty to 50 percent of newborns born to mothers with primary herpes simplex virus (HSV) infections are infected at birth and present at about 6 weeks of age. Less than 10 percent of infants who are born to mothers with recurrent infection or are exposed to infected caregivers develop infections.

Other viral causes of encephalitis include enteroviruses (echoviruses and Coxsackie virus) and arboviruses (St. Louis encephalitis, eastern equine encephalitis, western equine encephalitis, and West Nile virus). Mortality is highest with the arboviruses, which also are more likely to have neurologic consequences such as seizures or developmental delay.

## SEIZURES

The clinical presentation of childhood seizures is highly variable. The history (see Table 26-2) from an observer and the patient is very important in distinguishing between seizures and other movement disorders. Loss of consciousness with movements that are symmetric and equal from one side to the other are termed generalized seizures. Focal seizures are limited to one area of the body: to an arm or the face most commonly. Partial and focal seizures may impair consciousness and the ability to communicate but usually do not result in complete loss of consciousness.

### FEBRILE SEIZURES

Febrile seizures are the most common seizure disorder in pediatrics, occurring in 2 to 5 percent of children. Over 50 percent of febrile seizures are reported in children between 1 and 2 years of age. Febrile seizures can be diagnosed when the seizure is brief (usually 2 to 5 min and < 15 min) and generalized, and the patient returns to usual health quickly. Often the

Table 26-1 **Important Causes of Meningitis by Age Group**

| Age | Glucose | Protein | Cell Count |
|---|---|---|---|
| 0–3 months<br>Common: | | | |
| Group B streptococci | <40 | 100–500 | 100–10K, > 80 percent PMN |
| Escherichia coli | <40 | 100–500 | 100-10K, > 80 percent PMN |
| Enterococcus sp. | <40 | 100–500 | 100–10K, > 80 percent PMN |
| Listeria monocytogenes | 20–80 | >45 | 5–1000, 50–80 percent PMN |
| 3 months–5 years<br>Common: | | | |
| S. pneumoniae | <30 | >100 | 1K–10K, >80 percent PMN |
| N. meningitidis | <30 | >100 | 1K–10K, >80 percent PMN |
| Haemophilus influenzae B | <30 | >100 | 1K–10K, >80 percent PMN |
| 5–18 years<br>Common: | | | |
| Streptococcus pneumoniae | <30 | >100 | 1K–10K, >80 percent PMN |
| Neisseria meningitidis | <30 | >100 | 1K–10K, >80 percent PMN |
| Enterovirus spp. | 50–90 | 20–80 | <1000 PMN, then shift to lymphocytes |
| Less Common to Rare:<br>Rickettsia (Lyme disease) | | | |
| Mycobacterium tuberculosis | varies | >100 | 10–500, PMN and lymphocytes |
| Coccidioides immitis | 10–40 | 50–1000 | 50–1000 lymphocytes or eosinophils |
| Candida albicans | | | |
| Cryptococcus neoformans | <40 | >40 | > 20 lymphocytes |

PMN = polymorphonuclear leukocyte.

Table 26-2 **Distinguishing Features of Possible Seizures**

| Feature | How It Helps |
| --- | --- |
| Aura | Rarely found in problems other than seizures and migraines |
| Focal? | Gives clues to where in the brain the activity is |
| Precipitant? | Head trauma *immediately* preceding makes recurrence risk low |
| | Hypoglycemia and hypoxia make recurrence risk low; vasovagal syncope has low risk of seizure recurrence |
| Length | Seizures lasting > 30 min are usually epilepsy; seizures lasting < 15 min may be febrile seizures |
| Incontinence | Increases the chances that the episode is a seizure |
| Behavioral change | |
| Loss of development | Increases the risk of a mass precipitating the seizures |
| Family history of seizures | Increases the risk that this is epilepsy |

seizure occurs as the fever is first rising, and so the family does not know that the child is ill until seeing the seizure. Febrile seizures usually occur in children 6 months to 5 years of age, with the majority occurring in toddlers. Many of these patients have a family history of febrile seizures.

The cause of the fever must be determined in children who present with fever and seizures. The neurologic examination of a child with a febrile seizure should be completely normal. The practitioner must be certain that the child does not have an intracranial infection such as meningitis or encephalitis as the underlying cause of both the seizure and the fever. In children less than 18 to 24 months of age, the lack of a stiff neck does not exclude meningitis. A bulging, hard fontanel may be present in a child with meningitis. Children who have experienced a seizure with fever usually have a fever caused by a viral infection, with very few fevers being due to a serious bacterial infection such as meningitis, pneumonia, sepsis, or urinary tract infection. Herpes encephalitis can present with seizures, fever, and mental status changes. Laboratory evaluation usually is needed only to evaluate the source of the fever. Routine imaging of the head or an electroencephalogram (EEG) is not indicated. The source of the fever should be treated with appropriate antibiotics or antivirals when the cause is discovered. In all cases, treatment must include antipyretics for the expected duration of the fever. Anticonvulsants are not administered routinely in patients with febrile seizures.

In general, febrile seizures are innocent. There is no evidence that febrile seizures cause any long-term problems or developmental delay. They can recur with other episodes of fever, either during the initial illness or with other illnesses. Rarely do they continue after age 5 years. Patients who have complex febrile seizures, a family history of epilepsy, or developmental delay have a higher likelihood of epilepsy.

## GENERALIZED SEIZURES WITHOUT FEVER

Without a fever, generalized seizures can have many causes. Metabolic, traumatic, mass effect, and cardiovascular causes must be sought and corrected if present. The questions in Table 26-2 help point the examiner toward or away from the diagnosis of idiopathic epilepsy. This diagnosis is one of exclusion, however, and must await at least a second seizure. Seizures are more likely to occur when a patient with epilepsy is ill with a fever, sleep-deprived, sobering after intoxication, dehydrated, falling asleep, or awakening.

Metabolic etiologies are most commonly hypoglycemic, but electrolyte abnormalities, hepatic or renal insufficiency, and problems of oxygen delivery also can cause seizures.

Traumatic seizures that occur immediately after head injuries have no prognostic significance for the development of further seizures. Seizures that occur minutes to hours later usually are caused by swelling or bleeding within the closed space of the skull and should be investigated promptly. Posttraumatic and postinfectious seizures are thought to result from a disruption of the CNS that leaves a potential seizure focus. They can recur many times over months to years.

If there is any focality or asymmetry to the neurologic examination or there has been a loss of developmental milestones, the CNS must be imaged to look for a tumor, a structural abnormality, or a bleed. Many neurologists recommend imaging for any first prolonged nonfocal seizure. If it is not done with the first generalized, afebrile seizure, imaging should be considered if a second seizure occurs.

Any cause of poor CNS perfusion deprives the CNS of its required fuels: glucose and oxygen. Thus, hypoglycemia, hypoxia, hypotension, and many toxins or ingestions can cause generalized seizures. Many medications, when taken in excess, are epileptogenic, some by the metabolic derangements they cause and others by their precipitating hypoperfusion of the brain or by creating acute hypertensive episodes. Thus, a thorough search must be made for any possible underlying cause of a first generalized seizure.

Infantile spasms are a type of seizure seen only in the first few months of life. The seizure consists of flexion at the neck, hips, and back while a child raises the arms above the head. They often are associated with a particular

EEG pattern called hypsarrhythmia and carry a poor developmental prognosis. These seizures do not respond to conventional anticonvulsants. Adrenocorticotropic hormone (ACTH) and steroids often are used, with modest success.

### FOCAL MOTOR AND PARTIAL COMPLEX SEIZURES

Focal motor and complex partial seizures can be difficult to diagnose. Focal motor seizures most commonly involve the arm, hand, or face but can affect any motor group. The patient is conscious and able to describe the involved area. Complex seizures usually involve a partial loss of consciousness such that the patient is not able to communicate as usual. The patient may be able to talk but does so incoherently or nonsensically.

Absence seizures are similar, though they do not necessarily involve a visible moving body part. They are often quite brief, but these patients lose some of the auditory and/or visual information they normally would receive from the world around them.

## HEADACHE

Headache is a common complaint in children. The timing, duration, and pattern of a headache can help determine the etiology of the headache. The most common causes of *acute* headache are infectious and traumatic. Headache with fever and/or myalgias usually results from upper respiratory infections, sinusitis, or otitis. These causes are self-limited and should be treated symptomatically once meningitis and encephalitis have been excluded clinically. Rarely, patients who present acutely with headache and possibly with a low-grade fever have an intracranial bleed from trauma, an aneurysm, or an arteriovenous malformation. Patients presenting with these bleeds commonly describe "the worst headache of my life," which started quickly. Ingestion of toxins such as carbon monoxide, inhaled hydrocarbons, and even caffeine, tobacco, or alcohol can cause acute or withdrawal headaches.

Recurrent episodes of acute, severe headache may result from toxin ingestion. Commonly, acute, recurrent headaches are vascular in origin. Migraines are the most common, run strongly in families, and are seen in patients of virtually all ages. Classic migraines are the easiest to diagnose, as they present with an aura, develop unilaterally, and decrease or resolve with rest, quiet, and analgesia. Common migraines are more common in children. They present acutely, with or without an aura, and resolve with analgesia or rest. Headaches that last for longer periods—days to weeks—are cluster headaches. The initial treatment for both migraine and cluster headaches consists of acetaminophen or nonsteroidal anti-inflammatory drugs (NSAIDs) and sleep. Vasoconstrictors and stronger pain medications are sometimes necessary. If the frequency of headache becomes more than weekly or if the headaches are very severe and difficult to treat, a preventive medication can be considered. Preventive medications decrease the frequency and severity of headaches. Most antidepressants, including tricyclic and tetracyclic antidepressants and selective serotonin reuptake inhibitors (SSRIs), have been used for the prevention of vascular headaches. Vasodilators such as the calcium channel blockers also have been used with some success. Recently, many of the antiepileptic medications, such as carbamazepine, valproate, and Trileptal, have been used successfully.

Another common etiology for acute, recurrent headaches is tension headaches. These headaches often are school- or work-related, develop as the day progresses, and are not present during vacations, weekends, or other days off from the tension-producing activity. Recurrent episodes of headache can be due to viral, bacterial, or allergic sinusitis. The underlying etiology should be sought and treated to relieve these sinus headaches. Rarely, atypical seizures can present as acute recurrent headaches. This is more likely if there is amnesia for the headache, an olfactory aura, or accompanying behavior changes.

Trauma-induced headaches may result from the covering soft tissues, shearing forces to the brain, or damage to the brain itself. After a brain injury, the damage may cause prolonged headaches, neurologic disability or dizziness, and the postconcussive syndrome.

Headaches that become progressively more frequent and/or severe are concerning as they are likely to be due to a growing space-occupying lesion or increasing pressure. Benign and malignant tumors, the most common solid tumors in children, can grow. Two-thirds of brain tumors are infratentorial, and these tumors are likely to cause obstruction to cerebrospinal fluid (CSF) flow. Subdural bleeds slowly increase in size; subarachnoid bleeds evolve more rapidly. Vascular malformations often grow or worsen because of bleeding into the lesion. Infections such as brain abscesses and meningitis cause swelling and mass effect. Blocking of the third or fourth ventricle or the arachnoid granulations causes an increase in the amount of CSF and a secondary increase in pressure. Idiopathic increases in pressure and pseudotumor cerebri are not rare, especially in peripubertal girls. The cause has not been identified clearly, but several possibilities are under investigation. Patients with progressive and frequent headaches warrant imaging studies to exclude tumors.

## INCREASED INTRACRANIAL PRESSURE

Depending on the age of the child, rapid head growth and the symptoms of headache and sixth cranial nerve palsies are the markers of increased intracranial pressure (ICP). Infants up to 2 years of age, whose head grow rapidly compared with their bodies, should have large sutures and open fontanels. Genetic, metabolic, and Chiari-type malformations and aqueductal abnormalities are most common in term infants. Preterm infants are more likely to have intracranial bleeds, infections, or meningoencephalitis as the cause.

## ATAXIA

The diagnosis of ataxia is based on the time course. Acute ataxias result from acute intoxications (e.g., benzodiazepines, anticonvulsants, ethanol, tricyclic antidepressants, and some antihistamines), recent head trauma, infectious or postinfectious complications [e.g., viral infections such as Epstein-Barr virus (EBV), varicella, and influenza], or a migraine. Rarely, a brain tumor or paraneoplastic syndrome presents acutely. More likely, ataxia will develop gradually over weeks.

The chronic or slowly developing ataxias usually involve brain tumors or have metabolic causes (e.g., abetalipoproteinemia, Wernicke encephalopathy, mitochondrial diseases) or result from inherited diseases (e.g., Friedreich ataxia, adrenoleukodystrophy, Niemann-Pick disease, Rett syndrome).

## MASSES

Three types of masses can present in the cranial vault: cancers and benign tumors, abscesses, and vascular malformations. All present as a result of their mass effect, causing headaches or neurologic defects. They are differentiated by imaging studies. About 50 percent of tumors are supratentorial (mostly gliomas), about 40 percent are in the posterior fossa (evenly split among gliomas, medulloblastomas, and astrocytomas), and the remainder are below the brainstem. For most, the treatment of choice is resection that sometimes is followed by radiation.

Cerebral abscesses are usually bloodborne in patients with cardiac disease. Vascular malformations are mostly congenital and present when they bleed or when they shunt blood away from some areas of the brain.

## WEAKNESS

Children who present with weakness can be divided into two categories: those with weakness with a congenital or genetic cause and those who present with the relatively acute onset of weakness.

Congenital and genetic forms of weakness can have central or peripheral etiologies. They usually present in the first months of life and may progress.

The central weaknesses usually result from a brain abnormality such as cerebral palsy or a structural abnormality such as schizencephaly. The remainder are chromosomal abnormalities such as Prader-Willi syndrome and Down syndrome. Systemic diseases such as hypothyroidism, adrenal insufficiency, and hypoparathyroidism also can cause diffuse muscle weakness.

Much more common are presentations of weakness after the first year of life. The acute-onset weaknesses are often disorders of the peripheral nerves (Guillain-Barré syndrome, Lyme disease, or traumatic injury) of the cranial nerves (Bell palsy), or of the spinal cord (trauma, vascular accident, spinal dysraphism, transverse myelitis, or spinal cord abscess).

The slower-onset presentations of weakness are the muscular dystrophies, congenital myopathies, metabolic abnormalities, and inflammatory myopathies.

---

### "Don't Miss" Diagnoses for the Central Nervous System

---

Meningitis
Headache secondary to brain tumor
Ataxia
Increased intracranial pressure

---

### BIBLIOGRAPHY

Fenichel GM. *Clinical Pediatric Neurology: A Signs and Symptoms Approach*, 5th ed. Philadelphia: Saunders, 2005.

Forsyth R, Farrell K. Headache in children. *Pediatr Rev* 20:39–45, 1999.

Provisional Committee on Quality Improvement, Subcommittee on Febrile Seizures. Practice parameter: The neurodiagnostic evaluation of the child with a first simple febrile seizure. *Pediatrics* 97:769–771, 1997.

# SELECTED TOPICS

# CARDIOLOGY

## Joseph Gigante

● LEARNING OBJECTIVES

1. Describe the differences between a benign murmur and a pathologic murmur.
2. Describe the difference between central cyanosis and peripheral cyanosis.
3. List the common causes of chest pain in children.
4. Describe the steps involved in identifying the correct diagnosis of syncope.

## MURMURS

Murmurs occur because of turbulent flow within the heart or large vessels. Many children (approximately 50 percent) have murmurs. The majority of those murmurs, approximately 90 percent, are benign and require no further evaluation. It is important to distinguish between a benign murmur and a pathologic murmur, since a pathologic murmur commonly is associated with a congenital heart malformation.

### HEART SOUNDS

The first and second heart sounds are best heard with the diaphragm of the stethoscope. The first heart sound, $S_1$, is due to closure of the mitral and tricuspid valves. It typically is heard best at the apex and the lower sternal border. The second heart sound, $S_2$, is due to closure of the aortic valve, followed by closure of the pulmonary valve. It is heard best at the left and right upper sternal borders. The time between the closures of the aortic and pulmonary valves varies with respiration; it is normally shorter with expiration and longer with inspiration. The third and fourth heart sounds ($S_3$ and $S_4$) are low-pitched and are heard best with the bell of the stethoscope. $S_3$ occurs because of sudden filling of the ventricles and may be heard in a normal child. $S_4$ is a diastolic murmur caused by atrial contraction and is always pathologic.

## HISTORY

Most children with murmurs are asymptomatic. Those who have pathologic murmurs often present with respiratory symptoms such as tachypnea, wheezing, grunting, flaring, and retractions. They also may have constitutional complaints such as diaphoresis, tiring with feeding, poor weight gain or failure to thrive, and cyanosis, which are symptoms that may be seen in patients with congestive heart failure. There are also certain underlying diseases or syndromes that have a known association with congenital heart disease, including trisomy syndromes, connective tissue diseases, and metabolic disorders. A family history of congenital heart disease is important, as there is a 1 to 4 percent risk of congenital heart disease in the sibling of an affected child.

## PHYSICAL EXAMINATION

The physical examination should begin by obtaining a complete set of vital signs, including weight, height, heart rate (regular versus irregular), respiratory rate (tachypnea), and blood pressure (upper and lower extremities). Next, the general appearance of the patient should be assessed. One should evaluate for the presence or absence of cyanosis, respiratory distress, edema, weight loss, or any phenotypic features suggestive of a syndrome with a known association with congenital heart disease, such as Down, Turner, or Marfan syndromes. Important physical findings to look for include respiratory findings such as wheezing and rales.

The cardiac examination begins with inspection. Because many children have thin chest walls, the point of maximal impulse may be visualized. Palpation of the chest wall may reveal the presence of a thrill. With palpation of the femoral and brachial pulses simultaneously, one may detect coarctation of the aorta. After inspection and palpation have been completed, the stethoscope can be used to auscultate the chest. One should auscultate the chest in a routine manner each time so that a key finding is not missed. First listen to the rate and rhythm and then listen for $S_1$, $S_2$, $S_3$, and $S_4$ and for extra sounds, such as a systolic click, that often are associated with minor valve abnormalities such as a bicuspid aortic or pulmonary valve. End the examination by listening for murmurs during both systole and diastole. Murmurs are graded on the basis of their intensity. Table 27-1 summarizes the six different murmur grades.

Conditions that increase cardiac output, such as anemia, fever, and exercise, can accentuate murmurs. Murmurs also can vary in intensity by alterations in respiration or by position change (lying down versus sitting up).

The abdominal examination should include the size and location (right-sided, midline, or left-sided) of the liver. Ascites may be present in children

*Table 27-1* **Grading Murmur Intensity**

| Grade | Intensity |
|-------|-----------|
| 1 | Soft, barely audible |
| 2 | Easily audible |
| 3 | Loud; easily audible but not accompanied by a thrill |
| 4 | Loud and associated with a thrill |
| 5 | Loud, audible with stethoscope partially off the chest |
| 6 | Loud, audible with stethoscope off the chest |

with congestive heart failure. Examination of the extremities should include an assessment of capillary refill, peripheral perfusion, and peripheral pulses. Cyanosis, edema, and/or digital clubbing may be present in children with underlying cardiac disease.

## INNOCENT MURMURS

As was noted at the beginning of this chapter, most murmurs in children are benign. These murmurs, also commonly referred to as innocent or functional murmurs, are not due to a cardiac abnormality but are caused by an abnormality of flow through the heart. A few of the more common innocent murmurs are peripheral pulmonary stenosis, Still's murmur, pulmonary flow murmur, and venous hum. Peripheral pulmonary stenosis is a murmur heard in early infancy that is caused by the bending and branching of the pulmonary artery. Still's murmur, the most common innocent murmur of early childhood, is thought to be due to the harmonic vibrations of the left ventricular outflow tract. Pulmonary flow murmur is the most common innocent murmur in older children. It is caused by the normal turbulence across the pulmonary valve and right ventricular outflow tract. Venous hum is the most common continuous murmur noted in children. It is caused by the normal, turbulent flow patterns at the junction of the innominate vein drainage into the superior vena cava. The murmur is less audible when the patient is supine or if the jugular vein is compressed. The characteristics of these innocent murmurs are summarized in Table 27-2.

## PATHOLOGIC MURMURS: ACYANOTIC VERSUS CYANOTIC

Roughly 5 to 10 percent of murmurs are pathologic. Among these murmurs, only approximately 1 percent are hemodynamically significant. The hallmark of a pathologic murmur is an abnormal cardiovascular examination, in contrast to the normal cardiovascular examination in children with innocent murmurs. Some of the characteristics of pathologic heart murmurs are listed in Table 27-3.

Table 27-2 *Characteristics of Innocent Murmurs*

| Innocent Heart Murmurs | Stills | Pulmonary Flow | PPS | Venous Hum |
|---|---|---|---|---|
| Age | Not common before age 2 years, usually seen at age 3–6 years | Common in 8- to 14-year-olds | Newborns, usually disappears by 3–6 months of age | Common at 3–6 years of age |
| Location | Loudest at LLSB | LUSB, usually with little radiation | LUSB with radiation to chest, axillae and even back | Infraclavicular/supraclavicular areas |
| Timing | Usually short and midsystolic | Short, early to midsystolic | Early to midsystolic | Continuous; diastolic louder than systolic |
| Intensity | Usually 2–3/6 | 1–3/6 | 1–2/6 | 1–2/6 |
| Quality | "Twangy," musical, or vibratory ("washing machine") | Grating or blowing | Blowing | Medium frequency |
| Physical examination | Best heard when patient is supine; increased in fever, exercise | Normal $S_2$; louder when supine | Normal $S_2$; louder when supine | Heard only in upright position; generally disappears when supine or head rotated |

LLSB = left lower sternal border;  LUSB = left upper sternal border;  PPS = peripheral pulmonic stenosis.

*Table 27-3* **Characteristics of Pathologic Heart Murmurs**

- Presence of cyanosis
- Abnormally strong or weak pulses
- Loud murmur (grades 4–6)
- Diastolic murmur
- Other abnormal heart sounds (i.e., clicks, fixed split $S_2$)
- Chest x-ray: abnormal cardiac size/silhouette or abnormal pulmonary vascularity
- Abnormal electrocardiogram

## ACYANOTIC MURMURS

Some of the more common acyanotic murmurs and the clinical features associated with them are listed below:

*Patent ductus arteriosus (PDA):* The ductus arteriosus is a normal fetal vessel that shunts blood away from the lungs to the descending aorta. It typically closes at 1 to 5 days of age in healthy term infants. When the ductus remains open, it causes a murmur that results from the pressure difference between the aorta and the pulmonary artery, leading to continuous left-to-right shunting during the cardiac cycle. This results in a characteristic continuous murmur described as "machinery-like" that is heard best inferior to the left clavicle as well as along the left second and third intercostal spaces.

*Coarctation of the aorta:* Coarctation usually occurs at the junction of the ductus arteriosus and the aortic arch, just distal to the left subclavian artery. The murmur is a systolic murmur that is heard along the left sternal border, left axilla, and back. A common finding in this diagnosis is diminished femoral pulses, along with a discrepancy between the femoral and brachial pulses, that is confirmed by a difference in upper and lower extremity blood pressures. Infants with this diagnosis often have signs of low cardiac output and poor peripheral perfusion and may be thought to have sepsis before being diagnosed with coarctation.

*Ventricular septal defect (VSD):* VSD can vary in size from small to large. The size of a VSD will determine the volume of left-to-right shunting across the ventricle. The murmur is systolic and is heard best in the left lower sternal border. As pulmonary vascular resistance decreases over the first few months of life, a greater amount of blood flow occurs across the defect, resulting in a louder murmur. Most small VSDs close spontaneously in the first 1 to 2 years of life. Interestingly, because of the turbulent blood flow that occurs across a small closing VSD, the murmur may get louder as the patient gets older.

*Atrial septal defect (ASD):* An ASD allows for passive low-pressure flow of blood from the left atrium to the right atrium. This results in increased flow across the pulmonary valve, resulting in a systolic murmur in the left upper sternal border. One of the classic findings in patients with ASD is a fixed, widely split $S_2$ caused by the large right ventricular ejection fraction.

*Aortic stenosis:* Aortic stenosis often is due to a bicuspid aortic valve. It results in a systolic, sometimes harsh murmur that is heard best at the right upper sternal border. An ejection click in early systole, just before the murmur, may be heard in mild to moderate cases.

*Pulmonary stenosis:* A bicuspid or dysplastic pulmonary valve may cause pulmonary stenosis. Children with pulmonary stenosis typically have systolic murmurs that are heard best at the left upper sternal border and often radiate to the left shoulder and back.

### CYANOTIC MURMURS

Several congenital heart diseases commonly present with cyanosis in the immediate newborn period or shortly afterward. These cyanotic congenital heart lesions are referred to commonly as the "terrible T's" or the "5 T's." These lesions are transposition of the great vessels, tetralogy of Fallot, tricuspid atresia, truncus arteriosus, and total anomalous pulmonary venous return (TAPVR). In addition to the lesions listed here, other heart lesions, such as hypoplastic left heart syndrome, can present with cyanosis. The characteristics of these lesions are listed in Table 27-4.

## CYANOSIS

Cyanosis can be defined as greater than 5 g/100 mL of desaturated hemoglobin regardless of the actual $PO_2$. An anemic patient may have a very low $PO_2$ before becoming cyanotic.

Clinically, *cyanosis* loosely means a blue or dusky color. It is a physical finding that can occur at any age but most often is a problem in neonates. It is important to differentiate between two types of cyanosis.

*Peripheral cyanosis* is blue discoloration visible only over extremities. It is common in normal newborns. It is seen commonly in infants who are exposed and become cold. It also can occur because of polycythemia and local venous obstruction.

*Central cyanosis* is a blue discoloration that involves the mouth, tongue, and mucous membranes. There are multiple etiologies for central cyanosis in the newborn. These etiologies include the following:

- Congenital heart disease with right-to-left shunt or decreased pulmonary blood flow

Table 27-4 *Characteristics of Cyanotic Congenital Heart Disease*

| Disorder | Time | Auscultation | CXR | EKG |
|---|---|---|---|---|
| TOGV | Cyanosis occurs early and is progressively severe. The degree of cyanosis depends on the degree of mixing of the two circulations | Single S₂ Murmur is usually absent unless a VSD or PS is present | Mediastinum is narrow; pulmonary vasculature may be increased | RVH with occasional RAD |
| Tricuspid atresia | Cyanosis occurs early and is intense | Single S₁, single S₂ May have loud holosystolic murmur along LSB if VSD or PS present. | Decreased pulmonary vasculature | LAD because of decreased RV forces; LVH with strain occasionally Bilateral atrial enlargement; RA may be massive LVH or BVH |
| Truncus arteriosus | Cyanosis occurs early and depends on the size of the pulmonary arteries. (Better pulmonary blood flow – less cyanosis) | Single S₂; loud pansystolic murmur is consistently present at LSB | Wide mediastinum Frequently associated with right aortic arch cardiomegaly Increased pulmonary vasculature | |
| Tetralogy of Fallot | May present at birth if PS severe or significant right-to-left shunt | Single S₂ (if P₂ soft) Loud pansystolic murmur at LSB and pulmonary ejection murmur | Boot-shaped heart Decreased pulmonary blood flow | RVH |
| TAPVR | May present early if venous return obstructed; suspect if minimal cyanosis but marked respiratory distress | Single S₂, no murmurs | Pulmonary edema with small heart, increased pulmonary blood flow | RVH |

BVH = biventricular hypertrophy; LAD = left axis deviation; LSB = left sternal body; LVH = left ventricular hypertrophy; PS = pulmonic stenosis; RA = right atrium; RAD = right axis deviation; RVH = right ventricular hypertrophy; TAPVR = total anomalous pulmonary venous return; TOGV = transportation of the great vessels; VSO = ventricular septal defect;

- Pulmonary diseases such as hyaline membrane disease, meconium aspiration, or pneumonia
- Central nervous system diseases such as intracranial hemorrhage or meningitis
- Hematologic diseases such as polycythemia or methemoglobinemia
- Infectious diseases that lead to sepsis and shock
- Metabolic disorders such as hypoglycemia

The determination of the cause of cyanosis in a neonate may be easy or exceedingly difficult. A careful history and physical examination may aid in the diagnosis.

## HISTORY

Answering the following questions will provide information that will help the clinician make the correct diagnosis. Were there any maternal/prenatal problems? Was the delivery route vaginal or caesarean? Were there any delivery problems or complications? Is the infant term or preterm? When was the cyanosis first noted? Is it worsening?

## PHYSICAL EXAMINATION

The clinician should review the vital signs. Tachypnea and/or tachycardia are suggestive of either pulmonary or cardiac disease. Fever or hypothermia is seen in infants with sepsis. Grunting, flaring, and retractions alone suggest pulmonary disease. A heart murmur or hepatosplenomegaly may be present in infants with congenital heart disease. Infants with hypotonia, lethargy, periodic shallow breathing, or apnea may have a central nervous system disorder, sepsis, or an electrolyte abnormality.

## LABORATORY AND RADIOGRAPHIC EVALUATION

The following evaluation should be considered in a newborn with cyanosis: pulse oximetry and arterial blood gas on both room air and 100% oxygen. If the oxygen tension is greater than 150 mmHg, cyanotic heart disease can be excluded. A congenital heart lesion should be strongly suspected if there is little or no change in the oxygen tension with the administration of 100% oxygen. An echocardiogram then should be performed to determine the anatomic abnormality. Other laboratory evaluation should include hematocrit, white blood cell count with differential, blood culture, chest radiograph, glucose determination, and computed tomography of the head if an intracranial hemorrhage is suspected.

## MANAGEMENT

The management of cyanosis is dependent on the identified cause of the cyanosis. The most common cause of cyanosis in a newborn is a cyanotic congenital heart defect, with treatment being dependent on the type of lesion. Many pulmonary problems that result in cyanosis will resolve partially, if not completely, after the administration of oxygen. The other causes of cyanosis should be treated appropriately once the diagnosis has been determined.

## CHEST PAIN

Chest pain is a common complaint in pediatrics. Although parents and patients often are concerned that the chest pain is due to a heart problem, previously undiagnosed cardiac disease is a rare cause of chest pain in children.

The most common diagnosis made in children with chest pain is idiopathic chest pain (no specific diagnosis can be determined). When a cause for chest pain is diagnosed, a musculoskeletal condition is the most common etiology. A history of direct trauma, exercise, or activity leading to chest muscle strain often can be elicited. Costochondritis, which often is associated with a recent viral respiratory infection, is a common disorder in children. Respiratory disorders also can be causes of chest pain. Children with asthma (especially exercise-induced asthma), pneumonia, or chronic severe cough may complain of chest pain that often is caused by overuse of chest wall muscles. Psychogenic causes of chest pain also should be considered. It is important to determine during the history whether there have been any recent stressful events at home or at school, such as illness, divorce, or school failure. It is not uncommon to elicit a recent history of a family member or friend with chest pain or cardiac disease.

Gastrointestinal disorders such as reflux esophagitis can cause chest pain that is described as burning in nature. It is worsened by reclining or eating spicy foods. Cardiac causes of chest pain, as was mentioned earlier, are rare. A family history of sudden unexpected death points toward hypertrophic cardiac myopathy or prolonged QT syndrome. Chest pain associated with syncope warrants an evaluation for a possible cardiac cause of these symptoms.

### HISTORY

The patient and/or parent should be questioned about the frequency and duration of chest pain, location, radiation, relationship with meals, and the presence of aggravating or relieving factors.

The duration and intermittency of chest pain may be useful in distinguishing significant causes of chest pain. Benign chest pain tends to be recurrent and of brief duration, often lasting seconds, and rarely persisting longer than a few minutes. For this reason, it is unusual for children to be brought for medical evaluation until the symptom has recurred a number of times. A typical history often includes episodes of brief, sharp chest pains that occur at rest and are punctuated by days or weeks of no symptoms. If patients report a more troublesome recurrence of pain and the chest wall tenderness can be reproduced, costochondritis often is diagnosed.

The past medical history may reveal a history of asthma. Previous heart disease or conditions such as Kawasaki disease may put the patient at increased risk for cardiac pathology. The family history may reveal a history of sudden death, which may be suggestive of a cardiac cause of chest pain.

## PHYSICAL EXAMINATION

The presence of fever in a patient with chest pain should raise the suspicion that the pain may be due to an infection such as pneumonia or pericarditis. The chest should be examined for signs of trauma or tenderness. Costochondritis is the probable cause of the chest pain if the tenderness is reproducible by applying pressure on the chest wall. Auscultation of the chest may reveal wheezing, rales, or decreased breath sounds if there is pulmonary pathology. Findings such as murmurs, rubs, gallops, and muffled heart sounds may be present in patients with cardiac pathology. The abdomen should be examined carefully, as it may be the source of referred chest pain.

## LABORATORY AND RADIOGRAPHIC EVALUATION

Extensive laboratory or radiographic evaluation rarely is needed for children with chest pain. It should be possible to diagnose most patients with chest pain by using the information obtained from the history and physical examination. A patient with a normal history and physical examination rarely has pathology, and routine tests and referrals are not necessary. A chest radiograph may be indicated in patients with suspected pulmonary or cardiac disease. An electrocardiogram may be indicated in patients with suspected cardiac disease but, unlike the case in adult patients, is not performed routinely on all patients presenting with chest pain. Chest pain associated with syncope, physical activity, or palpitations or a racing sensation should be referred to a pediatric cardiologist for further evaluation.

## MANAGEMENT

The mainstay of therapy in patients with chest pain is reassurance since most of these patients will not have any pathology causing the pain. Patients and their families often want to hear that the patient's heart is normal, and so it is important to address this with the family members and counsel them on the often benign course of pediatric chest pain. Follow-up visits may be necessary as chest pain is often recurrent. Chest pain related to a specific organic cause should be treated appropriately (e.g., rest and analgesics for costochondritis, antacids for reflux esophagitis).

# SYNCOPE

Syncope can be defined as a brief loss of consciousness and muscle tone as a result of a transient decrease in cerebral perfusion. It is a common complaint, as 15 percent of children experience syncope before the end of adolescence. Although there are many causes of syncope, the etiologies can be grouped into three main categories: neurocardiogenic, cardiogenic, and noncardiogenic. Neurocardiogenic (vasovagal) syncope is thought to account for approximately three-quarters of children with syncope. The other causes include cardiac syncope resulting from structural heart disease (hypertrophic cardiomyopathy, anomalous coronary artery) and arrhythmias (prolonged QT syndrome, Wolff-Parkinson-White syndrome). Other noncardiac causes include migraines, seizures, metabolic causes (hypoglycemia), toxins and drugs, hyperventilation, and conversion reactions.

## PATHOPHYSIOLOGY

Regardless of the cause, the pathophysiology of syncope usually results from cerebral perfusion that is compromised by a transient decrease in cardiac output caused by vasomotor changes that decrease venous return. With regard to neurocardiogenic syncope, the physiologic basis for the event is decreased venous return that results in decreased left ventricular volume, increased contractility, and stimulation of the cardiac vagal fibers, which can cause hypotension, bradycardia, and vasodilation. Thus, hypotension, the bradycardia, or a combination of the two can lead to decreased cerebral perfusion and syncope. Nausea, sweating, pallor, light-headedness, and shortness of breath typically precede such episodes. Prolonged standing, pain, fear, exhaustion, a recent illness, dehydration, anemia, the sight of blood, pregnancy, and temper tantrums (breath-holding spells) are among the many triggers for neurocardiogenic syncope.

## HISTORY

The information obtained in the history is often the key in diagnosing the cause of a syncopal event. It should be obtained not only from the patient but also from anyone who was present and witnessed the event. Specific questions should be asked pertaining to the following:

- Presence of any presyncopal symptoms, such as dizziness, light-headedness, weakness, pallor, and sweating (suggestive of neurocardiogenic syncope)
- The situation and antecedents of the episode (an event associated with exercise suggests cardiac syncope; a syncopal event at rest suggests seizures or arrhythmias)
- The duration of the event (syncope is transient and usually resolves with a recumbent position)

The past medical history may reveal an associated disease that may predispose the patient to syncope. A medication history may reveal prescription, over-the-counter, or illicit drugs that may have precipitated the event. The patient should be asked about any family history of sudden death or seizures.

## PHYSICAL EXAMINATION

The physical examination of patients with syncope often is normal. The physical examination should focus on vital signs, a cardiac examination, and a neurologic examination. Measurement of vital signs is important. Approximately 90 percent of cases of orthostatic hypotension occur within 2 min of standing upright. The cardiac examination may reveal a murmur or arrhythmia; a neurologic examination immediately after the event may reveal a postictal state consistent with a seizure.

## LABORATORY AND RADIOGRAPHIC EVALUATION

The laboratory and radiographic studies ordered in patients with syncope will be guided by the results of the history and physical examination. The tilt table test has become the test of choice for diagnosing neurocardiogenic syncope. An electrocardiogram is recommended for cases of unexplained syncope, especially in patients in whom an arrhythmia is suspected. A cardiology consultation may be warranted to help guide further testing if a cardiac cause of syncope is suspected. Serum electrolytes and glucose may be useful in an acute episode. An electroencephalogram (EEG) or neuroimaging may help with suspected seizures.

## MANAGEMENT

Management is based on the specific cause for syncope. Those with neurocardiogenic syncope often can be managed with changes such as increasing salt and water intake, eating regularly, avoiding noxious stimuli that precipitate syncope, and lying down before losing consciousness. Occasionally these patients also are treated with a mineralocorticoid such as fludrocortisone. Cardiac disease may require antiarrhythmics or surgery. Seizures may require anticonvulsants. There are a variety of medications available for the treatment of migraines.

## BIBLIOGRAPHY

Brumund MR, Strong WB. Murmurs, fainting and chest pain: Time for a cardiology referral? *Contemp Pediatr* 19:155–159, 2002.

Cava JR, Sayger PL. Chest pain in children and adolescents. *Pediatr Clin North Am* 51:1553–1568, 2004.

Willis J. Syncope. *Pediatr Rev* 21:201–204, 2000.

# PEDIATRIC ENDOCRINOLOGY

*Aida Yared*

## LEARNING OBJECTIVES

1. Know that diabetes mellitus (DM) is common in children.

2. Recognize the clinical presentation of DM and the clinical and laboratory findings in diabetic ketoacidosis.

3. Know the management of DM acutely (fluids, insulin) and chronically (insulin, diet, monitoring)

4. Know the causes and clinical findings of congenital and acquired hypothyroidism.

5. Understand that untreated congenital hypothyroidism can cause permanent mental retardation.

6. Know the highlights of adrenal steroidogenesis and the most common congenital enzymatic deficiencies.

7. Recognize that ambiguous genitalia most commonly are due to congenital adrenal hyperplasia.

8. Know the side effects of corticosteroids. Know that intake of oral steroids (prednisone) is the most common cause of Cushing syndrome in children.

9. Plot and interpret a growth chart. Differentiate normal variants (familial short stature, constitutional delay) from medical problems (growth hormone deficiency, hypothyroidism).

10. Know the sequence and timing of changes in normal puberty (Tanner stages) and the possible abnormalities.

11. Recognize the clinical features and causes of rickets.

## INTRODUCTION

### COMMON MEASUREMENTS

*Length/height, weight, and head circumference:* These parameters are plotted sequentially on *growth curves*. Length is measured in infants still unable to stand, and height is measured in older children.

*Growth rate:* Increase in length or height per unit time. It varies with age, with three phases being recognized: infantile (30 to 35 cm in the first year of life), childhood (5 to 7 cm per year), and pubertal ("growth spurt" of 7 to 14 cm per year).

*Arm span:* Used in assessing body proportions. In a normal child, arm span equals height. If arm span is longer than height, it suggests Marfan or Klinefelter syndrome; if it is shorter, it suggests an osteochondrodysplasia such as hypochondroplasia or achondroplasia.

*Height of both parents:* Used to calculate *midparental height,* a rough predictor of the genetic height potential of a child. The formula is as follows:

$$\text{Boy's predicted stature} = \frac{(\text{mother's height} + 13 \text{ cm}) + \text{father's height}}{2}$$

$$\text{Girl's predicted stature} = \frac{\text{mother's height} + (\text{father's height} - 13 \text{ cm})}{2}$$

Commonly, the parents' heights are averaged, and 6.5 cm is added for a boy or subtracted for a girl.

*Tanner stages:* Used for the staging of pubertal changes. It assigns a stage (1 through 5) for breast development in girls, external genital development (testes, scrotum, and penis) in boys, and pubic hair in both sexes. A child thus is assigned two Tanner stages. Tanner 1 is prepubertal.

### COMMON DEFINITIONS

*Hypoglycemia* is a blood sugar < 40mg/dL in a newborn and < 70 mg/dL thereafter.

*Hyperglycemia* is a blood sugar > 120 mg/dL.

*Diabetic ketoacidosis (DKA)* is the decompensated picture of diabetes mellitus. DKA is present when there is hyperglycemia (glucose > 300 mg/dL), acidosis (pH < 7.25, bicarbonate < 15 mEq/L), and ketosis (ketones in blood and urine). DKA can be the presentation of diabetes mellitus (DM), can occur in a diabetic patient who skipped insulin dosing, or can be precipitated by infection, stress, or pubertal changes.

*Congenital adrenal hyperplasia (CAH),* or *adrenogenital syndrome,* is a set of congenital enzymatic deficiencies in the adrenal steroid pathways that have in common deficient production of cortisol, the only steroid that feeds back on (i.e., suppresses) adrenocorticotropic hormone (ACTH). ACTH is high, causing hyperplasia of the glands and increases in all the pathways proximal to the enzyme defect.

*Glucocorticoids* are hormones that are elaborated in the zona fasciculata of the adrenal gland, such as cortisol. They have potent anti-inflammatory action, promote fat deposition and protein and glycogen breakdown, and help maintain blood sugar. They are important under stress.

*Mineralocorticoids* are hormones that are elaborated by the zona glomerulosa of the adrenal gland, such as deoxycortisol (DOC) and aldosterone. They cause sodium retention and potassium secretion and thus help maintain volume and blood pressure (BP). Their excess leads to hypertension.

The *adrenal sex hormones* androstenedione, dehydroepiandrosterone (DHEA), and its sulfate DHEA-S are weak androgens that are elaborated by the zona reticulata of the adrenal gland.

*Short stature* is height below the 5th percentile, or 2 standard deviations (SD) below the mean, for age and sex.

*Tall stature* is height above the 95th percentile, or 2 SD above the mean, for age and sex.

*Projected height* is an estimate of the expected adult height of a child. A rough estimate is height at 2 years of age × 2.

*Growth failure* is a suboptimal growth rate. In childhood, it is defined as < 5 cm per year.

*Adrenarche* is the maturational increase in adrenal androgen production, which represents a change in the adrenal secretory response to ACTH, with 17-OH pregnenolone and DHEA increases relative to cortisol. It clinically manifests with pubic and axillary hair.

*Pubarche* is the appearance of pubic hair. Premature pubarche is four times more common in girls than in boys.

*Puberty* is the sequential development of secondary sex characteristics. The first sign in boys is testicular enlargement, followed by penile enlargement (12 to 18 months later), a growth spurt, and pubic hair growth; spermatogenesis occurs at a mean age of 13.5 years. In girls, the first sign is breast enlargement, followed by pubic hair, a growth spurt, and then menarche (2 years later).

*Premature* or *precocious puberty* traditionally is defined as < 8 years in girls and < 9 years in boys. Recently, the definition has been revised, and workup is warranted in a Caucasian girl with breast development or pubic hair < 7 years, an African-American girl < 6, and a boy < 9 years.

*Thelarche* is breast development in a girl.

*Gynecomastia* is breast development in a boy.

## COMMON LABORATORY STUDIES

*Hemoglobin A1c (Hb A1c)*, or glycosylated hemoglobin, reflects the state of glycemia over the life span of a red blood cell. It usually is measured every 3 months in a child with DM to assess control over that time span.

Normal is < 6 percent; the target level in DM patients is 7 to 8 percent; a level > 9 percent indicates poor control.

*Insulin and C-peptide.* Insulin and C-peptide can be measured to differentiate type 1 from type 2 DM. C-peptide is formed during the conversion of proinsulin to insulin and reflects the availability of insulin. An insulin level <5 μU/mL or a peptide level <0.6 ng/mL indicates type 1 DM.

*Thyroid function tests (TFTs).* The thyroid hormones measured are $T_4$ (the one in the largest amount in circulation) and $T_3$ (more potent, derived mostly from the peripheral conversion of $T_4$). $T_4$ (or free $T_4$), $T_3$, and thyroid-stimulating hormone (TSH) usually are measured. High TSH is expected in primary (thyroid) as opposed to central (pituitary) hypothyroidism.

*Antithyroid antibodies* are measured in the workup of suspected thyroiditis.

*17-OH progesterone* is a key compound in steroidogenesis. It is the crossroad for many enzymatic deficiencies that lead to CAH, including the most common 21-OHase deficiency.

The *DHEA level* is measured as a marker of adrenal sex hormone production. The *testosterone level* is measured as a marker of testicular sex hormone production.

*Follicle-stimulating hormone (FSH)* and *luteinizing hormone (LH)* are measured to differentiate precocious puberty (high) from pseudo-precocious puberty (prepubertal).

A *karyotype* may be ordered in the workup of short stature (to rule out Turner syndrome) or tall stature (to rule out Klinefelter syndrome) or as part of sex assignment in CAH.

## COMMON PROCEDURES

*Growth hormone (GH) stimulation tests* measure serum levels of GH in response to stimuli (sleep, insulin, exercise, arginine, L-dopa, growth hormone-releasing hormone) in the evaluation of GH deficiency. The diagnosis of GH deficiency requires two abnormal provocative tests. The usefulness of provocative tests in the workup of GH disorders is controversial.

*Insulin-like growth factors 1 and 2 (IGF-1 and IGF-2)* and *insulin growth factor binding protein 3 (IGFBP-3) radioimmunoassays* are replacing provocative tests in the diagnosis of GH disorders. IGF-1 is a hormone secreted by the liver that largely mediates the action of GH on its target cells. IGFBP-3 is the major carrier protein for IGFs.

*ACTH stimulation test* is used to study the responsiveness of the adrenal gland to stimulation by ACTH, including the relative ratios of various adrenal products, in the workup of pubertal disorders. It also is used to assess adrenal responsiveness in suspected Addison disease.

The *dexamethasone suppression test* is used to determine whether high levels of cortisol are autonomous (e.g., adrenal tumor) and in the evaluation of premature adrenarche.

## COMMON IMAGING STUDIES

*Bone age (BA):* X-rays of the left hand and wrist are obtained. BA commonly is determined by comparing various parameters (appearance of ossification centers, contour of bones, and thinning of growth plates) to an atlas of standards for the same sex and finding the closest overall match. BA is normal if it is within 2 SD of chronologic age (CA).

*Brain magnetic resonance imaging (MRI):* Brain MRI is used for imaging of the brain, pituitary, and hypothalamus in suspected pituitary disorders.

*Adrenal ultrasound:* Adrenal ultrasound is used to image the adrenal glands, for example, for CAH. Normal adrenals are visualized as thin lines overlying the kidneys; a hyperplastic gland is visible as a plump triangular structure.

*Pelvic ultrasound:* Pelvic ultrasound is used to image the ovaries (e.g., in the evaluation of precocious puberty or in suspected polycystic ovary syndrome) and in the workup of ambiguous genitalia.

*Knee x-ray:* An anteroposterior view of the knees is the best radiologic test for diagnosing rickets in a child < 3 years old.

## COMMON TREATMENTS

*Insulin:* Recombinant insulin is given in the treatment of DM. It is available in four forms—ultra short (Lispro or Humalog), short (regular), intermediate (NPH), and long-acting (ultralente)—with the onset of action gradually lengthening from 10 min to 4 h, and the duration of action from 1 to 2 h to 24 h. DM is treated by trying to replicate insulin's physiologic release with a once-a-day longer-acting dose or twice-a-day NPH to establish a basal level and shorter-acting doses added three or four times a day with meals.

*Insulin pump:* An insulin pump may be used in motivated teenagers. It provides better control of DM but requires more frequent monitoring of blood sugar (six to eight times a day). It is about the size of a beeper and is worn with a belt around the waist.

*Glucagon:* Glucagon is part of the "emergency kit" of a diabetic child for the treatment of hypoglycemia when oral intake of sugar is not an option (e.g., an obtunded child). It can be administered intramuscularly (IM), subcutaneously (SC), or intravenously (IV) at 1 mg per dose.

*Thyroxin ($T_4$):* Thyroxin is used as replacement therapy in hypothyroidism. $T_4$ is never given as a suspension, as the effective dose may vary. It is available in pills of various doses, color-coded for ease of recognition, and crushed for administration to infants.

*Hydrocortisone:* Hydrocortisone is used as glucocorticoid replacement in patients with Addison disease or CAH. It is given as a physiologic dose under normal circumstances and doubled during stress such as infection or surgery.

*Florinef* or *fludrocortisone:* Fludrocortisone is used as mineralocorticoid replacement in Addison disease and in salt-losing CAH.

GH. Available as a recombinant, GH is approved for the treatment of growth failure resulting from growth hormone deficiency, Turner syndrome, chronic renal failure, Prader-Willi syndrome, and (controversially) idiopathic short stature. It is given SC at 0.3 mg/kg weekly or divided into daily doses.

*Gonadotropin-releasing hormone (GnRH) antagonist:* A synthetic analog of the amino acid sequence of natural GnRH, GnRH antagonist blocks the effect of endogenous GnRH and is used to counter precocious puberty.

*Vitamin D:* The Recommended Daily Allowance (RDA) is 400 U a day in children; pharmacologic doses are used in the treatment of rickets. *Calcitriol* is 1,25(OH)$_2$ vitamin D, the active form sometimes used orally in the treatment of rickets.

## COMMON SIGNS AND SYMPTOMS

### HYPOGLYCEMIA

In newborns, the findings are nonspecific: jitteriness or seizures, cyanosis, apnea, poor feeding, and hypothermia. In older children, the signs and symptoms are hunger, perspiration, light-headedness, and weakness. Nocturnal hypoglycemia may present with disordered sleep or nightmares.

*Neonatal hypoglycemia* can be due to the following:

- Lack of (glycogen) substrate. This is common and transient, often resulting from prematurity, prolonged delivery, or sepsis.
- Insulin excess. In an infant of a diabetic mother, because of the high blood sugar of the mother when the infant is in utero, there is pancreatic release of insulin and islet cell hyperplasia in the fetus.
- Deficiency in hormones that counter insulin, such as GH and cortisol.
- Metabolic disorders such as glycogen storage diseases or galactosemia.

### HYPOGLYCEMIA IN AN OLDER CHILD

Ketotic hypoglycemia is seen between 6 months and 6 years of age; it is basically the inability to adapt to normal fasting. It is managed with frequent feeding of high-carbohydrate foods during "at risk" periods. Reactive hypoglycemia may occur in otherwise normal individuals (especially well-trained athletes) within 4 h of eating and also is managed with dietary modification. Hypoglycemia can occur in a diabetic patient who skipped meals, exercised, or took too much insulin. It rarely is due to (accidental) ingestion of oral hypoglycemics or alcohol.

## HYPERGLYCEMIA

Hyperglycemia usually raises the concern of DM. However, it can be a transient finding after a carbohydrate meal, during IV infusion of glucose-containing fluids, or after steroid administration.

## SHORT STATURE

Nutritional and genetic, environmental, and hormonal factors affect growth.

- Nutritional deficiency is a common cause of growth failure in infants. Typically, weight is affected more than is height or head circumference.
- Familial short stature. The annual growth rate is normal, height follows a curve at a low percentile, BA = CA, and the parents are short.
- Constitutional delay. These children are smaller than their peers during adolescence and then catch up in high school ("late bloomers"). A family history in the parents is often present. Height is at the lower percentiles, growth rate is < 5 cm a year, and puberty and BA are delayed. The ultimate height is normal.
- Endocrine causes (GH deficiency, hypothyroidism).
- Metabolic causes and any chronic disorder (congenital heart disease, chronic lung disease, renal failure, renal tubular acidosis).
- Genetic causes (Turner or Noonan syndrome, osteochondrodysplasia, or other forms of genetic dwarfism).

The workup includes growth curves, parental height, family history (helpful for familial short stature, constitutional delay, and some genetic causes), and review of systems (crucial in hypothyroidism). Physical examination includes height and weight; blood pressure; body proportions; examination of the skin and hair (hypothyroidism), hands, feet, and jaw (GH); distribution of fat (GH deficiency, Cushing syndrome); skeletal anomalies (skeletal disorders, rickets, Turner syndrome); cardiac examination (Turner, Noonan, Marfan syndromes); and Tanner staging. Laboratory tests may include complete blood count (CBC), electrolytes, calcium, phosphorus, creatinine, bone age, TFTs, karyotype, GH testing, and head imaging.

## TALL STATURE

This may be a normal variant: familial tall stature. Hormonal causes include GH excess (gigantism) and sex steroids excess (precocious puberty or adrenal hyperplasia). Genetic and metabolic causes include Klinefelter or Marfan syndrome and homocystinuria (clinically very similar to Marfan syndrome). Cerebral gigantism causes tall stature with mental retardation.

## DELAYED PUBERTY

Delayed sexual maturation is lack of puberty in a girl > 13 years or a boy > 15 years. The most common cause is constitutional delay, which often is familial. Hormonal deficiencies can occur but are uncommon.

## PREMATURE SEXUAL CHARACTERISTICS

*Thelarche* is the appearance of breasts in a girl < 3 years old. If there are no other changes (growth acceleration, estrogen effect on vaginal mucosa), it is termed *benign premature thelarche*. Exposure to estrogens (e.g., topical Premarin in the treatment of labial adhesions) must be ruled out. Follow-up is required to ascertain that no other features of premature puberty develop later.

*Gynecomastia* is normal and common around puberty, affecting, usually transiently, 40 percent of boys; it may be unilateral.

*Isolated premature pubarche* is the appearance of pubic hair in a girl < 8 years old. This is quite common and is benign as an isolated finding. If, however, other signs of androgen excess are present (enlargement of the clitoris, acne, acceleration in growth, voice change), endocrine problems must be ruled out.

*Precocious puberty* is puberty at < 8 years in girls and < 9 years in boys. This should be investigated thoroughly, although the chances of finding a cause in a girl are very small and are around 50 percent in a boy. A hypothalamic tumor or other endocrine problem must be ruled out.

*Precocious pseudo-puberty*, or "false puberty," can occur with intake of hormones or with tumors (ovarian, adrenal, or testicular) that secrete sex hormones.

Workup of premature sexual characteristics includes BA, FSH, and LH levels; TFTs; sex hormone levels; pelvic ultrasound; and brain MRI.

## AMBIGUOUS GENITALIA

In a female, this is due to exposure to androgens in utero (e.g., CAH, maternal intake of androgens). In a male, it can be due to CAH or testicular feminization (a rare disorder with lack of receptors for androgens). The workup includes karyotype, pelvic ultrasound, and 17-OH progesterone and other adrenal hormone levels. Treatment is of the adrenal disorder if present, early sex assignment, corrective surgery as needed, and hormone replacement as needed.

## BONE METABOLISM DISORDERS

*Hypocalcemia.* Manifestations are neuromuscular irritability: tetany, jitteriness, or seizures. Hypocalcemia in a newborn can be a transient finding resulting from birth stress, maternal DM, or maternal hyperparathyroidism; it also can be due to absence of the parathyroid glands (Di George syndrome). Older children can have primary hypoparathyroidism or pseudohypoparathyroidism. The workup includes blood studies [serum creatinine, calcium and phosphorus, alkaline phosphatase, parathyroid hormone (PTH) level, vitamin D levels], and a chest x-ray to ascertain the presence of a thymus. Treatment consists of calcium replacement and vitamin D as needed.

*Hypercalcemia.* Hypercalcemia is rare in pediatrics and can be due to immobilization (accidents, casts), parathyroid problems, or a malignancy.

*Rickets.* Bone mineralization depends on adequate plasma concentrations of calcium and phosphorus; throughout childhood, serum phosphorus levels and the product [calcium × phosphorus] are relatively high. Rickets develops if serum calcium or phosphorus is low. Growing bone is not well mineralized; hence, bones are soft and growth plates are wide. A common initial presentation is hypotonia. Skeletal manifestations in an infant are a box-shaped head (caput quadratum), large fontanels, prominent costochondral junctions (rosary beads), and wide wrists and ankles (double malleoli). In an older child, poor growth and bowing of the legs can become evident. X-rays show poor mineralization. The causes of rickets include nutritional vitamin D deficiency. Chronic renal failure can lead to a lack of active vitamin D. Less common causes are vitamin D–resistant rickets, vitamin D–dependent rickets, and familial hypophosphatemic rickets. The workup includes serum creatinine, electrolytes, calcium, phosphorus, alkaline phosphatase, and vitamin D levels. Rickets can be confirmed by x-rays. Treatment consists of supplementation of vitamin D and calcium/phosphorus as needed.

## COMMON DISEASES

### DIABETES MELLITUS

DM is the most common pediatric endocrine problem. Type 1 (insulin deficiency) is the usual childhood form, with a prevalence of 1 in 500 and an incidence of 15 per 100,000 new cases per year in children <18 years old. It is more common in whites than in other ethnic groups. Type 2 (insulin resistance) is an emerging concern in overweight teenagers.

*Insulin* is a hormone secreted by the beta cells of the islets of Langerhans in the pancreas that permits glucose to enter into cells. Lack of insulin leads to hyperglycemia, with osmotic diuresis (polyuria) and hence polydipsia, hunger, and polyphagia with weight loss. When unrecognized or untreated, DM progresses to vomiting, abdominal pain, and mental changes, culminating in coma (DKA).

DM is associated with autoimmune disorders (Hashimoto, Graves', Addison diseases). It has a genetic predisposition: Over 90 percent of these patients have specific human leukocyte antigen (HLA) antigens. Siblings have a 5 percent risk of DM, and 50 percent if they are identical twins. Immunity, environment, viruses, and "stress" also may play a role.

## PATHOPHYSIOLOGY

Normally, blood glucose level is tightly regulated at around 80 to 100 mg/dL. After a meal, the serum level of insulin increases, allowing glucose to enter the cells and be used as fuel or stored as glycogen. During "fasting," a variety of hormones (GH, steroids, catecholamines, glucagon) help maintain serum glucose by inducing glycogenolysis and gluconeogenesis, and fat is broken down. The same mechanisms are activated in DM, even though glucose is present, because glucose is unavailable to cells. Despite hyperglycemia, the child is hungry and polyphagic but loses weight. Fats are broken down, producing ketoacids.

## HISTORY AND PHYSICAL EXAMINATION

Most of these patients present with polyuria, polydipsia, polyphagia (with weight loss), and lassitude. Blood glucose is high, and glucosuria is present. Ten percent of patients with new onset DM present in DKA (most commonly 2- to 3-year-olds). DKA usually develops over several days: The child gradually becomes dehydrated and lethargic, with vomiting and abdominal pain. Acidosis leads to hyperventilation with deep rapid (Kussmaul) breathing. Laboratory tests show hyperglycemia and glucosuria, ketosis, acidosis, hyponatremia, and azotemia. The white blood cell (WBC) count is often high even when there is no infection. Treatment of DKA consists of initial replacement of fluid and electrolytes (normal saline with potassium added as the serum potassium level decreases). Insulin is given IV at an initial dose of 0.1 unit/kg per h. Bicarbonate is rarely needed; it may be used if the pH is < 7.10. The metabolic disturbances gradually correct over 24 to 36 h. Too rapid a correction may lead to brain edema. When serum glucose reaches 200 to 300 mg/dL, glucose is added to the IV as D5 or D10. Once ketosis is resolved, IV insulin is discontinued and SC insulin is started.

## MANAGEMENT

A new diabetic must be taught about the disease, the dosage and administration of insulin, monitoring of blood and urine glucose levels and logging them in a "diabetes diary," and diet. The mainstay of chronic treatment is insulin administration. A typical stable diabetic patient receives 1 unit/kg per day divided into three or four daily doses. The insulin requirement decreases with exercise and increases during puberty and infections. The goal of control is a glucose level 100 to 200 mg/dL in a younger child, 80 to 180 at 5 to 11 years, and 70 to 150 above 12 years. The family is instructed that serum glucose values < 70 or > 180 mg/dL require attention. Hypoglycemia may manifest with sweating, tremor, anxiety, or mental status changes; it may follow exercise, lack of oral intake, or an excessive insulin dose. It should be treated immediately with oral sugar (glucose tablet, soft drink, or hard candy); in a child unable to receive glucose, glucagon is administered. Caloric requirements for DM are the same as those for a normal child. Calories should come 55 percent from complex carbohydrates, 30 percent from fat, and 15 percent from protein. Food intake is divided into three meals and three snacks.

Follow-up includes review of home monitoring diaries, growth (height and weight), pubertal development, recognition of infections (at insulin injection sites, vulvovaginitis in a girl), and complications. Chronic control is assessed by Hb A1c, which is followed every 3 months. Long-term complications of DM, though rarely seen in pediatrics, include nephropathy (high blood pressure, proteinuria, and chronic renal failure), retinopathy, and vascular complications.

## THYROID DISORDERS

Thyroid hormone plays a major role in metabolism and heat production and is important for skeletal growth and maturation and for neurologic development. A deficiency of thyroid hormone before 2 years of age may result in severe and permanent mental retardation.

### CONGENITAL HYPOTHYROIDISM

Congenital hypothyroidism affects 1 in 4000 births. In over 90 percent of cases, there is an absent or poorly formed gland; hence, $T_4$ is low and TSH is high. Less frequently (5 percent), congenital hypothyroidism is due to an enzymatic defect in the synthesis of $T_4$ (associated with a goiter) or to maternal thyroid problems. Its clinical manifestations can be missed easily. A "typical" hypothyroid baby is full term and large in size (> 4 kg), with a large posterior fontanel, lethargy, an umbilical hernia, mottling, a large tongue, dry skin, and a hoarse cry. Symptoms are constipation, hypothermia, and prolonged physiologic jaundice. However, most of these babies appear normal, which validates neonatal screening for hypothyroidism. Breast-feeding has a mildly protective effect in hypothyroid newborns.

### ACQUIRED HYPOTHYROIDISM

The most common cause of acquired hypothyroidism in the United States is thyroiditis. Its incidence is around 1 in 500, peaking in adolescence and affecting females more than males. These patients will have a goiter. A less common cause is iodine deficiency (as table salt often is supplemented with iodine). Manifestations include a slowing in linear growth (with no weight loss), dull facies, a large tongue, dry skin, and coarse brittle hair. Symptoms may include cold intolerance, constipation, and developmental delay. Physical examination may reveal hypotonia, delayed relaxation of reflexes, myxedema, carotenemia, and a hoarse voice. Teenagers may present with weight gain or menstrual irregularities (precocious or delayed puberty). BA is delayed.

## Hyperthyroidism

The manifestations of hyperthyroidism in children include nervousness, palpitations, tachycardia, atrial arrhythmia, increased sweating, heat intolerance, fatigue, weight loss, increased appetite, and increased bowel movements. Examination may reveal systolic hypertension, fine tremors, brisk reflexes, proptosis, and stare. The most common cause is Graves' disease caused by antibodies and thyroid-stimulating immunoglobulins (TSIs) that stimulate the thyroid. The gland is often enlarged and palpable. Since the TSI antibodies can cross the placenta, a mother with Graves' disease can have a baby with transient hyperthyroidism (irritability, tachycardia, heart failure); treatment of the baby with antithyroid drugs may be needed for 2 or 3 months. Tumors of the thyroid are rare, presenting as hard painless nodules, mostly in girls at a mean age of 9 years.

## ADRENAL DISORDERS

### Addison Disease

Addison disease involves adrenal insufficiency. Most causes of adrenal insufficiency are acquired and include severe infection with shock or disseminated intravascular coagulation (e.g., neonatal asphyxia, meningococcemia), local infection (tuberculosis), and autoimmune disorders. Prolonged courses of oral steroids may suppress the adrenal glands and lead to adrenal insufficiency if they are discontinued abruptly.

### Congenital Adrenal Hyperplasia

The clinical manifestations depend on the enzyme that is lacking.

- Deficiency in glucocorticoids leads to weakness, hypoglycemia, low stress tolerance, and hypotension/shock.
- Deficiency of mineralocorticoids leads to hypotension, vomiting, weakness, hyponatremia, hyperkalemia, and acidosis. An excess leads to hypertension and hypokalemia.
- Deficiency or excess of adrenal androgens manifests differently in a boy versus a girl. An excess leads to ambiguous genitalia (virilization) in a girl but no genital abnormalities in a boy. A deficiency leads to ambiguous genitalia in a boy but no abnormalities in a girl. An excess leads to growth acceleration.

The most common deficiency is 21-hydroxlyase deficiency, which accounts for 95 percent of cases of CAH. It is an autosomal recessive disorder. This is a neonatal emergency. There are no mineralocorticoids or glucocorticoids; therefore, there is salt wasting, hyponatremia, hyperkalemia, acidosis, vomiting, dehydration, and shock, which start soon after birth. There is excess adrenal androgens, and so a female will have ambiguous genitalia. Laboratory data reveal low cortisol and aldosterone and high 17 OH-progesterone. Treatment consists of hormone replacement and sex assignment and surgery as needed. A deficiency of 11-OHase causes salt retention and hypertension in addition to the effects of androgens.

## CUSHING SYNDROME

Cushing syndrome involves adrenal excess. It manifests with truncal obesity and moon facies, plethora, striae, and growth and pubertal delay. It is rare as a primary disorder in children and results from an adrenal tumor or a pituitary adenoma. Most commonly, it is iatrogenic, resulting from the use of prednisone in conditions such as nephrotic syndrome, asthma, allergies, organ transplantation, and chemotherapy. The side effects of prednisone, in addition to the ones listed above, include hirsutism, acne, hypertension, osteoporosis, aseptic necrosis of the hips, cataracts, and hyperglycemia. They can be minimized if prednisone is given as a single morning dose on alternate days and gradually tapered after a prolonged course.

## GROWTH DISORDERS

### GH DEFICIENCY

GH deficiency has an incidence of 1 in 10,000, can be inherited or sporadic, and can be due to anatomic defects in newborns or craniopharyngioma in older children. It presents with growth failure and mild adiposity. Additional findings may be hypoglycemia and a small phallus. The workup reveals decreased GH to stimulation (or decreased IGFs and IGFBPs) and delayed BA. Treatment consists of GH replacement.

### TURNER SYNDROME

The karyotype is XO. Short stature is the most common feature; others are webbing of the neck, a low posterior hairline, cubitus valgus, and left-sided (aortic) cardiac anomalies. If untreated, the average ultimate height is 140 to 145 cm.

### NOONAN SYNDROME

Noonan syndrome is an autosomal dominant disease that occurs in both sexes. It manifests with growth failure and features similar to those of Turner syndrome except that cardiac anomalies are primarily right-sided (pulmonary valve).

Other growth disorders include the following:

*Prader Willi syndrome* is characterized by hypotonia neonatally; with age, growth failure and hyperphagia with obesity are the hallmarks of the syndrome. Cryptorchidism and microphallus are often present.

*Beckwith-Wiedemann syndrome* presents neonatally with macrosomia, omphalocele, a big tongue, hepatomegaly, and hypoglycemia.

*GH excess* in childhood is rare and usually is due to a pituitary tumor. It leads to gigantism or acromegaly (tall stature with overgrowth of bones and soft tissues, a prominent jaw, and large hands and feet).

*Marfan syndrome* includes tall stature with increased arm span and dislocation of the lenses; it carries a risk of later aortic regurgitation.

## PUBERTAL DISORDERS

*Klinefelter syndrome (XXY)* is the most common chromosomal disorder associated with male hypogonadism and infertility. It is characterized by hypogonadism (small testes, later oligospermia) and gynecomastia during puberty. Infants and children initially have normal height, weight, and head circumferences; then height velocity increases (by age 5). Adult height is usually taller than average. Affected individuals have disproportionately long arms and legs.

*Premature adrenarche* is a benign condition, though its association with future polycystic ovary syndrome or type 2 DM is increasingly recognized.

*McCune Albright syndrome* in females is characterized by the triad of precocious puberty, polyostotic fibrous dysplasia. and café-au-lait spots.

## BONE METABOLISM DISORDERS

*Di George syndrome* presents neonatally with hypocalcemia and a peculiar facies; the thymus is absent.

*Vitamin D deficiency* can be nutritional. It occurs typically in a breast-fed infant with a dark complexion who is not exposed to sunlight and not supplemented with vitamin D, especially in rapidly growing premature babies.

*Vitamin D resistance* denotes end-organ resistance to vitamin D, requiring pharmacologic doses.

*Hypophosphatemic rickets* is a genetic renal tubule disorder with urinary phosphorus loss.

*Pseudohypoparathyroidism* manifests with growth failure and hypocalcemia; it is due to end-organ resistance to PTH. Truncal obesity and short metacarpals are common findings.

## BIBLIOGRAPHY

American Academy of Pediatrics. Evaluation of the newborn with developmental anomalies of the external genitalia. *Pediatr* 106:138–142, 2000.

American Diabetes Association. http://www.diabetes.org.

Juvenile Diabetes Research Foundation. http://www.jdrf.org.

Little People of America. http://www.lpaonline.org.

National Institute of Diabetes & Digestive & Kidney Diseases. http://www.niddk.nih.gov

Prevention of rickets and vitamin D deficiency: New guidelines for vitamin D intake. *Pediatr* 111:908–910, 2003.

# CHAPTER 29

# GENETICS

*Aida Yared*

## LEARNING OBJECTIVES

1. Describe the approach to the evaluation of a child with a suspected genetic disorder.
2. List some of the minor and major anomalies that may be present at birth.
3. Recognize some of the common chromosomal disorders.
4. List several of the common single-gene disorders.

## INTRODUCTION

Genetics is more than the identification and classification of syndromes and the study of obscure metabolic diseases. A syndrome is not always due to a genetic cause; it can be due to a chromosomal anomaly (e.g., Down syndrome), a teratogen (e.g., fetal alcohol syndrome), or a deformation (e.g., oligohydramnios syndrome). Conversely, a "genetic" disease is not always associated with anatomic birth defects; for example, newborns with inborn errors of metabolism are normally formed. Increasingly, it is recognized that diseases and malformations are due to a combination of genetic and environmental factors.

The scope of genetics has expanded tremendously: Genetics has become an integral part of hematology, oncology, and organ transplantation; it also provides useful tools in the identification of infectious organisms [e.g., polymerase chain reaction (PCR) detection of herpes simplex virus (HSV), *Neisseria*, and *Chlamydia* organisms]. The definition of a genetic disease also has expanded in that, with improved methods of studying genetic material at the molecular level, many diseases now are known to have a genetic component. With advances in cell and molecular biology, genetics is making strides in the management of metabolic disorders. With systematic study of the human genome and the possibility of cloning, genetics also is mingling with ethics and politics.

## GENERAL PRINCIPLES

The most common problems that trigger a genetic evaluation are dysmorphism (see Table 29-1 for definitions), unexplained short stature, failure to thrive or developmental delay, recurrent episodes of lethargy, and unexplained or repeated miscarriages or neonatal deaths. This chapter presents snapshots of the most common or most recognizable disorders. The following general principles apply in all cases.

### HISTORY

The medical history should include details of the pregnancy, including maternal age, parity, complications of pregnancy, exposures (medications, alcohol, drugs), and supplementation with vitamins (folic acid), as well as details of perinatal events. The child's history should include a detailed and

---

*Table 29-1* **Definitions of Terms Commonly Used in Genetics**

*Congenital anomaly:* an abnormality of structure or function that is present at birth even if it is not evident till later in life or at all, e.g., single kidney.

*Minor anomaly:* an anomaly of no functional significance that does not require medical intervention, e.g., simian line.

*Major anomaly or birth defect:* a medically or socially significant anomaly, e.g., tetralogy of Fallot, cleft palate, large cavernous hemangioma.

*Syndrome:* a combination of anomalies that occur in a recognizable pattern and are ascribed to a single cause, e.g., Down syndrome.

*Association:* a combination of anomalies that tend to occur together more than by chance alone, e.g., CHARGE or VACTERLS association.

*Sequence:* a combination of anomalies resulting from a "domino effect," e.g., Pierre Robin sequence.

*Malformation:* anomaly in which the development of a structure is "programmed" to be abnormal, e.g., heart disease in Down syndrome.

*Disruption:* an anomaly resulting from external interference with a structure meant to develop normally, e.g., abnormal extremities with thalidomide exposure.

*Deformation:* an anomaly resulting from mechanical forces on a normally developing structure, e.g., clubfoot.

chronologic developmental history (e.g., acquisition and then loss of milestones suggests a degenerative or storage disease). If skin lesions are present, the timing of their appearance and their evolution over time are important (e.g., neurocutaneous syndromes). The family history should go back as many generations as are available, and a pedigree should be drawn for easy reference; consanguinity should be noted. Ethnic origin is relevant in some genetic disorders.

## PHYSICAL EXAMINATION

Growth charts for height, weight, and head circumference should be plotted. Body proportions should be noted. All minor anomalies should be noted (Table 29-2); although the presence of one or two minor anomalies is normal, the presence of three or more raises concern for a major anomaly or a syndrome. The whole skin should be examined, and all lesions charted (e.g., hemangiomas, pigmented lesions).

## LABORATORY EVALUATION

Serum α fetoprotein (AFP) often is obtained during pregnancy; high levels are found in neural tube or abdominal wall defects and congenital nephrosis, and low levels in Down syndrome. Many pregnant women get one or

*Table 29-2* **Major and Minor Anomalies**

MINOR ANOMALIES
Skin and hair: cutis aplasia, synophrys (unibrow), birthmarks
Eyes: hypertelorism or hypotelorism; upslanting or downslanting of eyes, small palpebral fissures, epicanthal folds, blue sclerae
Jaw: micrognathia
Ears: low-set ears, rotated ears, ear tag or pit
Chest: accessory nipple
Umbilical cord: single umbilical artery
Hands and feet: simian line, clinodactyly (incurving of fifth finger), hypoplastic middle pharynx of fifth finger, polydactyly, arachnodactyly, syndactyly not involving bone, wide space between first and second toes, "curly" toes

MAJOR ANOMALIES (2–3 Percent of Births)
Microcephaly, hydrocephalus
Cataracts
Cleft lip or palate
Congenital heart disease
Ambiguous genitalia
Neural tube defect

more fetal ultrasounds that can detect various birth defects. More specific prenatal diagnosis is available for a wide variety of diseases through the use of chorionic villus sampling (CVS) in the first trimester or amniocentesis in the second trimester. Postnatally, every state in the United States screens for a panel of congenital diseases, including at least phenylketonuria, galactosemia, and hemoglobinopathies.

### RADIOLOGIC EVALUATION

Echocardiography, renal ultrasound, or skeletal surveys are performed as indicated.

### MANAGEMENT

Management almost always includes neurodevelopmental and behavioral testing, early intervention services, and genetic counseling.

## CHROMOSOMAL DISORDERS

Normal humans have 46 chromosomes: 22 autosomes and 1 pair of sex chromosomes. Each chromosome has a short arm p and a long arm q. Chromosomal disorders are those associated with abnormalities that are demonstrable on a karyotype, such as an extra or a missing chromosome, a deletion, or a translocation. With improved detailing of chromosomal structure [karyotype with special banding, fluorescent in situ hybridization (FISH)], the definition of a chromosomal disorder has been expanding.

## ANEUPLOIDY (MONOSOMY AND TRISOMY)

### MONOSOMY X: TURNER SYNDROME

Turner syndrome should be considered in any girl with significantly short stature. It affects only females, with an incidence of 1 in 4000.

#### PATHOPHYSIOLOGY

Turner syndrome is due to the absence of genetic material from an X chromosome, with the majority of affected girls having a 45, XO karyotype, 25 percent having a significant X deletion, and 15 percent having mosaicism (XX and XO).

Physical examination reveals lymphedema of the hands and feet, a webbed neck, a shield chest, cubitus valgus, and pigmented nevi. Congenital heart disease is present in 20 percent, usually involving the left side of the heart (aortic stenosis or coarctation, bicuspid aortic valve). Renal anomalies are present in 40 percent.

Laboratory evaluation includes a karyotype to confirm the diagnosis and endocrine studies as indicated.

Radiologic evaluation may include pelvic ultrasonography. There is gonadal dysgenesis in all the patients.

The clinical course is notable for short stature, with an average (untreated) adult height of 135 cm. Lack of pubertal development is always present, and sometimes there are learning disabilities as well.

Management consists of hormone replacement, including estrogen and growth hormone.

## TRISOMY 21: DOWN SYNDROME

Down syndrome is the most common autosomal disorder and also the most common genetic cause of mental retardation. The risk increases with maternal age, being 1 in 1000 live births at age 30 years, 1 in 100 at age 40, and 1 in 10 at age 50. However, most babies with Down syndrome are born to young mothers. The overall incidence is 1 in 800.

### PATHOPHYSIOLOGY

Down syndrome is due to the presence of extra genetic material from chromosome 21. In 95 percent of cases, three chromosomes 21 are identified on karyotyping (i.e., trisomy 21), and in 5 percent, the extra chromosome 21 is translocated onto another autosome, commonly 14. Most translocations are accidental, but 25 percent are due to the presence of a balanced translocation in one of the parents.

### PHYSICAL EXAMINATION, LABORATORY AND RADIOGRAPHIC EVALUATION

Down syndrome consists of a pattern of minor anomalies, together with possible major anomalies, as well as functional defects. Minor anomalies consist of a combination of upslanting palpebral fissures, hypertelorism, low-set ears, flat occiput (brachycephaly), Brushfield spots (speckling of the iris), simian creases on the palms or soles, clinodactyly (incurving of the fifth finger), and a large space between the first and second toes. Major cardiac anomalies are present in 50 percent of cases (usually septal defects or endocardial cushion defects), eye disease in 60 percent (refraction errors, cataracts), and, less commonly, there are gastrointestinal conditions (e.g., duodenal atresia, Hirschsprung disease). Functional problems include hypotonia and mental retardation (average IQ is 50) and a cell-mediated immune deficiency.

Laboratory and radiographic evaluation consists of a karyotype. In older children with Down syndrome, thyroid function tests are followed regularly.

Echocardiography is indicated in every child with Down syndrome even if there is no evident cardiac problem. In older children, x-rays of the cervical spine are indicated for sports participation because of the frequency of atlantooccipital instability.

## MANAGEMENT AND CLINICAL COURSE

In addition to developmental delay, children with Down syndrome have a T-cell immune deficiency with increased infections (pneumonia) and often develop hypothyroidism. They are prone to chronic serous otitis media with subsequent hearing problems. With advancing age, they are prone to develop cataracts and have a higher risk of leukemia and early Alzheimer disease than does the general population.

Management of children with Down syndrome includes the surgical management of congenital anomalies if present. Early intervention services, treatment of infections, and screening for and treatment of hypothyroidism are also important.

## TRISOMY 13: PATAU SYNDROME

Trisomy 13 also is associated with advanced maternal age, though more loosely than is Down syndrome. Its incidence is 1 in 5000.

## PATHOPHYSIOLOGY, PHYSICAL EXAMINATION, LABORATORY AND RADIOGRAPHIC EVALUATION

Seventy-five percent of cases involve a trisomy, and 25 percent involve a translocation of an extra chromosome 13.

Physical examination reveals severe anomalies, including microcephaly with typical areas of cutis aplasia in the scalp, microphthalmia, cleft lip, and polydactyly. Congenital heart disease is common, and there often is severe mental retardation.

A karyotype establishes the diagnosis.

Echocardiography is indicated for cardiac disease, and head imaging may show central nervous system (CNS) anomalies (e.g., prosencephaly).

## MANAGEMENT AND CLINICAL COURSE

Fifty percent of these patients die by age 1 month, and 90 percent by 1 year of age. Mean survival is 6 months. Management is supportive.

## TRISOMY 18: EDWARD SYNDROME

Trisomy 18 also is loosely associated with advanced maternal age. Its incidence is 1 in 5000.

## PATHOPHYSIOLOGY, PHYSICAL EXAMINATION, LABORATORY AND RADIOGRAPHIC EVALUATION

Trisomy 18 usually is due to meiotic nondisjunction.

Babies born with trisomy 18 have significant intrauterine growth retardation. Examination reveals microcephaly with a prominent occiput, micrognathia, clenched fingers with fixed contractures and overlapping of the second and fifth fingers over the third and fourth fingers, dislocated hips, and "rocker bottom" feet. Congenital cardiac anomalies are common.

A karyotype establishes the diagnosis. Echocardiography is indicated for cardiac disease, and head imaging may show CNS anomalies.

## MANAGEMENT AND CLINICAL COURSE

Patients with trisomy 18 have severe hypertonia and mental retardation. The prognosis is poor, as 30 percent die by 1 month and 90 percent die by 1 year of age. Management is supportive.

### KLINEFELTER SYNDROME

Klinefelter syndrome initially was described in adult men with gynecomastia, sparse facial and body hair, small testes, and azoospermia. It affects only males, with an incidence of 1 in 1000.

## PATHOPHYSIOLOGY, PHYSICAL EXAMINATION, LABORATORY AND RADIOGRAPHIC EVALUATION

Klinefelter syndrome is due to the presence of an extra sex chromosome X, with 80 percent of patients having the karyotype 47, XXY, and the rest being mosaics.

Physical examination reveals tall stature with an increased arm span.

The laboratory and radiographic evaluation includes a karyotype to confirm the diagnosis and hormonal studies.

Echocardiography may be performed to detect mitral valve prolapse in older patients.

## MANAGEMENT AND CLINICAL COURSE

Klinefelter syndrome rarely is diagnosed during childhood, more often coming to attention during the teenage years, when males have evidence of testicular failure with small testes, a female body habitus, scant body hair, and often gynecomastia. There is mild mental retardation (mean IQ is 85) and often behavior problems. Many cases remain undiagnosed. Management includes androgen replacement therapy.

## DELETIONS AND REPEATS

Chromosomal deletions may lead to recognizable syndromes. The rare cri du chat, named for the peculiar catlike cry emitted by these patients, is due to 5p-deletion; it may include heart disease and eye problems (cataracts). Deletions also are associated with tumors: Deletions of 13q14 may lead to retinoblastoma, which at times is present at birth and bilateral; children with aniridia (absent iris) and a deletion in p11 are at risk for Wilms' tumor and are followed with renal ultrasounds every 6 months.

## PRADER-WILLI SYNDROME

Prader-Willi is a syndrome that is characterized neonatally by severe hypotonia and feeding difficulties and later by an insatiable appetite and obesity. Its incidence is 1 in 20,000.

### PATHOPHYSIOLOGY

Some 70 percent of patients are found to have a deletion in 15q, and the rest have other or no detectable findings. Prader-Willi is the first syndrome in which "imprinting" was described: the idea that a gene is expressed differently depending on whether it is of maternal or paternal origin. The same deletion at 15q11-13 leads to Prader-Willi if paternal and to Angelman syndrome if maternal.

### PHYSICAL EXAMINATION, LABORATORY AND RADIOGRAPHIC EVALUATION

Dysmorphic features include a narrow face, almond-shaped palpebral fissures, a downturned mouth, and hypogonadism. After the first year, there is significantly short stature and obesity.

The laboratory and radiologic evaluation includes chromosomal studies with FISH to detect the q15 deletion and evaluation of hypogonadism. Skeletal x-rays may be performed for osteoporosis or femoral head abnormalities in symptomatic patients.

### MANAGEMENT AND CLINICAL COURSE

These patients may be noted to have severe hypotonia and failure to thrive in infancy. At around age 4, they develop an insatiable appetite. Mental retardation is a major feature, along with behavior problems. Complications related to obesity (e.g., slipped capital femoral epiphyses, sleep apnea, diabetes mellitus) and behavior problems contribute to morbidity and mortality. Management consists of special education services, dietary control, and behavior intervention, as well as growth hormone replacement.

## WILLIAMS SYNDROME

Williams syndrome (WS) is a rare genetic disorder with characteristic facial features, cardiovascular anomalies, and neonatal hypercalcemia. Its incidence is 1 in 20,000. In 95 to 98 percent of individuals, a deletion on chromosome band 7q11.23 that includes the elastin gene can be identified.

### PHYSICAL EXAMINATION

Children with WS have facial features that include a short upturned nose, a flat nasal bridge, a long philtrum, a flat malar area, a wide mouth, full lips, dental malocclusion, micrognathia, and stellate irides. Some 60 percent have cardiovascular anomalies, most commonly supravalvular aortic stenosis, but peripheral pulmonary branch stenosis, mitral valve prolapse, and renal artery stenosis leading to hypertension also may be found.

## LABORATORY AND RADIOGRAPHIC EVALUATION

The laboratory and radiologic evaluation includes serum calcium neonatally. FISH is used to detect the genetic deletion. Echocardiography and renal ultrasound may be indicated.

## MANAGEMENT AND CLINICAL COURSE

Newborns with WS generally are full-term infants and may come to medical attention because of supravalvular aortic stenosis (an otherwise uncommon cardiac anomaly). Hypercalcemia may be found at that time but resolves later. During childhood, WS may present with failure to thrive, short stature, or developmental delay. It also comes to the clinician's attention in an examination for the evaluation of the physical features or because of renal anomalies. Many children with WS have a gregarious and friendly personality. In addition to special education services, management may include cardiac and renal treatment if necessary.

## *DI GEORGE SYNDROME AND CATCH 22*

Di George syndrome is characterized by absence of the thymus and parathyroid glands, together with cardiac defects and subtly abnormal facial features. It overlaps with several other syndromes that now are termed collectively CATCH 22, an acronym for cardiac defects, abnormal facies, thymic hypoplasia, cleft palate, and hypocalcemia.

All CATCH 22 syndromes are associated with a deletion on 22q.

## PHYSICAL EXAMINATION

Facial anomalies include hypertelorism, low-set ears, a short philtrum, micrognathia, and cleft palate. Cardiac anomalies are varied and include tetralogy of Fallot, ventricular septal defect (VSD), and truncus arteriosus.

## LABORATORY AND RADIOLOGIC EVALUATION

A deletion is detected by FISH analysis in 90 percent of patients with Di George syndrome. Evaluation of calcium metabolism and parathyroid function is done. A chest x-ray or computed tomography (CT) may be obtained to ascertain the presence or absence of thymus. Echocardiography is done, looking for cardiac defects.

## MANAGEMENT AND CLINICAL COURSE

The diagnosis is suspected when a newborn with heart disease also develops jitteriness or seizures and is found to have hypocalcemia. Patients with Di George syndrome have a T-cell-mediated immune deficiency and hence are at risk for recurrent infections. The most common causes of death are cardiac disease and infections. Management includes calcium replacement and vitamin D.

## FRAGILE X SYNDROME

Fragile X syndrome is the most common inherited cause of mental retardation and should be suspected in any boy with unexplained mental retardation. It is an X-linked disorder with a prevalence of 1 in 4000 in males and 1 in 8000 female carriers.

Fragile X syndrome is due to the presence of hundreds of unnecessary repeats in the DNA of the X chromosome (long arm) of the sequence CCG; this causes fragile sites, which are detected on karyotyping.

These infants may be large at birth but otherwise have no notable anomalies. Later, they may be noted to have a prominent forehead, large ears, and macrognathia. Macroorchidism typically is noted after puberty.

The laboratory evaluation includes a karyotype in the appropriate medium,

### MANAGEMENT AND CLINICAL COURSE

Most of these children reach expected milestones during the first year of life. Fragile X syndrome comes to medical attention during later childhood because of progressing mental retardation (IQ 20 to 70), autistic behavior (e.g., hand flapping, avoidance of eye contact), attention deficit, and aggressive tendencies. Life span is normal. Management consists of special education, behavior intervention, and pharmacologic management of attention deficits.

## SINGLE-GENE DISORDERS

Over 3000 single-gene disorders have been described, classified by their mode of inheritance into autosomal dominant, autosomal recessive, or X-linked. Following are the most common of these diseases.

## CYSTIC FIBROSIS

Cystic fibrosis (CF) is a common autosomal recessive disorder that manifests with chronic pulmonary infections and pancreatic insufficiency. Its incidence is 1 in 2000 white births; the incidence is lower in other races.

### PATHOPHYSIOLOGY

CF is caused by defects in the CFTR gene, which encodes for a chloride channel protein. This results in abnormalities of chloride transport across epithelial cells on mucosal surfaces, with associated water transport abnormalities and thus viscid secretions in the respiratory tract, pancreas, gastrointestinal tract, sweat glands, and other exocrine tissues.

## PHYSICAL EXAMINATION

Physical Examination may be normal in a newborn unless meconium ileus is present. A parent may notice a salty taste when kissing the baby. Later, there is frequent failure to thrive as well as findings related to chronic pulmonary disease.

## LABORATORY AND RADIOLOGIC EVALUATION

The diagnosis can be made by measuring the concentration of sweat chloride: Values > 60 mEq/L establish the diagnosis, and values of 40 to 60 are equivocal. Indications for testing include a family history of CF, unexplained failure to thrive, recurrent sinopulmonary infections, throat colonization with *Staphylococcus aureus* or *Pseudomonas*, nasal polyps, chronic diarrhea/steatorrhea, and recurrent dehydration with metabolic alkalosis. Sweat chloride testing may not be feasible in small babies. Alternatively, DNA testing can be done on a buccal smear; it provides confirmation of the diagnosis in 85 percent of patients, as it detects only the most common of a large number of CFTR mutations. Evaluation of pulmonary and pancreatic function is essential in patients with CF.

Chest x-rays are frequently obtained in children with pulmonary disease.

## MANAGEMENT AND CLINICAL COURSE

Some 15 percent of newborns with CF have meconium ileus, (partial or complete intestinal obstruction with thick inspissated meconium), presenting with delayed passage of meconium, abdominal distention, or vomiting. Later manifestations of CF are related to recurrent pulmonary infections or sinusitis or to steatorrhea with failure to thrive. Management consists of early treatment of infections, intensive chest physical therapy, and dietary management that includes a high caloric intake, digestive enzymes, and vitamin replacement. The most common cause of death is end-stage lung disease.

## *PHENYLKETONURIA*

Phenylketonuria (PKU), an autosomal recessive disorder, is the most common amino acid disorder. It is the first genetic disorder for which widespread neonatal screening became available, and it provides a clear illustration of how early detection can make a remarkable difference in outcome. Its incidence is 1 in 14,000 births.

## PATHOPHYSIOLOGY, PHYSICAL EXAMINATION AND LABORATORY EVALUATION

PKU is due to a deficiency of the enzyme phenylalanine hydroxylase, which converts the (essential) amino acid phenylalanine into tyrosine, resulting in hyperphenylalaninemia and accumulation of the neurotoxic metabolite phenylacetic acid.

Because tyrosine is a precursor to melanin, children with PKU have blue eyes and fair skin and hair but are otherwise normal at birth.

The neonatal screening is abnormal, and the phenylalanine level is elevated.

## MANAGEMENT AND CLINICAL COURSE

If undiagnosed, children with PKU do well initially but by 6 months of age seem to lose interest in their surroundings and by age 1 year have obvious developmental delay; they tend to have eczema, and 20 percent have seizures. If detected early and treated, children with PKU develop normally. Management consists of a phenylalanine-free diet, together with tyrosine supplementation. The artificial sweetener aspartame should be avoided by children with PKU as well as by pregnant women who may carry a child with PKU.

## GALACTOSEMIA

Galactosemia is an autosomal recessive disorder that is related to abnormal metabolism of lactose, the disaccharide sugar (glucose plus galactose) in milk. Its incidence is 1 in 40,000 to 60,000. Neonatal screening is available.

## PATHOPHYSIOLOGY

The most common form is caused by a deficiency of the enzyme GALT (galactose-1-phosphate uridylyl transferase), which converts galactose phosphate to glucose phosphate; this explains the accumulation of galactose. Other, less common enzyme deficiencies also cause galactosemia.

## PHYSICAL EXAMINATION

Physical examination is unremarkable at birth. Soon after milk is introduced, a newborn may develop vomiting, jaundice, hepatomegaly with ascites, and hypotonia.

## LABORATORY EVALUATION

A crude way to screen for galactose in the urine is to test for non-glucose-reducing substances. Galactosemia is included in neonatal screening tests, and a high galactose level has to be confirmed by enzyme assay. A benign variety of galactosemia is called Duarte variant and leads to no clinical disease.

## MANAGEMENT AND CLINICAL COURSE

Clinical manifestations occur soon after the introduction of lactose. The baby develops projectile vomiting and jaundice (conjugated hyperbilirubinemia with high liver enzymes) and is at risk for gram-negative sepsis. Older children have cataracts, developmental delay, and learning problems. Management consists of elimination of lactose from the diet and acute management of sepsis if present.

## SICKLE CELL DISEASE

Sickle cell disease involves a mutation that leads to a single amino acid sub-stitution (valine for glutamic acid) on the beta chain of hemoglobin. Its inci-dence is 1 in 500 live births in African Americans (see Chap. 31).

# STORAGE DISEASES

## GLYCOGEN STORAGE DISEASES

Glycogen storage diseases (GSDs, or glycogenoses) are a group of disorders caused by a deficiency in one of the enzymes involved in glycogen break-down or synthesis. Glycogen is the storage form of glucose in liver and mus-cle, and a particular GSD thus affects primarily the liver, the heart, or peripheral muscles.

### PATHOPHYSIOLOGY

There are 11 GSDs, all transmitted in an autosomal recessive fashion. The most common is GSD1 (von Gierke disease), which is caused by a deficiency of glucose-6-phosphatase and affects the liver. GSD2 (Pompe disease) is due to a deficiency of alpha-1,4-glucosidase (a lysosomal enzyme, also called acid maltase) and affects the skeletal and cardiac muscles. GSD5 (McArdle disease) is due to a deficiency of myophosphorylase and thus affects the skeletal muscles.

### PHYSICAL EXAMINATION

Most GSDs manifest with symptoms or signs related to the organ involved in the enzyme deficiency, with local glycogen accumulation. In GSD1, there is progressive and marked hepatomegaly; in GSD2, the main findings are hypo-tonia and cardiomegaly; and in GSD5, muscle may be noted to be prominent.

### LABORATORY AND RADIOLOGIC EVALUATION

In GSD1, laboratory evaluation reveals hypoglycemia, lactic acidosis, and hyperuricemia; there is no increase in plasma glucose with glucagon admin-istration. The diagnosis can be confirmed by liver biopsy. The diagnosis of GSD2 can be established by muscle biopsy; GSD2 also can be diagnosed less invasively (and prenatally) by measuring the enzyme in the lysosomes of cultured fibroblasts. The diagnosis of GSD5 is established by muscle biopsy. Abdominal ultrasound is helpful in diagnosing GSD1. Chest x-ray and echocardiography are helpful in GSD1 and GSD2.

### MANAGEMENT AND CLINICAL COURSE

Babies with GSD1 are unable to release glucose normally. Because of hypo-glycemia, they frequently are hungry and irritable; frequent feeds lead to adiposity with a "doll" facies. Hypoglycemia may become symptomatic with lethargy, jitteriness, or seizures. Babies with GSD2 present with hypotonia, muscle weakness, and findings of congestive heart failure; they often progress to respiratory insufficiency and heart failure and often die by 1 year of age. GSD5 presents in older children with severe muscle cramping and rhabdomyolysis after exercise. Management of GSD1 consists of providing a constant source of glucose (oral or tube feedings). Management of GSD2 is supportive. Management of GSD5 is also supportive and includes limiting exercise.

## LIPID STORAGE DISEASES

Lipid storage diseases are a group of disorders, mostly autosomal recessive, that are due to deficiencies in enzymes that break down lipids. The most common is Tay-Sachs disease, a severe neurodegenerative disease. It has a carrier rate of 1 in 250 in the general population and a higher rate (1 in 25) in Ashkenazi Jews, French Canadians, and Louisiana Cajuns. The incidence of the disease in the at-risk population is 1 in 3600.

### PATHOPHYSIOLOGY

Tay-Sachs disease is due to a mutation on chromosome 15 that leads to a deficiency of hexosaminidase A (Hex A), an enzyme necessary for the breakdown of GM2 gangliosides in brain cells. GM2 thus accumulates in brain cells.

### PHYSICAL EXAMINATION

Newborns with Tay-Sachs disease appear normal at birth. Later findings are macrocephaly, abnormal tone, inability to fixate, and a typical macular "cherry-red spot" on ophthalmoscopy.

### LABORATORY AND RADIOLOGIC EVALUATION

The diagnosis is established by measurement of Hex-A in blood or by DNA testing. Adults can be tested for a carrier state by enzyme levels (low in carriers) or by DNA testing (detects the majority of known mutations). Head imaging may be indicated.

### MANAGEMENT AND CLINICAL COURSE

Babies with Tay-Sachs disease start showing symptoms around 6 months of age, when they are noted to be easily startled (hyperacusis), their development slows down, and they lose milestones they had reached previously (e.g., ability to roll over, sit, or crawl). Hypotonia and blindness are present by age 1 year, seizures become a problem around age 2, and death occurs by age 4. A less severe form of Tay-Sachs disease has later manifestations. Management is supportive, including anticonvulsants.

## MUCOPOLYSACCHARIDOSES

Mucopolysaccharidoses (MPSs) are a group of storage diseases that are due to a deficiency of one of the enzymes involved in the lysosomal degradation of proteoglycans. Proteoglycans (protein moieties with polysaccharide, e.g., chondroitin sulfate, dermatan sulfate) thus accumulate in the lysosomes of tissues [skeleton, central nervous system (CNS), viscera, eyes].

### PATHOPHYSIOLOGY

Some seven types have been identified, with clinical features related to the enzyme (and organ system) involved. Except for MPS2 (Hunter disease, X-linked), they are autosomal recessive. Their overall incidence is 1 in 25,000.

### PHYSICAL EXAMINATION

Newborns with an MPS have a normal examination. Later, they have coarse facial features. Hunter (MPS2) and Hurler (MPS1H) syndromes have infantile kyphosis. Morquio (MPS4) syndrome also has significant orthopedic problems (short stature, kyphosis, and genu valgum). Maroteaux-Lamy (MPS6) presents with stiff joints and short stature.

### LABORATORY AND RADIOLOGIC EVALUATION

Urine proteoglycans are elevated as a screening test; confirmation of the diagnosis is provided by enzyme assay in white blood cells or fibroblasts. Prenatal diagnosis (by CVS) is possible. A skeletal survey defines bone involvement and may show findings typical for a specific MPS. The radiologic abnormalities are termed collectively "dysostosis multiplex" and become evident by 2 years of age.

### MANAGEMENT AND CLINICAL COURSE

Normal initially, patients with MPSs present during childhood with dysmorphic features, gradually worsening kyphosis (Hunter and Hurler syndromes), and hepatosplenomegaly. Eye involvement leads to cloudy corneas (in all MPSs except Hunter syndrome). Involvement of the respiratory tract leads to respiratory obstruction (sleep apnea) or infections. Cardiac involvement leads to cardiomyopathy or arrhythmias. CNS involvement leads to mental retardation, dementia, or behavior problems. Management is supportive.

## METABOLIC DISEASES

*Metabolic diseases* is the general term used to refer to three groups of disorders: Urea cycle disorders, aminoacidopathies, and organic acidemias often are lumped together because of common features in their presentation and initial management. The most common urea cycle disorder is ornithine carbamylase (OTC) deficiency, which is X-linked; other metabolic diseases are autosomal recessive.

## PATHOPHYSIOLOGY

Metabolic diseases are caused by defects in the structure or function of specific enzymes or by abnormalities in transport proteins; this results in the accumulation of unwanted precursors or alternate metabolites and a deficiency of the products necessary for normal metabolism. Most metabolic diseases present in the neonatal period with an overwhelming illness. The family history is often negative or may include a neonatal sibling death ascribed to sepsis or sudden infant death syndrome (SIDS). As soon as the diagnosis is suspected, intensive management should be implemented without awaiting a precise diagnosis.

## PHYSICAL EXAMINATION

Most babies with metabolic disorders are normal at birth, since the maternal side clears the majority of toxins during gestation. An unusual smell sometimes is noted (e.g., maple syrup urine disease).

## LABORATORY EVALUATION

The main findings are hyperammonemia and metabolic (high-anion-gap) acidosis. The workup of a child with suspected metabolic disease includes a complete blood count (CBC), serum electrolytes, glucose and blood gases and serum lactic acid level, urinalysis (including ketones, glucose, and reducing substances), plasma ammonia, serum amino acids, and urine organic acid. Infants with severe hyperammonemia in the first 24 h usually have a urea cycle disorder or organic acidemia.

## MANAGEMENT AND CLINICAL COURSE

These syndromes present soon after birth, when feeds are introduced, after an interval of hours to months. Typical symptoms include lethargy, poor feeding, apnea, and vomiting. Often sepsis is the initial consideration, and the baby gets a sepsis workup. When not treated, most metabolic disorders result in death or severe mental delay. The acute management of a child with a suspected metabolic disorder is supportive as appropriate (often intubation and assisted ventilation, hydration, antibiotics if sepsis is suspected, and glucose supplementation if needed) and includes stopping of the offending substrate (e.g., protein, galactose), removal of accumulated toxins (e.g., exchange transfusion, dialysis for hyperammonemia), and administration of cofactors (e.g., supplemental vitamin B, carnitine). Most of these children remain on lifelong dietary restrictions and may decompensate with intercurrent illnesses.

## BIRTH DEFECTS

Among all congenital anomalies, 15 to 25 percent are considered genetic in origin, 10 percent are due to environmental factors (Table 29-3), 20 to 25 percent are "multifactorial" (i.e., due to a combination of genetic and environ-

*Table 29-3* **Teratogens**

Acne treatment: tretinoin (Retin-A)
Anticoagulants: warfarin
Antipsychotics: lithium, haloperidol, thalidomide
Anticonvulsants: valproic acid, carbamazepine
Antimicrobials: tetracycline, chloramphenicol, amphotericin B
Chemotherapeutic agents: alkylating agents, folic aid antagonists
Hormones: progestins, diethylstilbestrol, androgens
Recreational drugs: alcohol, marijuana, narcotics,
Metabolic: glucose (maternal diabetes mellitus)
TORCH infections: toxoplasmosis, other infections, (e.g., syphilis), rubella, cytomegalovirus, and herpes simplex

mental factors), and the rest are of unknown cause. Below are some examples of birth defects, with illustrations of sequence, association, and syndrome.

## CLEFT PALATE OR LIP

This may be an isolated birth defect or part of a syndrome. The recurrence risk is 3 to 5 percent.

## PIERRE ROBIN SEQUENCE

Pierre Robin is the triad of micrognathia, retroglossia, and cleft palate. It is a sequence in that it is thought that a small jaw causes the tongue to push against the palate, preventing its midline closure. This leads to aspiration pneumonias, chronic otitis media, and obstructive sleep apnea. Management initially consists of promotion of optimal feeds and surgical correction of the cleft. It can occur alone or as part of multiple anomalies, with an incidence of 1 in 8500.

## NEURAL TUBE DEFECTS

A neural tube defect (NTD) is any anomaly involving failure of the neural tube (and its coverings) to close totally. The mildest form is spina bifida occulta, the most common is meningomyelocele (usually lumbar or sacral, more rarely cervical), and the most extreme is anencephaly. The sequence of NTD with hydrocephalus, vertebral anomalies, or clubfeet is commonly present. NTD is multifactorial in that it is associated with folate deficiency during pregnancy, but it also has a genetic predisposition. NTD can be prenatally suspected if the $\alpha$ fetoprotein level is high in a pregnant woman or may be diagnosed by prenatal ultrasonography. Treatment is surgical, with early intervention services as indicated.

## VATER OR VACTERLS ASSOCIATION

VACTERLS is the acronym for an association that includes vertebral anomalies, anal atresia, cardiac anomalies, tracheoesophageal fistula, esophageal atresia, renal anomalies, and radial dysplasia, limb anomalies, and a single umbilical artery.

## CHARGE ASSOCIATION

CHARGE is the acronym for an association that includes coloboma of the eye structures (iris, retina), heart defect [atrial septal defect (ASD), VSD, tetralogy of Fallot], atresia of choanae, retardation (physical or mental), genitourinary problems (small penis, undescended testicles, ureterovesical reflux), and ear abnormalities. Its incidence is 1 in 10,000. Treatment consists of surgery as indicated and early intervention services.

## FETAL ALCOHOL SYNDROME

Alcohol is a teratogen, and exposure to alcohol in utero leads to a spectrum of anomalies that range from subtle learning disabilities to the recognizable fetal alcohol syndrome (FAS). FAS has a variable geographic incidence in the United States, ranging between 0.2 and 1.5 in 1000 births. It is an important preventable cause of mental retardation.

### PATHOPHYSIOLOGY

It is estimated that an intake of four to six alcoholic drinks a day leads to FAS.

### PHYSICAL EXAMINATION

Newborns with FAS are typically low-birthweight infants (below the 5th percentile). Facial features include narrow palpebral fissures, a short upturned nose, a flat midface, a smooth philtrum, and a thin upper lip. These newborns also may have cardiac defects.

### LABORATORY AND RADIOLOGIC EVALUATION

There is no test to diagnose FAS; the diagnosis is clinical. Echocardiography is performed if indicated.

### MANAGEMENT AND CLINICAL COURSE

Newborns with FAS may exhibit poor feeding and growth. Later, they are at higher risk of coordination problems, developmental and learning disabilities, and behavior problems. Management is supportive.

## OLIGOHYDRAMNIOS SYNDROME

Also called fetal compression syndrome, oligohydramnios syndrome refers to multiple deformation anomalies consequent to a low volume of amniotic fluid and fetal cramming in utero. It can be due to renal agenesis (Potter syndrome), severe urinary tract obstruction, or chronic amniotic fluid leakage. The external findings are a flat facies, low-set or malformed ears, ridges under the eyes, micrognathia, and clubfeet. Importantly, there is pulmonary hypoplasia that often manifests as pneumothorax or pneumomediastinum immediately after birth. The prognosis is determined primarily by the degree of pulmonary hypoplasia and also by renal function.

## BIBLIOGRAPHY

Jones, KL. *Smith's Recognizable Patterns of Human Malformations,* 6th ed. Philadelphia: Saunders, 2005.

## GENETICS RESOURCES ON THE INTERNET

Alliance of Genetic Support groups
http://www.geneticalliance.org
American Academy of Pediatrics
http://www.aap.org
American Society of Human Genetics
http://www.faseb.org/genetics/ashg/ashgmenu.htm
Ethical, Legal, and Social Issues
http://www.ornl.gov/hgmis/elsi/elsi.htm
Family Village
http://familyvillage.wisc.edu
Gene Tests–Gene Clinics
http://www.geneclinics.org
National Coalition for Health Professional Education in Genetics
http://www.nchpeg.org
National Organization for Rare Disorders
http://www.rarediseases.org
Online Mendelian Inheritance in Man
http://www3.ncbi.nlm.gov/omim

# GASTROENTEROLOGY

## *Joseph Gigante*

LEARNING OBJECTIVES

1. List the primary clinical differences between Crohn disease and ulcerative colitis.

2. Describe the common symptoms seen in children with gastroesophageal reflux.

3. List the different causes of upper and lower gastrointestinal bleeding.

4. Describe the basic physiology of bilirubin metabolism and the classification of jaundice.

## INFLAMMATORY BOWEL DISEASE

*PATHOPHYSIOLOGY*

Inflammatory bowel disease (IBD) in childhood typically is categorized as two conditions: Crohn disease and ulcerative colitis. Crohn disease is characterized by transmural intestinal inflammation that may involve any portion of the gastrointestinal (GI) tract from the mouth to the anus. Ulcerative colitis is characterized by inflammation involving the mucosal layer of the colon. It can involve any portion of the colon or the entire colon. The rectum frequently is involved in ulcerative colitis, whereas in Crohn disease the terminal ileum and cecum are common regions of involvement. Perianal disease is not seen in patients with ulcerative colitis, but up to 30 percent of patients with Crohn disease have perianal disease, such as a perianal fistula or abscess. Growth failure is seen in up to 30 percent of patients with Crohn disease and 10 percent of patients with ulcerative colitis. Extraintestinal manifestations associated with both Crohn disease and ulcerative colitis include arthritis, uveitis, and erythema nodosum.

## HISTORY

Patients with IBD often present with vague, nonspecific symptoms, which can make the diagnosis of this disease difficult. These nonspecific symptoms can include abdominal pain, diarrhea (often bloody), nausea or vomiting, weight loss, fever, and arthalgias. Abdominal pain is usually more prominent in patients with Crohn disease. The pain can be severe, can occur at any time of the day, and may awaken the child from sleep. Those who have ileal or ileocecal disease may have more right lower quadrant pain, whereas those with colonic or generalized small bowel disease may have more periumbilical pain. Diarrhea is bloody in almost all patients with ulcerative colitis and in up to 50 percent of patients with Crohn disease. Nausea and vomiting can be present in either disease. Fever, more commonly associated with Crohn disease, can occur in the absence of gastrointestinal symptoms. Patients with Crohn disease may present with a fever of unknown origin.

## PHYSICAL EXAMINATION

A thorough physical examination may reveal gastrointestinal or extraintestinal findings that may aid in the diagnosis of Crohn disease or ulcerative colitis. Fever may be present in patients with IBD, especially those with Crohn disease. Measurement of growth parameters is important, as up to 30 percent of patients with Crohn disease and 10 percent of patients with ulcerative colitis may experience growth failure. In addition to weight loss and short stature, findings on physical examination may include oral ulcers, skin lesions (erythema nodosum), arthritis, or perianal disease (fissures or fistulas).

## LABORATORY AND RADIOGRAPHIC EVALUATION

A detailed history and physical examination often reveal clues to the diagnosis of IBD. Laboratory studies can be used to confirm the diagnosis. A complete blood count (CBC) may reveal anemia secondary to blood loss and iron deficiency and a thrombocytosis resulting from inflammation. The erythrocyte sedimentation rate is elevated in approximately 80 percent of patients with Crohn disease and 40 percent of patients with ulcerative colitis. Albumin levels are low, reflecting poor nutrition and enteric protein loss. Liver function tests may be elevated if there is hepatic involvement. Stool cultures should be considered to rule out enteric pathogens that may present with bloody diarrhea. The diagnosis is established by a combination of barium radiography, colonoscopy, and upper endoscopy. The terminal ileum should be evaluated, especially when one is looking for evidence of Crohn disease. Evidence of perianal involvement, small bowel disease, or granulomas on biopsy establishes the diagnosis of Crohn disease.

## MANAGEMENT

The management of IBD involves a combination of pharmacologic, nutritional, surgical, and psychological therapy. Pharmacologic therapy usually involves a combination of four different types of medications: aminosalicylates, corticosteroids, immunomodulators, and antibiotics. Nutritional therapy may be used as a primary or adjunctive therapy. It is typically more useful in Crohn disease than in ulcerative colitis. Mildly malnourished patients may benefit from high-calorie supplements or calorically dense diets. More severely malnourished patients may require nasogastric or gastrostomy feedings. Surgical therapies differ for ulcerative colitis and Crohn disease. Surgery (colectomy) is curative in ulcerative colitis; it is not curative in Crohn disease and is performed only to treat complications. The need for psychological therapy is important in IBD. Emotional support of the patient and family during the diagnosis and initial management of the disease is vital. Support groups and counseling help patients and their families deal with the stress and depression commonly seen with this disorder.

## GASTROESOPHAGEAL REFLUX

### PATHOPHYSIOLOGY

Gastroesophageal reflux (GER) is a common problem in pediatrics. It is estimated that up to 40 percent of infants spit up or regurgitate. Most infants outgrow reflux, but a small subset of children have persistent GER or develop complications. GER occurs as a result of the passive reflux of gastric contents into the esophagus because of an incompetent lower esophageal sphincter. Delayed gastric emptying also may play a role in GER.

### HISTORY

Children with GER may have a number of different symptoms. Infants most commonly have spitting up or vomiting, which may occur immediately or hours after feeding. Infants with excessive vomiting may lose weight. Infants with significant esophagitis may be irritable and have feeding problems. Older children may complain of chest pain. Anemia may be seen if there is erosive esophagitis. Painful esophagitis can cause Sandifer syndrome. Affected children arch the back and have torticollis and sometimes are mistakenly thought to be having a seizure. A number of respiratory symptoms can be seen with GER, including wheezing, cough, apnea, and pneumonia.

### PHYSICAL EXAMINATION

The physical examination should begin with a close look at the vital signs, including growth parameters. Children with respiratory complications resulting from GER may have tachypnea, whereas those with failure to thrive secondary to excessive GER may demonstrate weight loss. The physical examination typically is normal. These children may have wheezing noted on auscultation of the lungs.

## LABORATORY AND RADIOGRAPHIC EVALUATION

Many children are diagnosed with GER on the basis of their symptoms. Several studies can be performed to confirm the diagnosis. An overnight esophageal pH probe is the "gold standard" for diagnosis. Barium swallow with an upper gastrointestinal radiograph is an excellent test to evaluate anatomy. Scintigraphy involves the use of a radioactive marker mixed with food to measure gastric emptying and look for evidence of aspiration. Endoscopy can be performed to visualize the esophagus and obtain esophageal biopsies.

## MANAGEMENT

Most children with GER can be treated with conservative therapy. This includes changes in position and diet. Having the child avoid the supine position by staying prone or in the upright sitting position helps prevent GER. Dietary changes such as small, more frequent meals and thickening the formula of infants with rice cereal are also effective therapies. Medical therapy should be reserved for patients with complications secondary to GER. Several different categories of medications can be used, including antacids, H2 receptor antagonists, prokinetic agents, and proton pump inhibitors. Surgery (fundoplication) is indicated in patients who fail conservative and medical management.

## GASTROINTESTINAL BLEEDING

Gastrointestinal bleeding is a relatively common finding in children that is often very frightening to the child, family, and clinician. Fortunately, it is uncommon to see hemodynamically significant blood loss in children. A systematic approach is necessary in the care and management of this problem. First, one must determine if the child is hemodynamically stable. Second, one must ensure that the material visualized is really blood. Third, if it is blood, one must determine if it is blood from an upper or lower GI site. Fourth, once the bleeding site has been determined, one must outline the best treatment for the identified condition.

## PATHOPHYSIOLOGY

Blood in the GI tract can present in several different manners. Hematemesis is the vomiting of blood, which may appear bright red or may have a darker, "coffee ground" appearance if the hemoglobin has been denatured. Hematochezia is bright red blood per rectum or maroon-colored stool and is suggestive of a colonic bleed, although a brisk upper GI bleed also can present with hematochezia. Melena is a black, tarry stool that contains blood that has been in the GI tract for a prolonged period, allowing for denaturing of hemoglobin by colonic bacteria. It usually is seen in bleeding proximal to the ileocecal valve. Occult blood refers to the presence of blood in stool that is not grossly evident.

## HISTORY

Knowledge of the patient's age and condition is important for determining the cause of GI bleeding.

### UPPER GI BLEED

In the immediate newborn period, an infant may vomit maternal blood that was swallowed during the delivery. Mothers who are breast-feeding sometimes have cracked nipples and may bleed into the breast milk. In older children, a history of facial trauma or epistaxis may suggest blood originating from the nasopharynx. Excessive, forceful vomiting may cause a Mallory-Weiss tear. Epigastic abdominal pain may be due to gastritis or a peptic ulcer. The use of medications such as nonsteroidal anti-inflammatory drugs (NSAIDs) may cause a GI bleed.

### LOWER GI BLEED

Infants with a history of bloody diarrhea may have cow's milk protein intolerance or infectious enterocolitis. Anal fissures are also common in this age group. Older children can develop a rectal fissure after diarrhea or the passage of a large, hard stool. Infectious enterocolitis is also common in this age group. Impressive, painless rectal bleeding can be seen in patients with Meckel diverticulum and juvenile polyps. Patients with intussusception may present with intermittent colicky abdominal pain or changes in mental status (apathy) along with maroon-colored "currant jelly" stools. Abdominal pain and a purpuric rash are seen commonly in patients with Henoch-Schönlein purpura. A history of antibiotic use suggests the possibility of *Clostridium difficile* diarrhea. Patients with inflammatory bowel disease may present with abdominal pain, fever, or weight loss in addition to bloody stools.

## PHYSICAL EXAMINATION

In examining a child with a GI bleed, the vital signs should be assessed to evaluate for signs of shock. The clinician should determine whether the patient is hemodynamically stable before proceeding with the rest of the physical examination. Tachycardia is the most sensitive indicator of acute blood loss. Children often do not display hypotension unless they are in moderate to severe shock. If the patient is stable, a careful physical examination should be performed to look for clues to a potential diagnosis. Examination of the nose and mouth may reveal a nasopharyngeal source for the bleed. The presence of periorbital or facial petechiae suggests intense coughing or a retching episode. The presence of hepatosplenomegaly may indicate chronic liver disease and portal hypertension. Epigastric tenderness may suggest peptic ulcer disease. A right lower quadrant abdominal mass in an infant or toddler with hematochezia suggests intussusception, but Crohn disease is a more likely diagnosis in an older patient. An examination of the anal region may reveal an anal fissure or an anal skin tag or fistula, both of which are associated with Crohn disease. A purpuric rash on the buttocks or lower extremities is associated with Henoch-Schönlein purpura.

## LABORATORY AND RADIOGRAPHIC EVALUATION

The first consideration in evaluating a child with a possible GI bleed is to determine if the material observed is actually blood. A number of substances can mimic blood in vomitus and stool. Certain food-coloring agents in gelatins and juices can look like blood when vomited. Iron preparations, bismuth, and several fruits and vegetables may cause stools to be dark or melanotic in appearance. A positive guaiac test of stool will confirm the presence of blood. This test is not effective for detecting blood in emesis or a nasogastric aspirate. The Gastrocult test is used to confirm the presence of upper GI blood. A major upper GI bleed can present with bright red blood per rectum. If an upper GI bleed is suspected, nasogastric lavage may be performed to identify whether blood is present in the stomach. The most important test for a patient with a suspected upper GI bleed is esophagogastroduodenoscopy (EGD). EGD allows for direct visualization of the esophagus, stomach, and small intestine and is a safe and reliable means for diagnosing and treating most causes of upper GI bleeding. Flexible sigmoidoscopy (FS) and colonoscopy allow direct visualization of the colonic mucosa and provide an opportunity to obtain biopsies if necessary. With the increased use of flexible endoscopy, contrast radiography is used much less commonly. A Meckel scan, using technetium 99m pertechnetate, will localize within the functional gastric mucus cells that often are found in a Meckel diverticulum. Nuclear medicine techniques otherwise have a limited role in GI bleeding.

## MANAGEMENT

A patient who presents with a GI bleed and signs of shock will require aggressive fluid resuscitation with isotonic fluid and a transfusion with blood products if the bleeding is ongoing. If the patient is hemodynamically stable, management will be specific for the identified cause of the hemorrhage. For example, a child with a peptic ulcer may be treated with acid reduction therapy such as an H2 receptor antagonist. Use of medications, such as NSAIDs, that can induce ulcers should be discontinued. An infant with cow's milk protein intolerance should be switched to a hypoallergenic formula. Although there are many causes of GI bleeding in children, the majority of the causes are of low acuity and are self-limited.

## LIVER DISEASES AND JAUNDICE

### PATHOPHYSIOLOGY

Jaundice is defined by a yellow or yellow-green color to the sclera, skin, and mucous membranes caused by an increase in serum bilirubin. Jaundice can be detected clinically when the total serum bilirubin is higher than 5 mg/dL. Jaundice occurs much more frequently in neonates than in older children. The major source of bilirubin is the breakdown of heme pigment from degraded red blood cells (RBCs). Heme is converted to biliverdin by heme oxygenase and then bilirubin by biliverdin reductase in the reticuloendothelial system. After being produced in the reticuloendothelial system, unconjugated bilirubin, a lipophilic compound, is bound to albumin and transported to the liver. Once it is taken up in the liver, bilirubin is transferred through the hepatocytes into the endoplasmic reticulum, where it is conjugated into a water-soluble compound by uridine diphosphate (UDP)-glucuronyl tranferase. The conjugated bilirubin is excreted via the canalicular membrane into the bile duct system and into the intestine, where it is broken down to urobilinogen and stercobilin.

Total serum bilirubin consists of both unconjugated (indirect) bilirubin and conjugated (direct) bilirubin. Total bilirubin may be elevated because of an increased heme load (e.g., hemolysis, polycythemia, hematoma), a decreased capacity for excretion (e.g., hepatitis, liver failure), or obstruction to bile flow (e.g., biliary atresia, choledochal cyst).

In addition to bilirubin, there are several laboratory tests one can obtain to assess the liver for function and injury. Hepatocellular enzymes include aspartate aminotransferase (AST), alanine aminotransferase (ALT), and lactate dehydrogenase (LDH). Elevations of AST and LDH are sensitive but not specific markers for hepatocellular injury. AST and LDH also can be found in skeletal muscle, RBCs, and cardiac tissue. ALT elevation is a specific marker for liver injury. Alkaline phosphatase and gamma glutamyltransferase (GGT) are elevated more commonly in biliary tract disease. The synthetic function of the liver can be assessed by evaluating protein production [e.g., albumin, total protein, prothrombin time (PT)], serum chemistries (e.g., glucose, cholesterol), and toxin clearance (e.g., lactate, ammonia). Among these evaluations, the most sensitive test for synthetic function of the liver is the PT.

### DIFFERENTIAL DIAGNOSIS

The differential diagnosis for jaundice in older children is extensive. The first step is to classify the jaundice as unconjugated (indirect) or conjugated (direct) hyperbilirubinemia.

## UNCONJUGATED HYPERBILIRUBINEMIA

Unconjugated hyperbilirubinemia can result from increased production (e.g., hemolysis), decreased transport and uptake of bilirubin in the liver (e.g., hypoxia and acidosis), or decreased conjugation (e.g., Gilbert syndrome, Crigler-Najjar syndrome). In conditions that lead to excessive hemolysis, such as hereditary spherocytosis, a red blood cell enzyme defect (e.g., glucose-6-phosphate dehydrogenase, pyruvate kinase), or a hemoglobinopathy (e.g., sickle cell anemia, thalassemia), the hemolysis leads to excessive heme production and a consequent increased circulating unconjugated bilirubin load. Deficiency of UDP-glucuronyl transferase can lead to decreased conjugation of bilirubin. There are three diseases in which UDP-glucuronyl transferase function is impaired. Gilbert syndrome is an autosomal recessive disorder seen in approximately 5 percent of the population. Mild unconjugated hyperbilirubinemia is seen when affected patients have a mild infectious disease, fasting, or physical stress. The prognosis is excellent, with no long-term sequelae. There are two forms of Crigler-Najjar syndrome. Type I is an autosomal recessive disorder characterized by a complete absence of UDP-glucuronyl transferase. Affected patients develop marked elevated levels of conjugated hyperbilirubinemia in the first few days of life and are at risk for kernicterus. Crigler-Najjar syndrome type II is an autosomal dominant disorder characterized by partial activity of UDP-glucuronyl transferase. Affected patients typically have lower bilirubin levels because of the partially functioning enzyme.

## CONJUGATED HYPERBILIRUBINEMIA

A variety of different types of disorders can result in conjugated hyperbilirubinemia. They include viral infections, metabolic liver disease, biliary tract disorders, autoimmune liver diseases, hepatotoxins, and vascular diseases.

### VIRAL HEPATITIS

Infections with hepatitis A, B, C, D, or E can cause jaundice that is caused by conjugated hyperbilirubinemia resulting from intrahepatic cholestasis.

Hepatitis A virus (HAV) is an RNA virus that is transmitted via the fecal-oral route through contaminated food or water. It is the most common hepatitis virus that causes infection. Spread is common in schools and daycare centers. The majority of affected children, especially young children, are asymptomatic. Older children may have a prodrome that resembles a flulike illness (fever, headache, malaise) followed by predominantly GI symptoms (nausea, vomiting, diarrhea, abdominal pain). These patients have biochemical evidence of hepatitis (elevated AST, ALT, conjugated hyperbilirubinemia). The diagnosis is confirmed with serology [elevated immunoglobulin M (IgM) anti-HAV]. Chronic infection does not occur, and management is supportive as most clinical symptoms and biochemical abnormalities resolve within 4 weeks of the initial presentation.

Hepatitis B virus (HBV), a DNA virus, is transmitted in the perinatal period from an infected mother to the fetus; by the parenteral route through exposure to infected blood products, tattooing needles, and intravenous drug use or by exposure to infected body secretions, as is seen in adolescents who engage in high-risk sexual behavior with multiple partners and infrequent use of condoms. Symptoms are variable, ranging from asymptomatic infection to nonspecific symptoms to clinical hepatitis and fulminant liver failure, although most patients either are asymptomatic or have a limited, subclinical hepatitis. The diagnosis is based on serology, with HBV surface antigen being pathognomonic for active disease. Management consists of supportive care.

Hepatitis C virus (HCV) is an RNA virus that is transmitted via the perinatal route or by parenteral exposure. Acute infection is rarely symptomatic, although it can cause chronic infection that can take decades to progress to end-stage liver disease. The diagnosis is achieved by serology demonstrating HCV antibody. Hepatitis D virus (HDV, an RNA virus) infection is uncommon in the United States, occurring only in patients who already are infected with hepatitis B. Hepatitis E virus (HEV) is an RNA virus prevalent in developing countries that is transmitted via the fecal-oral route. It presents acutely with jaundice in a manner similar to that of hepatitis A.

## METABOLIC LIVER DISEASE

A number of different metabolic diseases may present with jaundice. Wilson disease may cause acute and chronic hepatitis and liver failure. It is an autosomal recessive disorder of copper metabolism that is characterized by accumulation of copper in the liver, central nervous system, kidney, eye, and other organs. Hepatic symptoms of Wilson disease can occur at any age but most frequently appear in late childhood or adolescence. Neurologic symptoms are unusual before adolescence. The hepatic presentation is typically not acute, and affected patients may present with recurrent episodes of hyperbilirubinemia that initially is misdiagnosed as viral hepatitis. The neurologic symptoms can include dysarthria and movement disorder, behavioral disturbances, and loss of intellectual function. Kayser-Fleischer rings, which represent deposits of copper, can be visualized as golden-brown pigmentation in the outer crescent of the cornea.

A number of hepatobiliary diseases can occur in patients with cystic fibrosis (CF). As children with CF are living longer with improved therapies for the disease, liver disease is now seen more commonly. $\alpha_1$-antitrypsin deficiency may present with pulmonary emphysema and chronic liver disease in infancy. Older children may develop jaundice, cirrhosis, or hepatic failure.

## BILIARY TRACT DISORDERS

Biliary tract disorders are not common in children and adolescents. These disorders can cause an obstructive type of jaundice that is manifested by conjugated hyperbilirubinemia, scleral icterus, acholic stools, dark urine, and pruritus. Among these disorders, cholelithiasis is the most common. These patients may complain of right upper quadrant pain, and in instances of cholecystitis, a fever may be present. Choledochal cysts (congenital cystic dilations of the intrahepatic or extrahepatic biliary ducts) and primary sclerosing cholangitis (chronic fibrosing of intrahepatic or extrahepatic bile ducts) are rare biliary tract disorders seen in children.

## AUTOIMMUNE HEPATITIS

Autoimmune hepatitis is a chronic, progressive liver disease. Two subtypes have been identified, based on circulating autoantibodies. Type 1 disease is characterized by the presence of antinuclear antibodies (ANA) or anti–smooth muscle antibodies (ASMA). It is more common than type 2 disease. Type 2 disease is characterized by anti-liver-kidney microsomal antibody. Both can present with acute hepatitis, fatigue, malaise, anorexia, jaundice, and abdominal pain. Type 1 is seen more commonly in adolescents; type 2, more commonly in younger children.

## HEPATOTOXINS

A number of drugs are hepatotoxic. Overdose with acetaminophen is the most common cause of hepatic failure in adolescents. Other drugs that can cause jaundice and hepatotoxicity include antibiotics (e.g., erythromycin, sulfonamides), anticonvulsants (e.g., valproate, phenytoin), oral contraceptives, antituberculous agents (e.g., isoniazid), anesthetics (e.g., halothane), and chemotherapeutic agents (e.g., methotrexate).

## VASCULAR DISEASES

Vascular diseases are rare causes of conjugated hyperbilirubinemia in children. In the first few weeks after bone marrow transplantation, recipients can develop venoocclusive disease, which results in hepatic congestion and jaundice.

### HISTORY

Patients with jaundice also may complain of abdominal pain. Those with gallstone disease often have sharp right upper quadrant or epigastric pain. Patients with hepatitis also may complain of right upper quadrant pain, but it is characteristically dull in nature. As was noted previously, nonspecific symptoms of nausea, vomiting, fatigue, malaise, and anorexia commonly are associated with hepatitis. A patient with jaundice and inappropriate behavior, personality changes, or worsening school performance is suggestive of hepatic encephalopathy or Wilson disease. Review of systems may reveal a history of dark urine, pale stools, and pruritus, suggestive of conjugated hyperbilirubinemia.

In obtaining a past medical history, it is important to ask about risk factors for viral hepatitis, including possible perinatal transmission, blood transfusions, intravenous drug use, high-risk sexual behavior, a history of infectious contacts, and travel history. One should inquire about the use of hepatotoxic drugs, especially acetaminophen. A family history that reveals family members with jaundice may suggest a metabolic disease such as Gilbert syndrome, cystic fibrosis, Wilson disease, or $\alpha_1$-antitrypsin deficiency.

## PHYSICAL EXAMINATION

The physical examination should focus on signs of liver disease. The general appearance of the patient may reveal malnutrition that is suggestive of chronic liver disease. Examination of the eyes may reveal Kayser-Fleischer rings that are suggestive of Wilson disease. The examination of the abdomen may reveal clues to a diagnosis. Abdominal distention or dullness on percussion may be present in a patient with ascites. A patient with an enlarged, tender liver may have acute hepatitis, whereas a shrunken liver is suggestive of cirrhosis. Splenomegaly may be seen in a patient with hemolytic anemia, Epstein-Barr virus (EBV) infection, or portal hypertension. Neurologic abnormalities (e.g., confusion, delirium, or hyperreflexia) may be present in patients with hepatic encephalopathy. The skin examination of a patient with hemolytic anemia may reveal pallor. Palmar erythema and spider nevi on the chest and abdomen suggest chronic liver disease.

## LABORATORY AND RADIOGRAPHIC EVALUATION

The first step in evaluating a patient with jaundice is obtaining fractioned bilirubin levels to determine whether the hyperbilirubinemia is unconjugated or conjugated. Unconjugated hyperbilirubinemia is most often due to hemolytic disease, and so tests such as a complete blood count, reticulocyte count, blood smear, direct and indirect Coombs test, and hemoglobin electrophoresis should be obtained. Conjugated hyperbilirubinemia is suggestive of hepatobiliary disease. The initial laboratory evaluation in these cases should include liver function tests (e.g., AST, ALT, GGT, alkaline phosphatase) and tests that measure synthetic liver function (e.g., PT, total protein, albumin, glucose, cholesterol, ammonia).

Further testing is dictated by the results of the initial laboratory results. Many patients with conjugated hyperbilirubinemia undergo an abdominal ultrasound to evaluate the liver and biliary tract. Serology for hepatitis A, B, and C should be considered in patients in whom viral hepatitis is suspected. A Monospot test or EBV serology should be obtained in patients in whom hepatitis resulting from EBV is suspected. A sweat chloride test is recommended in patients to rule out cystic fibrosis. A serum $\alpha_1$-antitrypsin level can help rule out $\alpha_1$-antitrypsin deficiency. Laboratory evaluation in patients with suspected autoimmune hepatitis should include ANA, AMSA, and anti-liver-kidney microsomal antibody. Patients with autoimmune hepatitis may have a high serum protein relative to the albumin, reflecting an increased globulin fraction. A decreased serum ceruloplasmin level is suggestive of Wilson disease. A 24-h urine collection for copper will reveal increased urine copper excretion in these patients. A liver biopsy may be performed to confirm the diagnosis of autoimmune hepatitis or Wilson disease.

## MANAGEMENT

Management depends on the specific cause of the liver disease. Those with hemolytic disease require close monitoring of their renal function and hyperhydration. Those with acute viral hepatitis often require supportive care for the acute infection. Patients with autoimmune hepatitis are treated with immunosuppressive agents (e.g., prednisone, cyclosporine). The drug of choice for patients with Wilson disease is penicillamine.

## BIBLIOGRAPHY

Fox VL. Gastrointestinal bleeding in infancy and childhood. *Gastroenterol Clin North Am* 29:37–66, 2000.

Hyams JS. Inflammatory bowel disease. *Pediatr Rev* 21:291–295, 2000.

Pashankar D, Schreiber RA. Jaundice in older children and adolescents. *Pediatr Rev* 22:219–226, 2001.

# HEMATOLOGY AND ONCOLOGY

*Joseph Gigante*

## LEARNING OBJECTIVES

1. Use the findings from the history, physical examination, and laboratory tests to help develop a differential diagnosis for anemia.

2. Outline the common signs and symptoms of iron-deficiency anemia.

3. List the clinical manifestations of bleeding disorders.

4. Describe the common presenting symptoms of acute lymphoblastic leukemia (ALL), neuroblastoma, and Wilms' tumor.

## ANEMIA

*PATHOPHYSIOLOGY*

Anemia is one of the most common laboratory abnormalities seen in pediatrics. Approximately 20 percent of children in the United States have anemia at some time before 18 years of age. Anemia is defined as a low hemoglobin (Hgb) concentration or red blood cell (RBC) mass compared with age-specific normal values. The Hgb of a term newborn is high at birth and then declines to a physiologic nadir between 6 and 8 weeks of age. After puberty, the Hgb values are similar to adult values. In thinking about the causes of anemia, one can classify the causes as secondary to decreased RBC production, increased RBC destruction, or blood loss. Another method of classifying anemia is based on the size of the RBC on a peripheral smear. In this scheme, there are three major morphologic categories: microcytic, normochromic, and macrocytic anemias.

A reticulocyte count also may be helpful in classifying anemias. The reticulocyte count is a measure of the activity of the bone marrow in producing immature RBCs. The normal reticulocyte count is 1 percent, reflecting the percentage of RBCs that are reticulocytes. The reticulocyte counts should rise in most anemias. A low reticulocyte count indicates an inadequate bone marrow response to low Hgb values, suggesting diminished hemopoiesis or bone marrow failure.

## HISTORY

The signs and symptoms of anemia vary with the degree of the anemia and the rate at which the anemia develops. Many children with mild anemia show few, if any, signs or symptoms. Pallor may be noted by the child's parents in instances of mild anemia. As the degree of anemia worsens, the child may develop more symptoms, such as weakness, fatigue, exercise intolerance, irritability, and anorexia. In severe cases, the child may have tachypnea and shortness of breath as a result of congestive heart failure. Other aspects of the history that may be helpful in patients with anemia include dietary history, family history, and social history. A child who has excessive milk intake (defined as more than 24 oz per day) is at risk for iron-deficiency anemia. A family history of splenectomy or cholecystectomy may indicate a hereditary hemolytic process (e.g., spherocytosis). With regard to social history, the ethnic background of the family may reveal clues to the diagnosis. Families of African descent have a higher risk of sickle cell disease. Families of Mediterranean or Asian descent have a higher risk of thalassemia. Children who live in older homes may be at risk for lead toxicity.

## PHYSICAL EXAMINATION

As was noted above, children with mild anemia may demonstrate few, if any, findings on physical examination. In patients with moderate to severe anemia, tachycardia may be noted when vital signs are obtained. Cardiac examination may reveal a systolic murmur, and in severe cases signs of congestive heart failure may be evident. Splenomegaly may be present in patients with a hemolytic anemia (e.g., spherocytosis). Hepatomegaly or lymphadenopathy may indicate a neoplastic process. The presence of pallor should be assessed by examination of the skin, conjunctiva, and mucous membranes.

## LABORATORY AND RADIOGRAPHIC EVALUATION

Children with mild anemia often present without symptoms. The condition is detected on routine screening, because of a low hemoglobin/hematocrit obtained for another reason, or because of pallor. Children usually are screened with hemoglobin or hematocrit at 9 to 15 months of age. The results of the hemoglobin and hematocrit should be interpreted in light of their variation with the patient's age. If anemia is suspected, the initial evaluation should include a complete blood count (CBC) with RBC parameters [e.g., mean corpuscular volume (MCV) and mean corpuscular hemoglobin concentration (MCHC)], reticulocyte count, and peripheral blood smear. The CBC is helpful in determining whether other cell lines are affected. The RBC parameters and peripheral smear will help determine if the anemia is microcytic hypochromic, normocytic normochromic, or macrocytic. The reticulocyte count measures circulating immature RBCs and is an indicator of erythropoiesis. It is decreased in patients with iron-deficiency anemia or bone marrow failure and increased in patients with acute blood loss or hemolytic anemia. If hemolysis is suspected, additional tests that may be useful include lactate dehydrogenase (LDH) and serum bilirubin, which will be elevated, and a Coombs' test. The direct Coombs' test will be positive when antigen binds antibody on the RBC surface, whereas the indirect Coombs' test will be positive when antigen binds circulating RBC antibodies.

Other tests can be ordered once a differential diagnosis has been formulated from the results of the history, physical examination, and initial laboratory tests.

## MANAGEMENT

The management of anemia depends on the underlying cause, the clinical status of the patient, and the degree of anemia. Most children who are affected have mild anemia and are not acutely ill, and so determining the cause of the anemia is the first step. However, in children who are ill, supportive care such as fluid resuscitation and blood transfusions may be necessary before one determines the cause of the anemia.

## COMMON ANEMIAS

### IRON-DEFICIENCY ANEMIA

Iron deficiency is the most common nutritional deficiency in the world, and iron-deficiency anemia is the most common cause of anemia in infants and children. In the United States, the most common cause of iron deficiency with or without anemia is insufficient dietary iron. Infants, toddlers, and adolescents are particularly susceptible because of their relatively rapid growth and increased demand for iron.

#### PATHOPHYSIOLOGY

Iron is critical for several vital functions, including oxygen transport. Most iron in the body is found in hemoglobin. Excess iron is stored in the liver, bone marrow, and spleen in the form of ferritin. A term infant is born with enough iron to last 6 to 9 months. Iron deficiency is common at 10 to 18 months of age because of inadequate iron stores and inadequate intake. It is also common in adolescent females because of rapid growth, poor diet, and loss of blood from menstruation.

## HISTORY AND PHYSICAL EXAMINATION

Many children with iron-deficiency anemia are asymptomatic. For those who are symptomatic, the signs and symptoms are those described in the section on anemia, above. Children who are started on cow's milk at an early age (younger than 1 year) and who drink large amounts of cow's milk (more than 24 oz per day) are at risk for iron deficiency because cow's milk contains little iron, replaces food with a higher iron content, and can cause occult intestinal bleeding. Iron-deficiency anemia in infancy and early childhood has been associated with developmental delays and behavior disturbances, which may be irreversible.

## LABORATORY AND RADIOGRAPHIC EVALUATION

Children with iron-deficiency anemia have levels of Hgb and hematocrit (Hct) below the 5th percentile for age, although these values are not specific for iron deficiency. The MCV is decreased, and the peripheral smear reveals a microcytic hypochromic anemia. Serum ferritin levels decline as iron stores are depleted. Total iron-binding capacity (TIBC) measures the amount of iron that can bind to serum proteins. As serum iron decreases, TIBC begins to increase. The red blood cell distribution width (RDW) measures the variation in size of RBCs and increases with iron deficiency. Impairment of hemoglobin synthesis results in accumulation of free erythrocyte protoporphyrin (FEP). FEP is elevated in iron deficiency but also is elevated in lead poisoning and chronic disease.

## MANAGEMENT

Iron-deficiency anemia is treated with 3 to 6 mg/kg per day of oral elemental iron. After 1 month of therapy, Hgb should be repeated, and an increase of 1g/dL confirms the diagnosis of iron-deficiency anemia. Therapy should be continued for 2 to 3 months to replenish iron stores. Dietary counseling also should take place to increase nutritional iron and prevent future iron deficiency. In children with anemia that does not respond to iron, further evaluation is needed to rule out other causes of anemia.

## SICKLE CELL DISEASE

### PATHOPHYSIOLOGY

Sickle cell disease is a hemoglobinopathy caused by the single amino acid substitution of valine for glutamic acid on the number 6 position of the beta chain of Hgb. Polymerization of Hgb occurs when RBCs are exposed to conditions such as low oxygen concentrations, acidosis, and temperature changes. This leads to distortion in the shape of the RBC (sickling), resulting in a decreased life span of the RBC (hemolysis), sludging, and organ ischemia and possible infarction.

## HISTORY

Many states have newborn screening programs that detect hemoglobinopathies such as sickle cell disease at birth. Beta-chain abnormalities such as hemoglobin S do not cause symptoms until the change from fetal hemoglobin to β hemoglobin, which occurs between the ages of 6 and 12 months. Symptoms therefore usually develop at 6 to 12 months of age. Symptoms of sickle cell disease often result from the occlusion of small vessels, but they also may result from infection or from the anemia itself. The vasoocclusive symptoms can occur in any organ. A common initial presentation is dactylitis (swelling and pain in the hands and feet). Painful crises as a result of vasoocclusion also occur in the extremities, joints, abdomen, and back. Vasoocclusive episodes also can cause priapism, stroke (the patient may have central nervous system complaints such as headache), and acute chest syndrome (infarction of the lung), with the possible complaints including chest pain, cough, and shortness of breath.

## PHYSICAL EXAMINATION

Fever in patients with sickle cell disease is always taken seriously because it may represent sepsis. Patients with sickle cell disease are susceptible to infection with encapsulated organisms such as pneumococci because of splenic dysfunction. There is also a susceptibility to osteomyelitis, possibly as a result of bone infections, with *Staphylococcus aureus* and *Salmonella* as organisms commonly causing infection.

Patients commonly have pallor and scleral icterus or jaundice. Those with severe anemia may have fatigue, exercise intolerance, lethargy, and limitation of activities. A heart murmur may be present. The spleen may be palpable during the first year of life, but it usually autoinfarcts and disappears after the first few years of life. Depending on the type of crisis these patients are experiencing, they may complain of joint, muscle, or abdominal tenderness. Those with acute chest syndrome may have consolidation on chest examination. Those with stroke may have neurologic signs such as dysarthria or hemiplegia, although some may be asymptomatic. Priapism may be noted on genital examination.

## LABORATORY AND RADIOGRAPHIC EVALUATION

Patients with sickle cell disease are anemic, and so the hemoglobin and hematocrit are decreased. The reticulocyte count, along with the white blood cell count and platelet count, is increased, reflecting heightened bone marrow activity caused by RBC destruction. Sickled cells, other abnormally shaped cells, and target cells are seen on the peripheral blood smear.

## MANAGEMENT

### Prevention

Patients with sickle cell disease should receive all the routine immunizations, including the 23-valent pneumococcal and meningococcal vaccine and a yearly vaccination for influenza virus. They also should be given daily penicillin prophylaxis to decrease the risk of pneumococcal infection. Daily folic acid is given to prevent folic acid deficiency.

### Infection

Because of the increased risk of infection, children with sickle cell disease and fever are managed with urgent assessment and appropriate cultures (blood and urine) along with CBC and chest radiographs to evaluate for pneumonia. Lumbar puncture and evaluation for osteomyelitis should be considered when there is a concern for meningitis or a bone infection. Parenteral antibiotics are administered until bacterial infection has been ruled out.

### Pain Crisis

Mild to moderate pain crises may be managed on an outpatient basis with increased hydration and oral analgesics. If the pain persists or worsens, inpatient treatment may be necessary. Hospital management of patients with severe anemia, vasoocclusion, or pain crises includes intravenous hydration, intravenous analgesia, oxygen, judicious transfusion, and exchange transfusion.

## HEREDITARY SPHEROCYTOSIS

### PATHOPHYSIOLOGY

Hereditary spherocytosis is the most common of the hereditary red blood cell membrane disorders and usually is inherited as an autosomal dominant trait. There is a deficiency or abnormality of the structural red blood cell protein spectrin that causes the RBCs to assume a spherical shape, which permits the cell to be destroyed prematurely in the spleen.

### HISTORY

Symptoms vary with the severity of the defect and the degree of compensation. Neonates can present with jaundice in the first day of life. Some children remain asymptomatic and are detected because they have splenomegaly or because of mild anemia noted on routine examination. The history may reveal jaundice or anemia. Familial history of splenectomy, gallbladder disease, or hereditary spherocytosis may be present (approximately 75 percent of these patients have a positive family history).

### PHYSICAL EXAMINATION

The physical examination may reveal pallor, fatigue, jaundice, and exercise intolerance. Splenomegaly may be present because spherocytes are trapped in the spleen and destroyed. These patients may complain of abdominal pain secondary to cholelithiasis caused by increased RBC turnover.

## LABORATORY AND RADIOGRAPHIC EVALUATION

A CBC and reticulocyte count may reveal anemia with a reticulocytosis that reflects increased RBC production. These patients are susceptible to aplastic crisis, most commonly caused by parvovirus infection. Those with aplastic crisis may have leukopenia and thrombocytopenia. The cardinal feature of this disorder is the presence of numerous spherocytes on the peripheral blood smear. The osmotic fragility test can detect spherocytes but is not specific for this disorder. In this test, spherocytic RBCs hemolyze more readily in hypotonic solutions.

## MANAGEMENT

Splenectomy is recommended after age 5 (to decrease the risk of infection with encapsulated organisms) in patients who cannot maintain an adequate hemoglobin level or have had aplastic crises. Transfusion therapy may be used in children younger than 2 years of age who have severe disease. Routine immunizations, including the 23-valent pneumococcal and meningococcal vaccine and a yearly vaccination for influenza virus, should be administered. Folic acid should be given daily to prevent secondary folic acid deficiency.

# BLEEDING AND BRUISING

## PATHOPHYSIOLOGY

Bleeding disorders may occur as a result of abnormalities of platelets, coagulation factors, or blood vessels. Dysfunction or deficiency of any of these elements may result in bleeding.

## HISTORY

A detailed history that includes the timing, location, and type of bleeding may give clues to possible causes of bleeding and bruising. An otherwise healthy child with the sudden onset of bruising and petechiae most likely has an acquired condition such as idiopathic thrombocytopenic purpura (ITP). In contrast, a history of repeated episodes of bleeding from surgical procedures (e.g., circumcision, dental extractions, tonsillectomy) or a family history of easy bruising or abnormal bleeding suggests a congenital disorder. A history of mucosal bleeding (e.g., bleeding gums) is suggestive of a platelet disorder or von Willebrand disease. Bleeding into muscles and joints suggests a coagulation disorder. Bleeding that is severe or persistent, occurs at more than one site, or requires treatment with a transfusion is suggestive of a bleeding disorder. A medication history is also important, since drugs such as aspirin and ibuprofen can cause platelet dysfunction.

### PHYSICAL EXAMINATION

A careful physical examination with attention to the skin and oral and nasal mucosa is important. The skin examination may reveal several different types of lesions. Petechiae are small (less than 3 mm), flat, nonblanching lesions. Ecchymotic lesions are large and can be flat, raised, or tender. Extensive ecchymotic lesions in various stages of resolution in areas of the body where children rarely experience trauma should raise the suspicion of child abuse. Deep hematomas or hemarthrosis suggests a coagulation disorder. Purpuric lesions are larger lesions that can vary in size that result from hemorrhaging in the skin. Purpura predominantly on the back of the legs and buttocks is suggestive of Henoch-Schönlein purpura. Purpura fulminans (purplish-black, well-demarcated lesions with central necrosis) usually is associated with sepsis and disseminated intravascular coagulation (DIC). Patients with significant lymphadenopathy and hepatosplenomegaly may have leukemia or a malignancy.

### LABORATORY EVALUATION

The following laboratory tests should be considered when one is evaluating a child for a bleeding disorder: CBC with platelets; peripheral blood smear to evaluate platelet morphology; prothrombin time (PT) to screen for clotting activity of factors II, V, VII, and X; and activated prothrombin time (aPTT) to screen for the clotting activity of factors V, VIII, IX, and XII. The PT measures the function of the extrinsic and common pathway, and the aPTT measures the function of the intrinsic and common pathways. Bleeding times are not obtained commonly but can provide information about the quality of platelet function and platelet interaction with the blood vessel wall.

## MANAGEMENT

Patients who have a life-threatening hemorrhage require immediate attention to their circulatory status. Fluid resuscitation with crystalloid solutions (e.g., normal saline, lactated Ringer's) or blood products will be needed for volume expansion. In instances in which the hemorrhage is not life-threatening, a diagnosis should be made and the appropriate treatment should be instituted.

## SPECIFIC BLEEDING DISORDERS

### IDIOPATHIC THROMBOCYTOPENIC PURPURA

Idiopathic thrombocytopenic purpura is the most common bleeding disorder of childhood. It occurs most frequently in children 2 to 5 years of age. The cause is not known, and a preceding viral illness 1 to 3 weeks earlier is common.

## HISTORY AND PHYSICAL EXAMINATION

Children with ITP are typically healthy and present with the appearance of multiple purpuric lesions. They may have petechiae of the lips and buccal mucosa. Significant bleeding is not common, but they may have epistaxis. A finding of lymphadenopathy or hepatomegaly should raise the suspicion for leukemia.

### Laboratory Evaluation

A CBC in a patient with ITP typically will reveal a markedly decreased platelet count (less than 50,000), with the platelets present being larger in size. The white blood cell count, differential, and hematocrit should be normal. Bone marrow aspiration is not performed routinely in patients who are thought to have typical findings of ITP. It should be performed before corticosteroids are administered to avoid masking a leukemic process.

## MANAGEMENT

Most children with ITP require no therapy. Those with acute ITP often have spontaneous resolution within 6 months of the diagnosis. In patients with significant bleeding, treatment with intravenous immune globulin (IVIG) or corticosteroids is indicated. IVIG is associated with a faster response in the platelet count than corticosteroids but is more expensive.

## HEMOPHILIA A (FACTOR VIII DEFICIENCY) AND HEMOPHILIA B (FACTOR IX DEFICIENCY)

Classic hemophilia (hemophilia A, factor VIII deficiency) is the cause of hemophilia in 85 percent of patients; the remaining 15 percent have hemophilia B (factor IX deficiency). Hemophilia A occurs in approximately 1 in 10,000 live male births. There is no racial predilection for this disorder, which typically occurs in males via an X-linked inheritance pattern.

## HISTORY AND PHYSICAL EXAMINATION

Most patients with hemophilia have a positive family history of bleeding disorders, but up to a third of cases are due to spontaneous mutations. Infants with hemophilia may experience excessive bleeding after a circumcision or bruising at injection sites. Older children may develop large hematomas, easy bruisability, and intramuscular hemorrhages. Recurrent hemarthrosis often leads to destruction of the affected joint. Those with severe factor deficiency have frequent episodes of spontaneous bleeding.

## LABORATORY EVALUATION

Laboratory evaluation should include a CBC with platelet count, PT, aPTT, and bleeding time. The aPTT will be prolonged with both factor VIII and factor IX deficiency, whereas the PT and bleeding time will be normal. Levels of factors VIII and IX can be measured. Factor VIII and factor IX levels less than 1 percent are classified as severe deficiency, whereas mild factor deficiency is seen in those with factor activity of 5 to 40 percent.

### MANAGEMENT

The aim of management is to correct the factor activity to normal to prevent or stop bleeding. The most severe hemorrhages are intracranial, abdominal, retropharyngeal, and in the extremities. Factors VIII and IX are available as concentrates from purified human plasma or as recombinant proteins. Much of the management of these patients is at home, with parents infusing factor.

## ONCOLOGY

### ACUTE LYMPHOBLASTIC LEUKEMIA

Acute lymphoblastic leukemia (ALL) is the most common malignancy seen in the pediatric population. It accounts for 80 percent of cases of acute leukemia, with acute myelocytic leukemia (AML) accounting for about 20 percent of cases. The peak age at onset is 4 years, although patients of all ages can be affected.

### PATHOPHYSIOLOGY

The cause of ALL is not known. Genetic factors play a role, as there is an increased incidence in twins and siblings. There is also an increased incidence of ALL in chromosomal abnormalities (e.g., trisomy 21) and immunodeficiencies (e.g., ataxia-telangiectasia).

### HISTORY

The symptoms most commonly seen in children with ALL are fever, fatigue, and bone or joint pain. The bone or joint pain may manifest as a limp or refusal to walk. The parents may note that the child appears pale or bruises easily. It is important to obtain a medication history and a thorough family history.

### PHYSICAL EXAMINATION

Signs on physical examination that are related to bone marrow infiltration of leukemic cells include pallor, bruises, petechiae, and purpura. Lymphadenopathy is common and may be localized or generalized to the cervical, axillary, and inguinal regions. A flow murmur secondary to anemia may be present. Hepatosplenomegaly can be seen in up to approximately one-half to two-thirds of affected patients. Testicular pain and swelling may be present secondary to leukemic infiltration. Epistaxis or evidence of bleeding elsewhere is common.

## LABORATORY EVALUATION

A complete blood count with differential is the most useful initial test in children with suspected ALL since it will reveal an abnormality in one cell line if not two or all three cell lines in 95 percent of patients. Anemia and/or thrombocytopenia may be seen. The white blood cell count (WBC) is variable: it may be low (<10,000 cells/mm$^3$), normal, or high (>50,000 cells/mm$^3$). Lymphoblasts may be seen on the peripheral smear, and sometimes are mistakenly reported as atypical lymphocytes. The definitive diagnosis of ALL is made by bone marrow examination, which reveals infiltration of lymphoblasts replacing normal marrow elements.

## MANAGEMENT

Management and treatment of children with ALL are determined by prognostic factors present at the time of diagnosis. Most patients with ALL are enrolled in clinical trials designed by the Children's Oncology Group, a worldwide organization whose members are committed to the development of new therapies for childhood malignancies. Management typically includes three stages: induction, consolidation, and maintenance. The goal of induction is to destroy as many malignant cells as possible to induce remission. The second phase of therapy—consolidation—is designed to destroy leukemic cells that may be present in the central nervous system. The final phase of therapy is maintenance, during which the patient is given daily and periodic chemotherapy during remission. The outlook for ALL is generally quite good. The survival rate for all patients with ALL is approximately 80 percent.

## NEUROBLASTOMA

Neuroblastoma is a malignant tumor that originates from neural crest tissue of the sympathetic ganglia or adrenal medulla. It is the most common malignancy of infancy and the most common solid neoplasm outside the central nervous system. Approximately half the cases are diagnosed before age 2, with 90 percent diagnosed by age 5.

## HISTORY

The presenting signs and symptoms of neuroblastoma vary with the primary site of the disease and metastasis. Patients with an abdominal primary tumor may present with abdominal pain, anorexia, weight loss, and abdominal distention. Patients with primary or metastatic neuroblastoma of the head and neck may present with Horner syndrome (e.g., miosis, ptosis, and anhydrosis). Neuroblastomas produce catecholamines, and so symptoms such as episodic sweating, flushing, pallor, headache, or palpitation may be reported.

## Physical Examination

Patients in whom catecholamines are secreted may have hypertension. Most of these patients have an abdominal primary tumor, and so a firm, non-tender abdominal mass that crosses the midline may be present. Patients with liver metastases may have hepatomegaly. Skin metastases may be suspected by the appearance of skin nodules with a "blueberry muffin" appearance. Neuroblastoma also is associated with paraneoplastic manifestations such as watery diarrhea as a result of the secretion of vasoactive intestinal peptides. Another paraneoplastic manifestation is opsoclonus-myoclonus (shooting eye movements and myoclonic jerking, commonly referred to as the "dancing eyes, dancing feet syndrome").

## Laboratory and Radiographic Evaluation

The initial evaluation of patients with suspected neuroblastoma includes a urine collection for catecholamines, along with imaging studies such as an abdominal ultrasound or computed tomography (CT).

## Management

Based on the staging of the tumor, a number of different treatments may be indicated. Surgery alone may be curative for stage I and stage II disease, whereas a combination of chemotherapy and radiation therapy may be used for metastatic or advanced disease. Interestingly, spontaneous regression without treatment may occur in infants with stage IV-S disease.

## WILMS' TUMOR

Wilms' tumor is the most common childhood renal tumor. It is the second most common abdominal tumor in children (after neuroblastoma). It occurs most commonly in children younger than 5 years of age.

## History

The most common presentation is increasing abdominal distention and/or an asymptomatic abdominal mass noted by a parent. Anorexia, weight loss, urinary retention, abdominal pain, or hematuria may be present.

## Physical Examination

As was noted above, patients with Wilms' tumor will have an abdominal mass on physical examination that is typically smooth and firm and rarely crosses the midline. Hypertension may be present secondary to pressure on the renal artery or increased renin secretion by the tumor. There are some congenital anomalies associated with Wilms' tumor, including aniridia, hemihypertrophy, and genitourinary malformations (hypospadias, cryptorchidism).

## LABORATORY AND RADIOGRAPHIC EVALUATION

Urinalysis may reveal gross blood or microscopic hematuria. If Wilms' tumor is suspected, an imaging study of the abdomen (ultrasound or CT) should be performed to establish the presence of an intrarenal mass.

## MANAGEMENT

Wilms' tumor typically is treated with a combination of surgical resection and chemotherapy. The prognosis is dependent on the staging and histology of the tumor.

## BIBLIOGRAPHY

Lanzowsky P, ed. *Manual of Pediatric Hematology and Oncology*, 4th ed. New York: Churchill Livingston, 2005.

Nathan DG, Orkin SH, eds. *Nathan and Oski's Hematology of Infancy and Childhood*, 6th ed. Philadelphia: Saunders, 2003.

Segel GB, Hirsh MG, Feig SA. Managing anemia in pediatric office practice: Part 1. *Pediatr Rev* 23:75–83, 2002.

# INFECTIOUS DISEASE

*Gregory Plemmons*

## LEARNING OBJECTIVES

1. Recognize the presenting signs and symptoms of meningitis.
2. List the treatments for common head and neck infections such as conjunctivitis, sinusitis, preseptal cellulitis, and cervical adenitis.
3. List the treatments for common skin infections such as impetigo, cellulitis, and skin abscess.
4. Describe the initial laboratory testing and imaging studies for osteomyelitis.
5. List the groups that are at high risk for tuberculosis.
6. Know the presentations of common viral infections such as erythema infectiosum and roseola.

## INTRODUCTION

Infectious disease plays more of a daily role in pediatrics than it does in any other primary care specialty. An overwhelming majority of visits for acute illness are for infectious diseases, ranging from ubiquitous rhinovirus "sniffles" to rare but life-threatening meningococcal sepsis. Each new edition of the *Red Book*, the pediatric infectious disease "bible" revised and updated every 3 years by the American Academy of Pediatrics (AAP) Committee on Infectious Diseases, is anticipated by many pediatricians almost as eagerly as a new *Harry Potter*. This chapter attempts to cover a spectrum of infectious diseases but is by no means exhaustive.

## BACTEREMIA AND SEPSIS

Sepsis is every pediatrician's nightmare. Within a matter of hours, a seemingly healthy child or infant can develop life-threatening complications from a variety of organisms as a result of immaturity or compromise of the immune system. Even with advances in immunization and antibiotic therapy, a pediatrician always must maintain a high index of suspicion for bloodborne pathogens and serious illness in any child who presents with fever in the outpatient setting. Although most illnesses in children are caused by viral infections and are usually self-limiting, clinicians often must weigh the likelihood of serious bacterial illness (SBI) with each child's presentation. Evidence-based guidelines developed over the last 20 years have helped guide the evaluation and management of fever in children and undoubtedly will continue to do so.

A landmark study in the management of pediatric fever published by Jaskiewicz and associates in 1994 often is referred to as the Rochester criteria. Historically, any infant less than 2 or 3 months of age presenting with fever underwent a full evaluation for sepsis, including blood and urine cultures as well as lumbar puncture for cerebrospinal fluid (CSF) cultures, usually was hospitalized, and empirically was begun on antibiotics for several days while awaiting culture results even though the majority of illnesses were suspected to be viral. Jaskiewicz and associates were able to show that the likelihood of SBI was minimal in infants less than 2 months of age who met the following criteria:

- Were well-appearing
- Had no evidence of focal infection
- Had a white blood cell (WBC) count between 5000 and 15,000 cells/L, a band count $\leq$ 5000 cells/L, $\leq$ 10 WBC per high-power field (HPF) on urinalysis, and/or $\leq$ 5 WBC per HPF on stool smear (if having diarrhea)

Subsequent studies have reexamined the criteria and will continue to refine the optimal way to evaluate fever in children. Evaluation and management of children with fever will keep changing as rapid techniques for identifying viral infections continue to evolve and the incidence of bacterial illness continues to decline as a result of the introduction of new vaccines.

## THE FEBRILE NEONATE

Infants are uniquely susceptible to sepsis. An organism as seemingly benign as group B streptococcus (*Streptococcus agalactiae*), which may colonize the reproductive tracts of up to 20 percent of women of childbearing age, may have devastating consequences in a neonate. An infant who presents with fever, even low-grade fever [38°C (100.4°F) or higher], often constitutes a pediatric emergency and frequently necessitates prompt evaluation and often hospitalization. Following is a list of the most serious pathogens in neonates:

- Group B *Streptococcus (Streptococcus agalactiae)*
- *Escherichia coli*
- *Listeria monocytogenes*
- Herpes simplex virus
- *Staphylococcus aureus*
- *Enterococcus* species

Most infants under 1 month of age generally undergo evaluation for sepsis, and urine and blood cultures are obtained as well as CSF culture. Empirical coverage of potential pathogens usually includes a β-lactam antibiotic such as ampicillin (for coverage of *Listeria* and group B streptococci) as well as an aminoglycoside (for coverage of gram-negative organisms such as *E. coli*). Antiviral coverage for herpes with intravenous (IV) acyclovir also may be a consideration.

*Bacteremia* simply refers to the presence of bacteria in the blood and is confirmed by a positive blood culture. Everyone has experienced transient bacteremia from something as seemingly benign as tooth cleaning. Although the human immune system provides constant surveillance to search for and destroy bloodborne intruders, these mechanisms are often immature or ineffective in neonates and young children. Bacteremia also may be common in children with central intravenous catheters and immunosuppressed children. A child with leukemia who becomes neutropenic from chemotherapy, for instance, usually is admitted automatically and treated with intravenous antibiotics at the onset of fever for fear of progression to sepsis.

*Occult bacteremia* refers to the presence of bacteria in the blood in children who are febrile with no obvious source of infection. Historically, *Strep. pneumoniae* and *Haemophilus influenzae* type B (HIB) were common causes, and they remain important pathogens, especially in the Third World. Widespread immunization against HIB and pneumococci undoubtedly will continue to affect etiology in children.

## Most Common Pathogens in Occult Bacteremia in Children 3 to 36 Months of Age (Ranked in Descending Order)

- *Streptococcus pneumoniae*
- *Haemophilus influenzae* type B
- *Neisseria meningitidis*
- *Salmonella* species

## SEPSIS

Septic shock is a common cause of admission to the pediatric intensive care unit (PICU). Organisms such as *Strep. pneumoniae, Neisseria meningitidis,* and historically *H. influenzae* type B can produce overwhelming infection in normal hosts, and even seemingly benign pathogens such as *Candida* spp. and *E. coli* may be life-threatening in an immunocompromised host. Increasingly, the host response to infection and the specific pathogen involved seem to play a crucial role in the survival and prognosis of children. Most children with sepsis demonstrate some variation in temperature (fever or hypothermia). In early sepsis, many children produce a high-cardiac-output state characterized by tachycardia, hypertension or normotension, and normal perfusion of tissue. In later stages, cardiac output decreases, often with notable changes in perfusion, marked by hypotension, decreased capillary refill time (often assessed at the bedside by blanching the nail beds), weakened peripheral pulses, and cool extremities. The WBC count may be elevated, normal, or even low, particularly in instances of overwhelming sepsis, when the body's reserves may be depleted. Airway management, volume resuscitation, and cardiovascular support (e.g., addition of medications such as dopamine and dobutamine) are crucial in the treatment of sepsis; antibiotic therapy may be useless unless it is given early in the course of disease.

## MENINGITIS

Any infection of the membranes overlying the spinal cord and the brain (meninges) and subarachnoid space may produce inflammation. The spectrum of acute clinical findings may range from headache to life-threatening cerebral edema, and postinfectious complications vary widely as well.

### CLINICAL PRESENTATION
- Fever
- Neck stiffness
- Rash (think viruses, rickettsial disease, and meningococcal disease)
- Headache
- Nausea and vomiting
- Focal neurologic abnormalities
- Seizures
- Mental status changes

### PHYSICAL EXAMINATION POINTERS
- *Always* assess vital signs and ABCs (airway, breathing, circulation).
- *Always* perform a careful and detailed neurologic exam, including a survey of the cranial nerves.

- The term *paradoxical irritability* often is used to describe a child with meningitis who is quiet at rest but cries when moved or comforted because of meningeal irritation.
- *Photophobia* may be present but is obviously difficult to detect in a non-verbal child.
- A *bulging fontanel* may be present in infants but is not entirely specific for meningitis.
- *Nuchal rigidity,* or "stiff neck," may be caused by torticollis or other non-infectious causes and is poorly sensitive in children, especially in those less than 18 to 24 months of age.

Additional maneuvers historically have been used to assess clinically for meningitis (sometimes called meningeal signs):

- *Kernig sign.* To perform the Kernig maneuver, have the patient supine with the hips flexed at 90 degrees. Extend the knee from this position. Any resistance or pain in the lower back or posterior thigh is considered a positive sign.
- *Brudzinski sign.* To perform this maneuver, have the patient supine and passively flex the patient's neck. Any flexion of the knees or hips is considered a positive sign.

These two signs are unreliable, especially in children under 18 to 24 months of age, and the diagnosis of meningitis still rests largely on studies and culture of CSF.

## LABORATORY STUDIES

As was mentioned above, clinical findings are frequently subtle and very nonspecific in children and often necessitate performing a lumbar puncture (LP), or "spinal tap." A frequently repeated axiom in pediatrics is "If you think about tapping a child, then you should do it," since the consequences of missing central nervous system (CNS) infection may be devastating. LP allows for rapid diagnosis and specific identification of pathogens through CSF analysis and culture and, increasingly, polymerase chain reaction (PCR) detection of pathogens. Most experts still recommend delaying the LP if signs of increased intracranial pressure (ICP) are present until further evaluation by computed tomography (CT) of the head, since LP may precipitate herniation in rare instances of increased ICP.

*CSF Findings in Infants and Children*

| Component | Normal Children | Normal Newborns | Bacterial Meningitis | Viral Meningitis | Herpes Meningitis |
|---|---|---|---|---|---|
| Leukocytes/μL | 0–6 | 0–30 | > 1000 | 100–500 | 10–1000 |
| Neutrophils (%) | 0 | 2–3 | > 50 | < 40 | < 50 |
| Glucose (mg/dL) | 40–80 | 32–121 | < 30 | > 30 | > 30 |
| Protein (mg/dL) | 20–30 | 19–149 | > 100 | 50–100 | > 75 |
| Erythrocytes/μL | 0–2 | 0–2 | 0–10 | 0–2 | 10–500 |

## BACTERIAL MENINGITIS

Bacterial meningitis is the most serious form of meningitis and fortunately is less common than viral meningitis. Group B streptococcus (*Strep. agalactiae*) and, less commonly, *E. coli* and *L. monocytogenes* are serious pathogens in infants in the first 3 months of life. Among older infants and schoolchildren, *Strep. pneumoniae* and *N. meningitidis* are important causes.

## VIRAL MENINGITIS

Viral meningitis may be caused by a variety of pathogens, including enteroviruses, arboviruses, and herpesviruses. The clinical presentation may be indistinguishable from that of bacterial meningitis, and frequently empirical therapy for suspected bacterial meningitis is begun while awaiting culture results or further CSF testing.

## ASEPTIC MENINGITIS

The term *aseptic meningitis* commonly is used to describe any instance in which CSF cultures do not yield bacterial growth and often is used interchangeably with *viral meningitis*. Less common causes of aseptic meningitis include fungal CSF infections (frequently in an immunocompromised host) and tuberculous infections.

### COMPLICATIONS

Most of the complications reported generally result from bacterial infection. In general, viral meningitis (with the exception of herpes) produces few postinfectious sequelae:

- *Deafness* is the most common complication that follows bacterial infection; up to a third of pneumococcal infections and 5 to 10 percent of meningococcal infections may result in sensorineural hearing loss.
- *Subdural effusions* and, less commonly, subdural empyemas may result from bacterial meningitis and the intense postinflammatory response

that may occur; this rarely may necessitate surgical drainage or shunt placement.

- *The symptom of inappropriate antidiuretic hormone (SIADH)* may occur rarely, and fluid status and urine specific gravity and electrolytes frequently are monitored.
- *Seizures* may occur during the initial presentation but also may persist after the infection and may require long-term anticonvulsant therapy.

## Prevention

There are currently four licensed vaccines against several serotypes of *Strep. pneumoniae* and *N. meningitidis*, the leading causes of bacterial meningitis in children. The pneumococcal conjugate vaccine (PCV7) and the meningococcal conjugate vaccine (Menactra) are routinely recommended in the childhood immunization schedule.

## Management

In patients with suspected bacterial meningitis, antimicrobial treatment is directed at the usual pathogens (*Strep. pneumoniae* and *N. meningitidis*). Empirical broad-spectrum treatment includes a third-generation cephalosporin (ceftriaxone or cefotaxime) in addition to vancomycin, which provides coverage for penicillin-resistant *Strep. pneumoniae*, pending the results of blood and CSF cultures. Antimicrobial therapy can be changed to more specific antibiotics once an organism has been isolated.

## ENCEPHALITIS

Encephalitis occurs with invasion of actual brain matter, in contrast to meningitis. Some pathogens may cause both encephalitis and meningitis. The most common causes of encephalitis in children are viral. Following are the infectious causes of encephalitis:

- Herpes (10 percent of all cases in the United States; most common cause of endemic encephalitis)
- Japanese encephalitis (important cause outside the United States; Asian children frequently are immunized)
- Arthropod-borne viruses (frequent outbreaks in summer corresponding to outdoor activity):
  - St. Louis encephalitis
  - Eastern equine encephalitis
  - La Crosse encephalitis
  - West Nile encephalitis

The presentation may be similar to that of meningitis in children except that mental status changes are frequently more common and diffuse rather than focal. Fever is almost always present as well. The diagnosis also largely depends on the collection of CSF, which typically shows a mononuclear pleocytosis and elevated protein. However, up to 5 percent of severely infected individuals may have normal CSF findings.

Although some children and adults may recover from encephalitis, *neonatal herpes encephalitis* can be devastating to a developing brain. Herpes infection always should be considered in any young infant presenting with fever or illness, particularly with mental status changes, focal seizures (which may be subtle), or vesicular rash. Acyclovir therapy may improve the outcome early in the course, but frequently the diagnosis is delayed because of initially subtle clinical findings. A specific electroencephalographic (EEG) pattern of periodic lateralizing epileptiform discharges (PLEDs) and characteristic magnetic resonance imaging (MRI) findings (necrosis or edema, particularly in the white matter of the temporal lobes) are suggestive but not diagnostic. Polymerase chain reaction testing is the most sensitive test currently available for CSF, since most CSF cultures are negative. If skin lesions are present, herpes cultures of the lesions also may be obtained and are fairly sensitive for diagnosis as well. Because of the devastating complications, therapy with acyclovir usually is begun while awaiting diagnostic results.

## HEAD AND NECK INFECTIONS

### INFECTIOUS CONJUNCTIVITIS

"Pinkeye" is a very common presenting complaint in the outpatient pediatric setting. Inflammation of the conjunctivae may be bacterial or viral, and there are few, if any, findings on clinical examination that help differentiate between causes. Purulent rather than watery discharge and lack of systemic illness (fever, respiratory symptoms) are suggestive but certainly not pathognomonic for bacterial causes. Among neonates, the most common infectious cause of neonatal conjunctivitis is *Chlamydia trachomatis*, although *N. gonorrhoeae* remains a common and destructive infection worldwide if untreated. Antibiotic prophylaxis against *Neisseria* shortly after birth is routine in most U.S. nurseries.

**Causes of Pediatric Conjunctivitis**

| Bacterial | Viral |
|---|---|
| *Haemophilus influenzae* (nontypeable) | Adenovirus |
| | Enterovirus |
| *Streptococcus pneumoniae* | Coxsackie virus |
| *Moraxella catarrhalis* | Herpes simplex |

Cultures are generally not helpful since conjunctivae may be contaminated with lid or transient flora but may be particularly useful in neonates. Many clinicians empirically treat with topical broad-spectrum antibiotics since it is currently difficult to distinguish between viral and bacterial causes.

## OTITIS-CONJUNCTIVITIS SYNDROME

Up to one-fourth of patients with conjunctivitis may have concurrent otitis media.

The pathogens often include nontypeable *H. influenzae* and *Strep. pneumoniae*. Physical examination of the ears always should be performed, particularly in young infants and children, before beginning empirical topical therapy. If otitis media is present and oral (systemic) antibiotic therapy is begun, topical therapy generally is not needed.

## SINUSITIS

Sinusitis in children is usually infectious, and bacterial pathogens often mirror those in otitis: *Strep. pneumoniae*, nontypeable *H. influenzae*, and *Moraxella catarrhalis*. Although the anterior ethmoid and maxillary sinuses are present at birth, the sphenoid and frontal sinuses do not develop until after early childhood. Clinical findings such as sinus tenderness and transillumination are often uncommon and unreliable in children and also, unfortunately, frequently overlap with those of the common cold (viral rhinitis). Thus, clinicians and evidence-based guidelines often use the duration of symptoms to help differentiate between the common cold and sinusitis. *Acute bacterial sinusitis* often is defined as upper respiratory symptoms (cough, nasal discharge) that are either

- *Persistent* (lasting longer than 10 to 14 days but less than 30 days) or
- *Severe* (high fever and several days of purulent discharge)

Evidence suggests that the majority of cases of acute bacterial sinusitis resolve spontaneously, and current evidence-based guidelines suggest that antibiotics for 10 days will produce modest short-term benefit, although approximately eight children must be treated to achieve one additional cure. The choice of empirical antibiotic therapy is often similar to that in the treatment for otitis media since the pathogens are often similar and typically include β-lactamase-resistant or high-dose penicillin derivatives.

## PRESEPTAL CELLULITIS

The terms *preseptal cellulitis* and *periorbital cellulitis* may be used interchangeably and generally refer to bacterial infection of the soft tissue surrounding the orbit. The orbital septum is an excellent barrier to the spread of infection. If infection spreads beyond this area, it is termed *orbital cellulitis* and patients may present with proptosis or even impairment of intraocular movement. This may necessitate surgical drainage to prevent permanent visual damage. In the pre-HIB vaccine era, *H. influenzae* type B was a common cause. The incidence of preseptal cellulitis has declined markedly since the advent of immunization.

### Bacterial Causes of Preseptal Cellulitis

| | |
|---|---|
| *Streptococcus pneumoniae* | Most often seen in toddlers; high fever usually present; rapid progression; may be bacteremic |
| *Staphylococcus aureus* | Often preceding event (insect bite, trauma, impetigo) |
| Group A *Streptococcus* | May be afebrile; bacteremia rare |
| Nontypeable *Haemophilus influenzae* | Often existing concurrent sinusitis |
| *Moraxella catarrhalis* | |

Since the decline of HIB disease, treatment has shifted to outpatient antibiotic therapy, although children with progressive disease frequently require hospitalization with IV antibiotics. Imaging studies may be needed to help differentiate between preseptal disease and septal disease, since physical examination findings such as disruption of ocular movement may be subtle or difficult to visualize, particularly with significant orbital swelling.

### CERVICAL ADENITIS

Swollen or enlarged cervical nodes are common in children, since the neck region is often the first defense against the multitude of pediatric upper respiratory infections. Part of the diagnostic challenge is to determine when to go "zebra hunting." Although infection is the most common cause of lymphadenopathy, it is important to remember that malignancies (lymphomas, leukemias) as well as congenital malformations (branchial cleft cysts) also may rarely present with cervical enlargement. It may be helpful to divide adenitis into subgroups of *bilateral, unilateral,* and *chronic* (more than 6 to 8 weeks) when formulating a diagnostic approach.

| | Causes | Comments |
|---|---|---|
| Unilateral | *Staphylococcus aureus* | Most common cause in newborns |
| | Group A *Streptococcus* | |
| | Anaerobic bacteria | May occur with dental abscesses |
| | Kawasaki disease | Of all diagnostic criteria, cervical enlargement is the least frequent finding |

*(continued)*

| | Causes | Comments |
|---|---|---|
| Bilateral (continued) | Adenovirus Influenza Respiratory syncytial virus | |
| | Epstein-Barr virus (EBV) | Adenopathy usually nontender and localized but may occasionally be tender, diffuse |
| | Cytomegalovirus (CMV) | Pharyngitis and adenopathy less common than with EBV |
| Chronic | EBV CMV Human immunodeficiency virus | |
| | Bartonella henselae | Causative agent of cat-scratch fever; cat exposure helpful but not always present |
| | Atypical mycobacteria | Purified protein derivative may be negative in up to 50%; may eventually cause sinus tract formation |
| | Mycobacterium tuberculosis | Usually accompanied by systemic findings of tuberculosis |
| | Francisella tularensis | Causative agent of tularemia; associated with animal exposure |
| | Brucellosis (Brucella species) | Caused by direct contact with infected animals or exposure to unpasteurized milk |

Since the majority of cases of cervical adenitis are usually infectious and self-limiting, a watch-and-wait approach and a minimal diagnostic workup may be acceptable with good follow-up if the clinical history does not suggest more serious causes. The initial diagnostic workup for worrisome nodes may include the following:

- Complete blood count with differential
- Erythrocyte sedimentation rate (ESR)
- Placement of purified protein derivative (PPD)
- Chest radiograph
- Serologies for Epstein-Barr virus (EBV) and cytomegalovirus (CMV)
- Serologies for Toxoplasma and human immunodeficiency virus (HIV)
- Lactate dehydrogenase (LDH) and uric acid (further evaluation for malignancy)

## MANAGEMENT

Viral adenitis requires no treatment. Treatment with antibiotics effective against *S. aureus* and *Strep. pyogenes* (group A streptococci) is recommended in children with suspected bacterial adenitis. Large suppurative lymph nodes also may require incision and drainage.

### *RETROPHARYNGEAL ABSCESSES*

Retropharyngeal abscesses usually result from the spread of upper respiratory illness (often staphylococcal or streptococcal). They often present with drooling or stridor and are less common in adolescents. In contrast, peritonsillar abscesses are more common in older children and adolescents and may present with dysphagia or "hot potato" voice, although these symptoms also frequently result from extension of infection with streptococci or staphylococci. Both illnesses generally require the administration of IV antibiotics and surgical consultation for management and often drainage.

## SOFT TISSUE AND SKIN INFECTIONS (IMPETIGO, ABSCESSES, CELLULITIS)

Bacterial skin infections may range from the superficial (impetigo) to the deep and even the life-threatening (necrotizing fasciitis). The two major bacterial pathogens most often implicated in pediatric skin infections are *S. aureus* and *Strep. pyogenes* (group A streptococci). Although the epidermis provides an excellent barrier against skin flora, minor trauma, insect bites, and other disruptions (eczema, varicella infection) often provide an opportunity for bacterial invasion.

*Impetigo* refers to a superficial infection that may progress from a small papule to a vesicular eruption that commonly is described as "honey-crusted." It is impossible to distinguish between staphylococcal impetigo and streptococcal impetigo on clinical findings alone. Both staphylococci and streptococci may produce exotoxins and vesiculation of skin. Topical antibiotics often are used, but when there are widespread cases, oral antibiotics may be administered.

*Skin abscesses* often evolve from untreated superficial infections and occasionally arise spontaneously in follicles or sebaceous glands, giving rise to folliculitis, boils, furuncles, or carbuncles. Treatment usually consists of local incision and drainage; systemic antibiotics may play a role if there are signs of systemic illness.

*Cellulitis* is an infection of subcutaneous tissue and dermis and usually presents with generalized redness, warmth, and tenderness in the infected area. Again, both staphylococci and streptococci commonly are implicated. Streptococcal cellulitis (sometimes called *erysipelas*) often is characterized by a rapid onset, a distinct border of erythema, and systemic findings, in contrast to staphylococcal cellulitis, which tends to be more localized and purulent. It is often impossible to distinguish between the two causes on the basis of clinical appearance alone. Treatment generally involves hospitalization and IV antibiotics, as well as culture of skin lesions and/or blood cultures if the child appears systemically ill.

### METHICILLIN-RESISTANT STAPHYLOCOCCUS AUREUS

Less than 25 years ago, simple β-lactam antibiotics such as amoxicillin often provided adequate coverage for both streptococci and staphylococci. Over the last two decades, many staphylococci have acquired the ability to produce β-lactamase as well, further limiting antibiotic selection to cephalosporins and amoxicillin-clavulanic acid (both of which counteract β-lactamase production).

As "superbugs" have continued to evolve, frequently in the hospital or nursing home setting, where antibiotic use is common, the recent emergence of methicillin-resistant *Staphylococcus aureus* (MRSA) has posed particular challenges. Historically, MRSA was reported only in immunocompromised or hospitalized individuals, but now it appears to have replaced methicillin-sensitive *Staphylococcus aureus* (MSSA) as the predominant organism in many communities in the United States. Further, the incidence of community-acquired MRSA infections appears to be rising among children. Clindamycin, trimethoprim-sulfisoxazole, and vancomycin may be the only alternatives against selected strains, although the loculations and high acidic environment of many soft tissue infections often make them impermeable to even systemic antibiotics. Surgical incision and drainage may be the only alternative in selected instances.

## INFECTIOUS ARTHRITIS

Infectious arthritis in children may be *acute* and related to actual invasion of joint space by bacteria or *postinfectious* and often related to the induction of cross-reactive antibodies (rheumatic fever being a classic example). Among children, acute arthritis may be caused by hematogenous seeding or, less commonly, extension of soft tissue infection.

| Common Causes of Acute Infectious Arthritis | Comments |
| --- | --- |
| Staphylococcus aureus | Most common cause of infectious arthritis in children |
| Streptococcus pyogenes (group A streptococci) | Arthritis associated with rheumatic fever is migratory and polyarthritic; generally larger |

*(continued)*

| Common Causes of Acute Infectious Arthritis | Comments |
|---|---|
| Neisseria gonorrhoeae | Common cause in adolescents and young adults; may spread hematogenously from mucosal infection |
| Kingella kingae | Generally monoarticular; usually knee |
| Neisseria meningitidis | Rare; may be accompanied by mild upper respiratory infection symptoms or life-threatening disease |
| Group B Streptococcus | Common cause in neonates |
| Haemophilus influenzae type B | Once a common cause in children; incidence markedly declined since vaccine introduction |
| Borrelia burgdorferi | Causative agent in Lyme disease; arthritis usually follows the initial characteristic rash, commonly referred to as erythema chronica migrans; arthritis may be acute or recurrent, chronic, and relapsing |

| Common Causes of Postinfectious Arthritis | Comments |
|---|---|
| Salmonella species | Often chronic; postinfectious arthritis caused by |
| Shigella species | enteric or venereal pathogens is often referred |
| Campylobacter | to as Reiter syndrome |
| Chlamydia trachomatis | |
| Parvovirus B19 (fifth disease) | Arthritis may follow systemic infection; more common in adults and usually self-limiting |
| Rubella | Up to a quarter of postpubertal females may experience arthralgia or arthritis after vaccination |

Although a red, swollen, and tender joint is a hallmark of arthritis, the diagnosis may be difficult in pediatrics, particularly if a less obvious joint such as the hip joint is involved, since infants and children may be unable to localize pain and swelling may go unnoticed. Frequently the diagnosis may be delayed. Suspicion usually warrants obtaining an aspirate of joint fluid for cell studies and bacterial culture as well as hospitalization and the administration of IV antibiotics, since, if untreated, infection may destroy the synovial structures and lead to long-term complications.

*Osteomyelitis* is defined as bacterial infection of the bone and, like septic arthritis, may be spread hematogenously or result from contiguous infection. Bacterial causes are very similar to those listed above for septic arthritis. Children with sickle cell disease are also uniquely susceptible to osteomyelitis from *Salmonella* species as well. *Staphylococcus aureus* continues to be the most common cause among all age groups.

| Aids in Diagnosis of Osteomyelitis | Comments |
| --- | --- |
| White blood cell count | May be normal or elevated |
| Erythrocyte sedimentation rate | Typically elevated |
| C-reactive protein | Typically elevated |
| Blood cultures | May be positive in up to 50% |
| Plain radiographs of affected area | May show periosteal reaction or new bone formation at site of infection; may be negative early (1–2 weeks) in the course of disease |
| Bone scan | More sensitive than radiographs; more helpful in early diagnosis |
| Magnetic resonance imaging | More sensitive than radiographs |

The definitive diagnosis of an organism may involve consultation with an orthopedic surgeon to obtain bone tissue for culture and pathology. Suspicion of osteomyelitis generally requires hospitalization as well, often not only for diagnosis but also for treatment with intravenous antibiotics. Historically, many patients were treated for long periods (6 to 8 weeks) with intravenous antibiotics. With specific identification of an organism, careful monitoring of antibiotic drug levels, and parameters such as sedimentation rate and C-reactive protein, completion of therapy with oral antibiotics may be appropriate provided that clinical improvement and family compliance with medication can be ensured.

## TUBERCULOSIS

Although the incidence of tuberculosis (TB) in the United States has declined steadily over the last few decades, *Mycobacterium tuberculosis* still remains an extremely important cause of disease worldwide. Indeed, up to one-third of newly diagnosed cases among children may represent foreign-born children or recent immigrants. Most children with tuberculosis are asymptomatic. The majority of disease spread throughout the United States and worldwide continues to be through adult vectors.

The most common easily employed method of screening for TB is the Mantoux skin test, or purified protein derivative (PPD). A small amount of material is injected subcutaneously under the skin. Individuals who have been exposed or have active infection generally respond with induration at the site of injection 48 to 72 h later provided that cellular immunity is intact. Historically, universal screening was recommended, but the Centers for Disease Control and Prevention (CDC) moved to targeted screening of high-risk populations in 1995 (rather than universal screening), since it appears to be more cost-effective to identify index cases and monitor completion of drug therapy.

The following are high-risk pediatric groups:

- Close contacts (those sharing a household with others with active TB)
- Foreign-born children recently arrived (within 5 years) from countries that have a high TB incidence or prevalence
- Persons infected with HIV
- High-risk substance abusers
- Residents and employees of high-risk settings (nursing homes, homeless persons, prisons, long-term facilities)
- Health-care workers
- Any child or adolescent exposed to an adult in one of the categories listed above

Interpretation of PPD results usually requires consulting the *Red Book*, since the size of induration and the clinical findings and history are often relevant. Children and adolescents with a positive PPD should undergo chest radiography to rule out pulmonary disease, but a positive PPD in a child or teenager also should provoke further investigation of potential adult index cases. This frequently is done in conjunction with the local health department. In the event of active pulmonary disease, consultation with pediatric infectious disease or pulmonary specialists may be helpful to obtain gastric aspirates for identification and culture and to guide therapy, since many mycobacterial strains are now resistant to multiple regimens.

## HUMAN IMMUNODEFICIENCY VIRUS

Although the incidence of HIV-infected children is decreasing significantly as a result of improved drug therapies and reduction of perinatal transmission, HIV disease has left a lasting imprint in the United States (an estimated 125,000 children and teens in the United States have lost mothers to AIDS as of this writing), not to mention the world. The number of children who have lost one parent or both parents to the disease in sub-Saharan Africa is expected to reach 18 million by the end of the decade.

Most HIV infections in children are acquired perinatally. Maternal, intrapartum, and postnatal treatment with retroviral therapy has reduced perinatal transmission from approximately 25 to 30 percent to less than 2 percent. Since maternal antibody may interfere with serologic testing in infants and young children, most children are followed closely for several years after birth. Risk factors in adolescent youth often parallel those in the adult population.

| Common Serologic Tests in the Diagnosis of HIV in Children | Comments |
| --- | --- |
| HIV antibody (ELISA) | Most common screening test; infants may be falsely positive due to transfer of maternal antibody |
| HIV Western blot | Generally more specific; confirmatory test usually done if HIV-ELISA is positive |
| HIV viral load (polymerase chain reaction) | Used to follow efficacy of therapy |
| p24 antigen | Used to detect early HIV infection; may be positive only during a short window of time |

Progression of disease from early asymptomatic infection to full-blown AIDS often relies on age-specific CD4 lymphocyte counts as well as the presence of opportunistic infections. Two clinical findings that often are unique to a child with HIV are failure to thrive (inability to gain weight at normal growth or even weight loss) and lymphocytic interstitial pneumonitis (LIP), an inflammatory lung condition related to primary EBV infection. Reverse transcriptase inhibitors such as azathioprine (AZT), as well as newer non-nucleoside agents such as nevirapine, remain mainstays of therapy in children as well as adults.

## KAWASAKI SYNDROME

Although specific infectious agents or triggers have not been identified, the diagnosis of Kawasaki syndrome often falls to the pediatric infectious disease specialist because its presentation frequently mimics that of many other childhood diseases. Fever is a hallmark of the syndrome and must be present for at least 5 days. For classic diagnosis, at least four of the following five characteristics also must be present:

- Conjunctivitis
- Mucous membrane changes (strawberry tongue, red cracked lips and oropharynx)
- Generalized, erythematous, and often nonspecific rash
- Hand and foot swelling
- Cervical lymphadenopathy (generally at least 1.5 cm in diameter)

Kawasaki syndrome produces a vasculitis of small and medium-size arteries. Up to 20 percent of these children may develop coronary aneurysms that obviously have long-term implications. Prompt therapy with aspirin and intravenous immunoglobulin reduces this risk to 2 to 4 percent, further implicating an inflammatory (possibly infectious) cause, although its mechanisms or pathogens have not been elucidated.

## PARVOVIRUS B19 (ERYTHEMA INFECTIOSUM, FIFTH DISEASE)

"Fifth disease," or parvovirus B19, historically referred to as one of the six classic infectious exanthems of childhood: measles, scarlet fever, rubella, Dukes' disease (now thought to be a variant of one of the other exanthems), and roseola. Fever may be present, and infection generally produces a characteristic "slapped cheeks" appearance of the face that often is followed by a more systemic lacy and reticular pattern that later erupts on the trunk and/or extremities. Interestingly, the rash may be reactivated weeks to months later upon exposure to sunlight.

Fifth disease is self-limiting in most healthy children. It occasionally may produce a mild postreactive arthritis and rarely may produce significant aplastic crises in children with hemolytic anemia or fetal death among nonimmune exposed pregnant women. Unfortunately, the period of highest transmission often coincides with the prodromal and often asymptomatic (rashless) phase of disease. Once the rash has erupted, the risk of contagion is generally low.

## HUMAN HERPES VIRUS 6 (HHV-6, ROSEOLA)

Although the majority of infections with human herpesvirus 6 (HHV-6) are asymptomatic, approximately one in five children may develop systemic signs of infection, often called roseola, "sixth disease," or, rarely, exanthem subitum. Unlike parvovirus, systemic infection with HHV-6 frequently produces fever that is often high [39.4 to 40°C (103 to 104°F)] and irritability. HHV-6 often is associated with the first manifestation of febrile seizures in children (10 to 15 percent of primary infections). As with parvovirus, rash often follows defervescence, although the erythematous maculopapular rash of HHV-6 is frequently nonspecific and may be mistaken for an allergic reaction. The often toxic and irritable appearance of affected infants and the degree of fever frequently provoke anxiety in both practitioner and parent. Unfortunately, rapid diagnostic techniques are not widely available in the outpatient setting to help differentiate roseola from other, more serious causes.

## FEVER OF UNKNOWN ORIGIN

Fever of unknown origin (FUO) is defined variably in pediatric literature but generally refers to fever lasting longer than 1 to 2 weeks or at least outside the scope of the duration of most common viral infections (typically 5 to 7 days). Unlike adults, in which case autoimmune disorders and malignancy often are listed in the differential diagnosis, FUO in children usually points to an infectious cause, either a "zebra" (a rare pathogen or zoonosis) or, more commonly, a "horse with stripes," that is, an unusual presentation of a common disorder. The following are the infections to consider in the diagnostic workup of children with FUO.

- Cat-scratch disease (*Bartonella henselae*)
- Tularemia
- Kawasaki syndrome
- Rickettsial infection (Rocky Mountain spotted fever, ehrlichiosis, Lyme disease)
- Viral infections (especially EBV, CMV)
- Urinary tract infections
- *Salmonella* infections
- Osteomyelitis
- Occult abscesses (hepatic or pelvic abscesses)
- Tuberculosis

Noninfectious causes that always should be included in the differential are juvenile rheumatoid arthritis (JRA) and neoplasms (leukemia and lymphoma being the most common malignancies presenting as FUO).

## BIBLIOGRAPHY

Allen CH, Patel B, Endom EE. Primary bacterial infections of the skin and soft tissue changes in epidemiology and management. *Clin Pediatr Emerg Med* 5(4):246–255, 2004.

Bloch A and the Advisory Council for the Elimination of Tuberculosis. Screening for tuberculosis and tuberculosis infection in high-risk populations: Recommendations of the Advisory Council for the Elimination of Tuberculosis. *MMWR Morb Mortal Wkly Rep* 44(RR-11):18–34, 1995.

Committee on Infectious Diseases. *Red Book: 2003 Report of the Committee on Infectious Diseases*, 26th ed. Elk Grove Village, IL, American Academy of Pediatrics, 2003.

Jaskiewicz JA, McCarthy CA, Richardson AC, et al. Febrile infants at low risk for serious bacterial infection—an appraisal of the Rochester criteria and implications for management. Febrile Infant Collaborative Study Group. *Pediatrics* 94(3):390–306, 1994.

Peters TR, Edwards KM. Cervical lymphadenopathy and adenitis. *Pediatr Rev* 21:399–405, 2000.

Subcommittee on Management of Sinusitis. Clinical practice guideline: Management of sinusitis. *Pediatrics* 108(3):798–808, 2001.

Wald ER. Periorbital and orbital infections. *Pediatr Rev* 25:312–320, 2004.

# PEDIATRIC NEPHROLOGY

## Aida Yared

## LEARNING OBJECTIVES

1. Know how to do a urinalysis to speed up the diagnosis and management of a child.

2. Know how to take blood pressure (BP) using different instruments. Interpret BP by plotting it on an age- and sex-appropriate chart.

3. Understand the various means of obtaining a urine specimen in a child and their reliability and limitations.

4. Use correct terminology. Commonly confused terms are azotemia and uremia, polycystic and multicystic, nephrotic syndrome and nephritic syndrome, and frequency and polyuria. Commonly confused diseases are HSP (Henoch-Schönlein purpura) and HUS (hemolytic-uremic syndrome), Fanconi syndrome (a renal tubule problem) and Fanconi anemia.

5. Know the differential diagnosis and workup of hematuria (gross and microscopic).

6. Know the differential diagnosis and workup of proteinuria.

7. Recognize the clinical presentation of urinary tract infection in children and its management and workup.

## INTRODUCTION

### COMMON DEFINITIONS

*Anasarca.* Generalized edema.

*Anuria.* No passage of urine. In babies anuria is a urine output of < 0.5 mL/kg per hour, and in older children it is a urine output <50 mL/m$^2$ per day.

*Azotemia.* High serum blood urea nitrogen (BUN) and creatinine.

*Cystitis.* Inflammation or infection of the urinary bladder.

*Dysuria.* Pain or burning on urination. Parents may notice that an infant screams when urinating.

*Enuresis (incontinence).* Involuntary passage of urine. Can be nocturnal (nighttime) or diurnal (daytime). Can be primary (the child was never toilet trained) or secondary (the child was trained and started wetting again).

*Frequency.* The feeling of wanting to pass urine when the bladder is not full so that "only a few drops come out."

*Glomerular filtration rate (GFR).* A measure of the filtration or clearance function of the kidney; often measured as creatinine clearance.

*Glomerulonephritis or nephritis.* Inflammation of the renal glomeruli, often immune-mediated, presenting clinically with the nephritic syndrome. Can be primary (e.g., poststreptococcal nephritis) or secondary to a systemic disorder (e.g., lupus nephritis).

*Hematuria.* Blood in the urine. Can be gross (visible to the naked eye) or microscopic (detected by dipstick or microscopy).

*Nephritic syndrome.* Renal inflammation manifesting with an abnormal urinalysis (hematuria, proteinuria) and a decreased GFR. If the decrease in GFR is severe, there will be azotemia, oliguria, edema, and hypertension.

*Nephrotic syndrome.* Massive proteinuria leading to hypoalbuminemia and edema.

*Nocturia.* Awakening at night to pass urine.

*Oliguria.* Low urine output. In babies, normal urine output is approximately 2 mL/kg per hour and oliguria is < 1 mL/kg per hour. In an older child, oliguria is a urine output < 300 mL/m$^2$ per day.

*Polydipsia.* Excessive drinking.

*Polyuria.* Passage of a larger urine volume per day than normal.

*Proteinuria.* Loss of protein in the urine.

*Pyelonephritis.* Infection of the kidney. In children, it is clinically defined as urinary tract infection with fever > 38.1°C (100.5°F).

*Pyuria.* White blood cells in the urine.

*Uremia.* Signs and symptoms resulting from chronic renal failure, such as poor growth, anemia, low exercise tolerance, anorexia, and tremors.

*Urgency.* Inability to hold urine for a reasonable time; the child feels the need to rush to the bathroom or wets herself or himself.

## COMMON LABORATORY TESTS

### BLOOD TESTS

*BUN* and *creatinine* are markers of filtration. Urea, a product of protein metabolism, increases with protein intake or gastrointestinal (GI) bleeding and is low in malnutrition. Creatinine issues from muscle, and its serum value is stable from day to day; serum creatinine is higher in an athletic adolescent boy than in a skinny girl of the same age. Creatinine increases with age. Both BUN and creatinine increase with dehydration and renal failure.

*Electrolytes* are sodium (Na), potassium (K), chloride (Cl), and total $CO_2$ ($TCO_2$). $TCO_2$ is a measure of plasma bicarbonate. In the absence of pulmonary problems, a decrease usually signifies metabolic acidosis.

The *anion gap* (AG) is calculated as $Na - (Cl + TCO_2)$. The AG is useful in the differential diagnosis of acidosis. A normal anion gap (<15 mEq/L) suggests bicarbonate loss (GI or renal); a high anion gap indicates the presence of unusual acids (e.g., lactic acid, ketoacids, salicylate).

*Serum protein and albumin* are important to measure in a child with proteinuria.

*Complement 3 (C3)* is obtained in a child with acute nephritis; a low value strongly suggests poststreptococcal glomerulonephritis.

*Creatinine clearance* (Ccr) is a common and convenient way to estimate GFR:

$$\text{Ccr (mL/min/1.73 m}^2) = \frac{\text{urine creatinine} \times \text{urine volume}}{\text{serum creatinine} \times 1440} \times \frac{1.73}{\text{BSA}}$$

In the equation, BSA is the child's body surface area in $m^2$ and 1440 is the number of minutes per day. The normal value in a child above 2 years of age is close to that of adults (80 to 100 for a girl, 100 to 120 for a boy).

### URINALYSIS

*Smell.* The urine may smell "strong" if it is concentrated. A foul smell may indicate a urinary tract infection (UTI). An unusual urine smell in a newborn suggests a metabolic disorder (organic or amino acid disorder).

*Appearance.* Urine is usually clear and straw-colored. Urine may be cloudy from white blood cells or crystals. In a newborn, pink urine is probably a benign and transient finding caused by the presence of large amounts of uric acid crystals. In an older child, pink urine may be due to pigments (beeturia, food colorings), myoglobin, free hemoglobin, or red blood cells. Urine can be tea-colored if it contains denatured hemoglobin. Urine that looks like water is dilute, usually because the child is well hydrated and rarely because of diabetes insipidus.

*pH.* The value is usually 5 to 6 (acidic) because the kidneys have to excrete the normal daily acid production. Alkaline urine suggests infection or renal tubular acidosis; intake of orange juice also may result in alkaline urine.

*Glucose.* Should be negative. If it is positive, diabetes mellitus should be ruled out. Glucosuria can occur as an isolated benign finding (renal glucosuria).

*Ketone.* Should be negative. Ketones can be positive in a dehydrated starving child (e.g., severe gastroenteritis). If both ketones and glucose are positive, diabetes mellitus should be ruled out.

*Protein.* See the section on proteinuria, below.

*Blood.* See the section on hematuria, below.

*Leukocyte esterase.* Indicates the presence of white blood cells in the urine; it is not diagnostic for a UTI, as it can accompany fever, recent immunizations, gastroenteritis, appendicitis, or sexually transmitted diseases (STDs).

*Specific gravity.* Indicates how concentrated the urine is and ranges from 1.000 to 1.035. There is no normal value since urine concentration depends on hydration status. In a dehydrated child, a low specific gravity raises the concern of diabetes insipidus.

*Microscopy.* The urine (3 to 10 mL) is spun for 3 min at low speed. A drop of the sediment is examined under microscopy. Normal sediment may contain mucus and squamous cells in a girl, along with occasional red blood cells (RBCs) or white blood cells (WBCs). White blood cells suggest infection but may be present with dehydration or fever. Red blood cells may be present in a menstruating girl or represent the trauma of catheterization. Visible bacteria denote infection. Uric acid crystals are common in neonates. Calcium oxalate crystals are usually of no significance. Hyaline casts may be found in patients with dehydration. Cellular casts indicate a glomerular disease.

## URINE CHEMISTRIES

*Urine calcium/creatinine ratio.* Screening test for hypercalciuria. A normal value is < 0.20.

*Urine protein/creatinine ratio.* Screening test for proteinuria. A normal value is < 0.20.

## COMMON PROCEDURES

### BLOOD PRESSURE MEASUREMENT

Blood pressure (BP) is an essential part of the physical examination of older children. The blood pressure cuff should cover at least two-thirds of the arm (a large cuff underestimates BP, and a small one overestimates it). BP should be compared to normal values for age and sex. It can be measured by using several instruments. The mercury sphygmomanometer is the oldest and still the gold standard; problems are that it relies on the observer, is inconvenient to use in small children, and is hard to use in a noisy environment. A spiral or digital sphygmomanometer often is used for home monitoring; it should be recalibrated periodically. Oscillometry gives a digital reading, and so there is no observer variability; it is convenient for use in small children or in a noisy environment.

## URINE CULTURE

There are several ways to obtain a urine culture (e.g. Dynamap).

*Clean bag.* This is used in babies and toddlers. After thorough cleaning of the perineal area, a sterile bag is applied. For reliability, it is very important that no cleanser be left on the skin, that the bag be taken off as soon as the child voids, and that there be no stool contamination.

*Clean catch.* Used in a toilet-trained child. The perineal area is cleaned. For a boy, the prepuce is retracted and the glans cleaned. For a girl, the labia are spread apart and cleaned. A midvoiding specimen is collected in a sterile container.

*Catheterization.* Saves time (especially in a dehydrated child) and is more reliable than a bag specimen. However, it can be traumatic (physically and psychologically).

*Suprapubic or bladder tap.* Is the most reliable (and most invasive) way of obtaining a urine culture. Urine is aspirated directly from the bladder by suprapubic puncture. It requires that the bladder be full.

UTI is diagnosed if growth of a single organism is obtained. A mixed growth usually indicates contamination. Interpretation should take into account the child's signs and symptoms, the presence of bacteria on microscopy, and the colony count. In a bag or clean catch specimen > 100,000 colonies/mm$^3$ is definite evidence of UTI; in a catheterized sample, >10,000 colonies; in a bladder tap, any growth. The laboratory usually performs a sensitivity profile.

## 24-HOUR URINE COLLECTION

A 24 h urine collection is used for measurement of creatinine (and calculation of its clearance). It also is used for total calcium (normal < 4 mg/kg per day) or protein (normal < 4 mg/kg per day). A specimen bottle usually is provided by the laboratory. For routine collection, a well-rinsed glass or plastic jug (e.g., a juice or milk jug) is adequate. The patient is instructed to discard the first morning void and collect all subsequent urine during the day and night and the first urine the next morning. The collection can be kept for 24 h in a refrigerator.

## CYSTOSCOPY

A cystoscopy is done by the urologist when an anatomic problem in the lower urinary tract is suspected. Under general anesthesia, an endoscope is introduced into the child's urethra to look at the urethra, bladder, and ureteral openings.

## RENAL BIOPSY

A renal biopsy is performed when a renal parenchymal disease is suspected; usually it is done percutaneously by a nephrologist under ultrasonic guidance. The risks are infection and bleeding. In high-risk patients, an "open" biopsy is performed in the operating room by a surgeon.

## DIALYSIS

This can be peritoneal dialysis (most commonly in children) or hemodialysis.

# COMMON IMAGING STUDIES

## RENAL ULTRASOUND

Renal ultrasound (U/S) is the safest way to image the urinary tract, as it entails no radiation. It is very useful for assessing the anatomy of the urinary tract for the presence or absence of kidneys, size, echogenicity, cysts, hydronephrosis, stones, or tumors. U/S is the best screening study for renal problems in a child.

## VOIDING CYSTOURETHROGRAM

A voiding cystourethrogram (VCUG) is used to assess bladder anatomy, suspected reflux, or urethral obstruction (e.g., posterior urethral valves). Contrast material is instilled into the bladder with a catheter, and voiding is followed under fluoroscopy. VCUG gives excellent images but entails a large amount of radiation. A nuclear cystogram is the same study, instilling nuclear material.

## COMPUTED TOMOGRAPHY

A noncontrast "spiral" computed tomography (CT) scan is the best study for kidney stones.

## RENAL SCAN

A renal perfusion scan is the best study for renal blood flow and function (including split function). A dimercaptosuccinic acid (DMSA) scan is the best study to image renal scars.

# COMMON SIGNS AND SYMPTOMS

In a pediatric patient, serious renal disease may present with nonspecific findings such as unexplained fever, irritability, chronic diarrhea, and failure to thrive. Common signs and symptoms are an abnormal voiding pattern, pain, systemic signs or symptoms, or an abnormal urine.

## ABNORMAL VOIDING PATTERN

Ninety-two percent of newborn infants pass urine in the first 24 h of life, and 98 percent do so within 48 h. In the first year of life, voiding is frequent and is both diurnal and nocturnal. Beyond school age, voiding is usually diurnal, occurs four to six times a day, and is voluntary. At all ages, voiding is effortless and painless, involves the passage of an adequate volume of urine, and leads to complete emptying of the bladder. An abnormal voiding pattern can involve any of these parameters.

### TIMING

Occasional nocturia can be normal, especially after copious intake of fluids around bedtime. Otherwise, nocturia can indicate an inability to concentrate the urine. Diabetes mellitus should be kept in mind.

### VOLUME

A normal urine void (i.e., bladder capacity) is equal in ounces to age (years) + 2 and plateaus by 9 years of age.

A newborn can come to medical attention because of a delay in the passage of urine. Renal agenesis and obstruction should be considered.

*Oligoanuria* can occur by two mechanisms. First, there may be elaboration of more concentrated urine while the GFR is normal, as may occur with dehydration. Second, there may be a decrease in GFR.

*Polyuria* is the passage of a larger daily urine volume than normal and should not be confused with *frequency*. If it is unclear whether a child has polyuria or frequency, a 24-h urine is indicated. Polyuria often is accompanied by *polydipsia*. Polyuria/polydipsia suggests diabetes mellitus (DM) and diabetes insipidus (DI); a quick way to differentiate the two is a urinalysis. DI may be central [low antidiuretic hormone (ADH)] or nephrogenic (unresponsiveness to ADH). Central DI can be congenital or can follow central nervous system (CNS) trauma, tumors, surgery, or infections (e.g., meningitis, mumps). Nephrogenic DI can be congenital (usually in boys) or secondary to a renal disease that impairs the concentrating mechanism. Polydipsia/polyuria is rarely psychogenic in children; a random specific gravity > 1.015 rules out DI.

### THE ACT OF VOIDING

*Urinary retention* or *dribbling* in a child with neurologic deficits (e.g., cerebral palsy, meningomyelocele) indicates a neurogenic bladder. In an otherwise normal male child, it suggests bladder outlet obstruction (posterior urethral valves, urethral stricture, or severe meatal stenosis). Acute difficulty in voiding also can occur with urethritis or cystitis and usually is accompanied by other signs and symptoms of inflammation. A weak urinary stream, or dribbling of urine, can be the presenting sign of obstruction.

*Dysuria* often is accompanied by frequency and urgency. This triad suggests urethral inflammation or UTI.

## VOLUNTARY CONTROL

*Enuresis* is very common in pediatrics. Its incidence is approximately 15 percent at 5 years of age, 10 percent at 8 years, and 5 percent at 10 years. Nocturnal enuresis is commonly benign and familial. Overall, a cause is found in fewer than 5 percent of cases. Diurnal enuresis, especially if secondary, is more likely to indicate pathology, whether infectious, anatomic, or emotional, and is an indication for urologic, neurologic, and psychosocial investigation. Enuresis frequently accompanies UTI in toddlers.

Urgency may be secondary to acute or chronic cystitis, occult neurogenic bladder, or uninhibited bladder contractions ("unstable bladder"), usually in a girl with recurrent UTIs. Overflow incontinence often is seen with neurologic problems.

## PAIN

*Flank pain* of renal origin most commonly results from infection or inflammation of the renal parenchyma that leads to stretching of the renal capsule. When accompanied by fever, nausea, and vomiting, flank pain strongly suggests acute pyelonephritis even in the absence of other symptoms of urinary tract infection. It also can be a prominent feature of immunoglobulin A (IgA) nephropathy (Berger disease) or poststreptococcal glomerulonephritis (PSGN). In both pyelonephritis and glomerulonephritis, the pain is described as dull with no radiation and often is accompanied by tenderness to percussion. Colicky pain suggests a renal stone; stones are relatively rare in children unless there is a family history. The pain of renal colic typically is described as excruciatingly severe, radiating to the groin, or migrating along the course of the ureter.

Dull abdominal, flank, or back pain is a common presentation of adult polycystic kidney disease, occurring in approximately 60 percent of cases.

*Suprapubic pain* with suprapubic tenderness suggests acute cystitis (bacterial or viral). Typically, it is accompanied by urinary frequency and urgency and often by hematuria.

## SYSTEMIC SIGNS OR SYMPTOMS

The systemic signs and symptoms of renal disease may be unrelated to the urinary tract. Thus, nausea, vomiting, and failure to thrive occur with uremia, acidosis, or urinary tract infection. Metabolic acidosis often is associated with vomiting and growth retardation. The three physical signs that strongly suggest renal pathology are edema, hypertension, and an abdominal mass.

## EDEMA

Proteinuria > 50 mg/kg per day defines the nephrotic syndrome, which typically presents with edema. Nephrotic edema tends to be prominent in the periorbital area because of the low tissue turgor; anasarca, or generalized edema, is common in younger infants. Edema also can be due to volume overload, which can occur when GFR is decreased. Typically, edema is present in 75 percent of children with acute glomerulonephritis. The parents may report that the child has a spontaneous tendency to remove his or her shoes or that socks leave their imprint when taken off. Edema typically changes position, involving the periorbital area in the morning and dependent areas such as the lower extremities after prolonged standing. In addition to the history and physical examination, the quickest screening test is a urinalysis.

## HYPERTENSION

Hypertension is defined as BP above the 95th percentile for age. Strictly, three values obtained 1 month apart are required before a child is labeled as hypertensive. Obviously, if the BP is very high or if the child has other findings (edema, hematuria, headache, nosebleeds), a single high reading is taken seriously.

Signs and symptoms of hypertension in children can be nonspecific, including irritability and failure to thrive. An older child may present with headache, low exercise tolerance, or recurrent epistaxis. In extreme cases, a child can present with heart failure, seizures, or neurologic deficits (e.g., facial palsy).

Hypertension can be primary (essential) or secondary. *Primary hypertension* is more common in African Americans and overweight adolescents, usually with a positive family history. *Secondary hypertension* can have a number of causes. Renal causes can be congenital (polycystic kidney disease), acquired, acute (pyelonephritis, glomerulonephritis), or chronic (chronic renal failure). It also can be vascular (e.g., coarctation of the aorta), renovascular (e.g., renal artery stenosis, or in babies, an embolus from an umbilical artery catheter), endocrine (rare, e.g., pheochromocytoma and some forms of congenital adrenal hyperplasia), neurologic (high intracranial pressure or Guillain-Barré syndrome), or iatrogenic (steroids).

The majority of cases of hypertension in infants below 1 year of age are of vascular or renovascular etiology. Coarctation of the aorta is a common cause; special attention should be paid to perfusion of the extremities, including temperature, femoral and dorsalis pulses, and BP in upper versus lower extremities.

Beyond the first year of life, most cases of hypertension in children are renal. The finding of hypertension in a child should prompt investigation of the kidney. Common nonrenal causes are coarctation of the aorta and iatrogenic factors (e.g., steroids).

The extent and invasiveness of the workup depend on age (more in younger children), severity of hypertension, presence of associated problems (retinopathy, cardiomyopathy), and response to treatment.

## ABDOMINAL MASS

A large proportion (55 percent) of abdominal masses in newborns are of renal origin. Most of these masses are benign; the majority represent hydronephrosis or cystic disease. Beyond the neonatal period, the majority of abdominal masses are retroperitoneal and renal in origin. An abdominal flank mass may represent an enlarged kidney (polycystic kidney disease, multicystic dysplasia, hydronephrosis), a tumor (Wilms' tumor or neuroblastoma), or a renal vascular accident (renal venous thrombosis). The incidence of malignancies (Wilms' tumor and neuroblastoma) increases with age to peak at age 2 to 3 years, when they become the leading cause of abdominal masses in a child. Wilms' tumor, the most common renal malignancy in children, peaks at age 2 to 3 years. It presents with hematuria, abdominal pain or mass, and hypertension.

The initial workup includes a detailed history, physical examination, and abdominal U/S.

## FAILURE TO THRIVE

Failure to thrive (FTT) is a common pediatric problem. The majority of cases are due to poor nutrition, parental ignorance, poverty, or neglect. The second most common causes are gastrointestinal (malabsorption and maldigestion, including cystic fibrosis, lactase deficiency, and gluten intolerance). The third most common causes are renal, including occult urinary tract infections, renal tubular acidosis, diabetes insipidus, and chronic renal failure.

# ABNORMAL URINE

## HEMATURIA

Not all red urine represents hematuria.

If a urine dipstick is negative for blood, the red color is likely to be due to pigments (beets or red food coloring), uric acid crystals (newborns), or drugs (rifampin). If a urine dipstick is positive for blood, after a history is taken and the patient is examined, there are three possibilities:

1. *Myoglobinuria.* It occurs with extensive muscle cell disruption such as crush injuries or prolonged seizures.

2. *Hemoglobinuria.* Hemoglobinuria is suspected if no red cells are seen in the urine and obviously if the child has anemia. This occurs with intravascular hemolysis, such as glucose-6-phosphate dehydrogenase (G6PD) deficiency.
3. *Hematuria.* Hematuria is suspected when red blood cells are seen in the urine.

## GROSS HEMATURIA

The most common pediatric cause of gross hematuria is UTI. Typically, the child also has fever, dysuria, frequency, or suprapubic tenderness. A urine culture will be positive if the infection is bacterial; however, viral cystitis can occur as well (adenovirus).

The next most common cause is perineal irritation or trauma. The external genitalia should be examined.

Hypercalciuria can be a cause of gross hematuria. Urinalysis may reveal crystals. Screening is done by the calcium/creatinine ratio on a random urine sample, and a high value is confirmed by a 24-h urine collection.

Gross hematuria can be the presentation of glomerulonephritis. Typically, the child also will have oliguria, edema, and hypertension, with a history of streptococcal infection in the preceding 2 to 3 weeks. Urinalysis will show casts. Blood studies will show azotemia, low complement, and evidence of streptococcal infection [high antistreptolysin O (ASO), Streptozyme].

Less common causes of gross hematuria in children include stones, tumors, cysts, and obstruction, which can be diagnosed by ultrasound. Sickle cell trait should be kept in mind, and a screening test should be obtained. A bleeding tendency should be considered if the child has other sources of bleeding (stools, nose, gums).

## MICROSCOPIC HEMATURIA

Microscopic hematuria is found commonly on a screening urinalysis. With a girl, one must make sure she is not menstruating. In an otherwise normal child, benign familial hematuria is the most common cause, and so one should do urine dipsticks on all family members.

Hematuria associated with proteinuria, casts, hypertension, or azotemia indicates significant underlying renal disease. One should evaluate for the presence of glomerulonephritis such as poststreptococcal nephritis; Berger disease (IgA nephropathy), which usually presents with recurrent gross hematuria during respiratory tract infections, can progress to chronic renal failure, and is diagnosed by biopsy; and Alport syndrome (familial nephritis, usually in males, accompanied by hearing loss).

Isolated hematuria can be the presentation of hypercalciuria. Many drugs can cause hematuria, including some antibiotics (penicillins, sulfas) and aspirin. It also is necessary to rule out a bleeding tendency or sickle cell anemia. U/S may be done to rule out tumors, cysts, stones, and congenital anomalies.

History and physical examination are essential to rule out a systemic disorder such as systemic lupus erythematosus (SLE) or Henoch-Schönlein purpura. A family history is very important for stones, deafness, and renal failure.

### PROTEINURIA

Proteinuria is found commonly during a routine urinalysis. It can be transient or persistent. Proteinuria is more likely to be serious if it is persistent or is accompanied by other abnormalities (e.g., hematuria). Also, the amount of protein spill is important and has to be measured on a 24-h urine.

The most common cause of proteinuria is orthostatic proteinuria, which is present in 10 to 15 percent of the normal population. In this condition, proteinuria occurs upon standing up. This condition is identified by testing the first morning specimen, by serially checking the urine throughout the day, or, more formally, by measuring protein on a split 24-h urine collection (day and night in separate bottles). Transient proteinuria can occur with infections, fever, exercise, seizures, and heart failure.

Persistent proteinuria may represent chronic renal disease (including chronic glomerulonephritis or pyelonephritis, reflux, and obstruction). Therefore, renal function and anatomy should be investigated. Proteinuria is much more serious if associated with other findings (e.g., hematuria, hypertension).

Severe proteinuria indicates glomerular disease. Protein excretion > 50 mg/kg per day is nephrotic syndrome.

## COMMON DISEASES

### CONGENITAL ANOMALIES

The urine that a baby passes in utero contributes to the amniotic fluid. Congenital anomalies in which urine output is low present with oligohydramnios. This can be due to the absence of both kidneys (bilateral agenesis, which has a frequency of 1 in 4000 births) or severe obstruction (e.g., posterior urethral valve). In extreme cases, the newborn has a typical appearance with a flat face, deep folds under the eyes, and clubfeet, as well as pulmonary hypoplasia, the so-called Potter syndrome.

Congenital anomalies can involve the number of kidneys (unilateral agenesis is the absence of a kidney), their size (hypoplasia is a small but otherwise normal kidney), their location (ectopic kidney), their shape (the two kidneys may be fused into a horseshoe kidney), or their architecture (dysplasia is abnormal organization and differentiation of renal parenchyma). Cystic diseases and obstruction are discussed below.

## CYSTIC DISEASES

*Multicystic kidney disease* is a form of dysplasia that usually affects only one kidney; it has equal frequency in boys and girls. It is not genetic. It often is detected by prenatal U/S or may present with an abdominal mass in a new-born. U/S shows a large cystic kidney, and renal scan shows poor or no function. The other kidney is usually normal. Indications for removal are infection, hypertension, or just big size. It carries a small potential risk of malignancy.

There are two types of *polycystic kidney disease (PCKD)*:

1. Infantile (autosomal recessive) PCKD presents with large spongy kidneys and oliguria/renal failure. There may be associated hepatic fibrosis. It progresses quickly to renal failure within 1 year of age.
2. The adult type (autosomal dominant) usually presents in adolescence or adulthood with masses, hematuria, flank pain, hypertension, UTI, or renal failure. It is associated with hepatic cysts (polycystic liver) and cerebral aneurysms.

The treatment for both forms is kidney transplantation. A correct diagnosis is important because of the implications for genetic counseling.

The *prune-belly syndrome* is the triad of (1) absent abdominal muscles, (2) hydroureters and hydronephrosis, and (3) undescended testicles. It occurs in boys; most cases are sporadic.

## OBSTRUCTION

Obstruction may present in a neonate with delay in passing urine or an abdominal mass. Later, it may present with UTI, pain, hematuria, or voiding dysfunction.

Obstruction can be unilateral. The most common location is the uretero-pelvic junction, with hydronephrosis on the affected site. With obstruction at the ureterovesical junction, there will be hydronephrosis and hydroureter on the affected side. If significant, it can lead to thinning of the renal cortex and a decrease in renal function. The treatment consists of surgery.

In a boy, bilateral obstruction can be due to a posterior urethral valve. It can present with UTI, abdominal mass, abnormal urine stream, or FTT. It is diagnosed by VCUG. The treatment consists of removal of the valve during cystoscopy.

Obstruction can be acquired, for example, from a stone. Obstruction can be functional rather than anatomic, such as neurogenic bladder in a child with a meningomyelocele or cerebral palsy.

## VESICOURETERAL REFLUX

Vesicoureteral reflux (VUR) is the most common abnormality in children investigated for UTI. It has a familial tendency (30 percent in siblings). It is important to diagnose VUR as early as possible because a kidney with VUR is at risk of function loss as a result of pressure and infection, leading to chronic renal failure or hypertension. VUR is diagnosed by VCUG. It is graded by severity, from I to V. Many children outgrow grades I to III reflux, and so management consists primarily of preventing UTIs (prophylactic antibiotics). Surgery (reimplantation of the ureter) is indicated for higher grades, poor follow-up risk, UTIs despite prophylaxis, and in older children. The success rate is > 95 percent.

## FAMILIAL NEPHRITIS (ALPORT SYNDROME)

Alport syndrome is a congenital disorder, transmitted as autosomal dominant, that presents in the second or third decade of life as a combination of nephritis and deafness. It tends to be more severe in males. It ultimately leads to chronic renal failure. It should be suspected in a boy with hematuria and a family history of renal failure or deafness. The diagnosis is made by renal biopsy, which shows an abnormal glomerular basement membrane on electron microscopy.

# GLOMERULAR DISEASES

## ACUTE POSTSTREPTOCOCCAL GLOMERULONEPHRITIS

Acute PSGN follows infection with a nephritogenic strain of group A streptococci, with 75 to 80 percent of cases occurring after pharyngitis (winter) and the rest after impetigo (summer and fall) after a latent period of 1 to 3 weeks. PSGN occurs mostly in children and young adults, peaking at age 2 to 8 years. PSGN is rare in the first year of life. Many cases are subclinical.

### PATHOPHYSIOLOGY

Acute PSGN is an immune-complex disease. Immune complexes (clumps of antigen, antibody, and complement) deposit along the glomerular basement membrane, leading to inflammation and cell proliferation. This results in a decrease in GFR, with consequent oliguria, fluid retention, and hypertension.

### HISTORY

Over 75 percent of these patients present with periorbital edema or hematuria (red or tea-colored urine); 30 percent note a decreased urine volume. Systemic symptoms such as malaise and anorexia are common. More seriously ill children present with heart failure (tachypnea, dyspnea) or with CNS symptoms of hypertension (headache, seizure).

## PHYSICAL EXAMINATION

The physical examination may show evidence of active streptococcal pharyngitis or impetigo. Edema (mostly periorbital puffiness) is noted in 75 percent of these patients. Hypertension is present in > 50 percent. Signs of heart failure occur with fluid overload (tachypnea, dyspnea, rales, tachycardia, cardiomegaly, gallop rhythm, hepatomegaly). Signs of encephalopathy occur in approximately 20 percent (headache, blurred vision, diplopia, seizure).

## LABORATORY EVALUATION

*Urine.* Red blood cells (gross or microscopic hematuria) are present in all cases; RBC casts are the hallmark of the disease (found in > 80 percent). Proteinuria is present in 60 percent.

*Chemistry.* BUN and creatinine are usually high. Hyponatremia may be seen from water overload. Hyperkalemia and acidosis may be seen with severe decrease in GFR.

*Serology.* ASO and Streptozyme are elevated. C3 is low in > 95 percent of these patients.

Pathology shows proliferation of glomerular cells and infiltration with neutrophils. Immune complexes are identified by immunofluorescence and electron microscopy. A biopsy is not done in uncomplicated cases.

## MANAGEMENT

Penicillin is given if indicated. Treatment is usually supportive, with fluid restriction, diuretics, or antihypertensives. Dialysis rarely is needed.

## CLINICAL COURSE

The prognosis in children is excellent. Typically, improvement starts within a week with a brisk diuresis, return of BP to normal, and decreases in BUN and creatinine. C3 normalizes within 3 months. Proteinuria resolves by 6 months. Hematuria can persist for 1 to 2 years.

### HENOCH-SCHÖNLEIN PURPURA (ANAPHYLACTOID PURPURA)

Henoch-Schönlein purpura (HSP) is the most common systemic vasculitis in childhood. The peak age is 3 to 10 years. A preceding URI is common. Four systems are involved: (1) the skin, with a typical purpuric rash over the legs and buttocks, (2) the joints with arthralgias (knees > ankles > upper extremities) and rarely arthritis, (3) the gastrointestinal tract (abdominal pain, nausea, vomiting, GI bleed in 5 percent, intussusception), and (4) the kidneys (nephritis).

Twenty-five to 50 percent of these children have renal involvement, which is noted days or weeks after nonrenal manifestations. There is usually mild proteinuria and hematuria. Rarely, there is acute renal failure. Complement is normal.

## PATHOLOGY

Immunoglobulin A can be found in the skin and kidney lesions and in circulating immune complexes.

## COURSE

Usually self-limiting over weeks to months, HSP rarely leads to chronic renal failure. Steroids or nonsteroidal anti-inflammatory drugs (NSAIDs) are used in the treatment.

## NEPHROTIC SYNDROME

Nephrotic syndrome is characterized by proteinuria (> 50 mg/kg per day) that leads to hypoalbuminemia (< 2.5 g/dL) and edema. The majority of pediatric cases are idiopathic. The peak is at 2 to 3 years of age.

## PATHOPHYSIOLOGY

There is urinary loss of protein of unknown cause. Liver synthesis of albumin increases but cannot keep up with the losses. This results in decreased plasma protein and albumin and hence to decreased oncotic pressure of plasma, fluid transudation to the extravascular space, and edema.

## HISTORY

During periods of edema, the child is prone to develop infections (e.g., spontaneous peritonitis) and intravascular clotting, most commonly of the renal vein, especially if dehydrated.

## LABORATORY EVALUATION

There is proteinuria of > 50 mg/kg per day. Microscopic hematuria may be present. Blood studies show a low protein and albumin; cholesterol and triglycerides are increased. Some laboratory values are low because of the low serum albumin, such as calcium. Hyponatremia is common, especially in children on diuretics.

## PATHOLOGY

There are four main forms that are differentiated by renal biopsy. Minimal change nephrotic syndrome (MCNS) is the most common (> 80 percent). Glomeruli are normal by light microscopy. The long-term prognosis is excellent in terms of preservation of renal function. The other three forms are membranoproliferative glomerulonephropathy (MPGN) in approximately 10 percent, focal segmental glomerulosclerosis (FSGS) in approximately 10 percent, and membranous glomerulopathy (rare).

## MANAGEMENT

Management entails a regular diet with salt restriction and cautious use of diuretics. There is daily home monitoring of urine protein (Albustix). Prednisone 2 mg/kg per day may be taken for a maximum of 1 month. If remission occurs (negative Albustix), prednisone is tapered. If steroids fail, biopsy is indicated. Ninety-five percent of children with MCNS respond to prednisone, though some two-thirds relapse, with the relapses often triggered by infections. Ultimately, most children outgrow it, maintaining good renal function. Patients with FSGS and MPGN are more likely to progress to chronic renal failure.

## HEMOLYTIC-UREMIC SYNDROME

Hemolytic-uremic syndrome (HUS) is the most common cause of acute renal failure requiring dialysis in pediatrics. The peak incidence is at 3 years of age. There is a triad of acute renal failure, microangiopathic hemolytic anemia, and thrombocytopenia.

## PATHOLOGY

The pathogenesis is thought to be endothelial cell damage, with consequent localized clotting in the small vessels of the kidney. The pathology entails thrombosed arterioles and glomeruli in the kidney, with fibrin deposition.

## HISTORY

The typical history is several days of acute gastroenteritis with bloody diarrhea and abdominal pain caused by toxin-producing *Escherichia coli* (*E. coli* O157:H7). Nephritis then develops, with anemia and a bleeding tendency (petechiae). Neurologic manifestations (lethargy, irritability, convulsions) are common.

## LABORATORY EVALUATION

The CBC reveals anemia with a high reticulocyte count and low platelets. The WBC count often is elevated. The peripheral blood smear shows fragmented red cells. Chemistries show azotemia, often with acidosis; hyperkalemia; and hyponatremia.

## MANAGEMENT

Any child with HUS should be referred to a nephrologist or a major medical center. The patient receives supportive care of renal function, and dialysis is instituted if the patient is anuric for more than 24 to 48 h. RBC or platelet transfusions are given as needed. Seizures are treated. Mortality is reported to be 5 to 45 percent. Long-term sequelae include hypertension and chronic renal failure.

## URINARY TRACT INFECTION

In the neonatal period, most UTIs occur in males, are bloodborne, and are part of generalized sepsis. An evaluation for an underlying congenital malformation should be performed. After the neonatal period, UTIs occur mostly in girls (10x) and uncircumcised boys. Many preschoolers with a febrile UTI have congenital anomalies (reflux or obstruction).

### PATHOGENESIS

There can be bladder infection (cystitis) or renal parenchymal infection (pyelonephritis). Pyelonephritis can lead to renal scars and ultimately loss of kidney function; the majority of scars appear very early (< 2 years of age). UTIs can be bloodborne (neonates) or, most commonly, ascending (this is why UTI is more common in girls).

### HISTORY

The symptoms can be typical of UTI (dysuria, urgency, frequency) or very nonspecific, especially in younger children (e.g., fever, low appetite, vomiting, diarrhea, abdominal pain, failure to thrive).

### LABORATORY EVALUATION

The urine often has a foul odor. The urinalysis may be positive for blood, leukocyte esterase, and nitrites. Urine culture is required for diagnosis. Bacteria are usually gastrointestinal flora: *E. coli* and other enteric gram-negatives (*Klebsiella, Proteus, Pseudomonas*). Because of the high incidence of associated anomalies, investigation of the urinary tract of any child < age 5 years with a febrile UTI > 38.1°C (100.5°F) should be done. The clinician is looking for reflux (girls) or obstruction (boys) so that the child can be followed up closely and surgical correction can be done if indicated. The usual workup is a renal U/S and VCUG.

### MANAGEMENT

Very young children and those with systemic symptoms of sepsis should be admitted and treated parenterally. Otherwise, the patient usually receives a 10-day course of oral antibiotics with careful follow-up. Some children need prophylactic therapy (Nitrofurantoin, Bactrim).

Parents and children should be instructed about hygiene, especially girls (cleanliness, wiping from front to back). Bubble baths are associated with UTIs and should be avoided.

In nonbacterial UTI, cystitis can be viral (adenovirus), typically with gross hematuria. Treatment is symptomatic.

## DISORDERS OF TUBULE FUNCTION

The functions of the proximal tubule (PT) include reabsorption of glucose, amino acids, phosphorus, and bicarbonate. Although the PT also reabsorbs water, sodium, potassium, and calcium, these are rarely relevant because more distal portions of the nephron can compensate for these compounds. Functions of the distal tubule include excretion of acid and urine concentration.

*Fanconi syndrome* is a generalized defect in PT function. All the compounds listed above are lost, with the clinical picture resulting mainly from phosphorus (growth failure, rickets, hypotonia) and bicarbonate loss (acidosis). It can be idiopathic or secondary to various systemic disorders.

*Renal glucosuria* is an isolated (genetic) defect in glucose reabsorption. Renal glucosuria is a benign condition.

*Familial hypophosphatemic rickets* is an inherited metabolic disorder with a specific defect in phosphorus reabsorption in the PT. It presents with short stature, bowing of the legs, and a low serum phosphorus level.

*Renal tubular acidosis (RTA)* is a common renal cause of failure to thrive. It results from decreased ability of the kidney to reabsorb bicarbonate or excrete acid. Serum electrolytes show hyperchloremic acidosis (normal anion gap). If, at the same time, the urine pH is inappropriately alkaline, the diagnosis is established. In unclear cases, acid or alkali loading tests may be helpful, though they are done only rarely in children. There are several forms of RTA (types 1, 2, 3, and 4); they are distinguished by the site of the nephron that is affected (proximal or distal) and the presence or absence of hyperkalemia. RTA can be congenital or acquired.

Distal RTA (type 1) is a defect in $H^+$ secretion by the distal tubule. Urine pH is always > 6 even with systemic acidosis. It is associated with hypercalciuria and the risk of nephrocalcinosis. Treatment is with alkali (Bicitra, Polycitra, Scholl's solution), usually in a dose of 1 to 3 mEq/kg per day. Type 1 RTA is usually a lifelong problem.

Proximal RTA (type 2) is a defect in bicarbonate reabsorption by the PT. The diagnosis is done by showing bicarbonaturia. Alkali losses can be massive, requiring 10 to 15 mEq/kg per day for treatment; often potassium must to be supplemented as well. Proper treatment optimizes growth. Many children outgrow it. When this form of RTA is diagnosed, Fanconi syndrome has to be ruled out.

Type 3 RTA is type 1 with associated bicarbonate loss.

Type 4 RTA is distal RTA with hyperkalemia. It can be idiopathic or secondary to obstruction.

*Diabetes insipidus* usually presents in older children with polyuria-polydipsia and in younger children with failure to thrive or recurrent hypernatremic dehydration.

*Bartter syndrome* is a rare tubule disorder that presents with failure to thrive and hypochloremic hypokalemic metabolic alkalosis.

## BIBLIOGRAPHY

American Society of Pediatric Nephrology. www.aspneph.com

National Institute of Diabetes, Digestive and Kidney Diseases. www.niddk.nih.gov

# FLUIDS AND

# ELECTROLYTES/

# DEHYDRATION

*Aida Yared*

## LEARNING OBJECTIVES

1. Recognize that children have proportionately more body water than adults and are at a higher risk of dehydration.

2. Know how to define the severity of dehydration in a child, using key components from the history and physical examination.

3. Be familiar with the composition of standard intravenous and common oral solutions used for hydration.

4. Be able to calculate maintenance fluid and electrolytes.

5. Be able to calculate fluid and electrolyte deficits in a child with hypernatremic, isonatremic, or hyponatremic dehydration. Be aware of special problems associated with hypernatremia and hyponatremia.

## INTRODUCTION

Acute gastroenteritis is a common problem with significant morbidity and mortality. Yearly, some 500 million children worldwide develop acute diarrheal disease, and 1.5 million die from it. This impressive number of fatalities is down from 3.5 million 20 years ago as a result of improved sanitation, education, and the availability of oral rehydration solutions. In the United States, acute gastroenteritis accounts for 5 percent of clinic visits, 10 percent of hospital admissions, and some 300 deaths per year in children under 5 years of age. Most of those deaths are due to dehydration.

The goal of rehydration therapy is twofold: first, to achieve euvolemia, with the endpoint usually considered as urine output of 1 to 2 mL/kg per hour, and second, to maintain or restore electrolyte homeostasis.

Fluid and electrolyte therapy can be divided into maintenance, deficits, and replacement of ongoing losses. All calculations are based on a child's weight in kilograms (kg). Fluids are considered isotonic if they have the tonicity of plasma, or an osmolality around 300 mEq/L.

In the majority of children with an acute illness, decision making is based clinically on the results of the history and physical examination. If the illness is unusually prolonged or severe, the levels of serum electrolytes are measured and followed periodically. The orders are written in the form of the composition of the solution and the rate in milliliters per hour.

## AVAILABLE SOLUTIONS

The ingredients of rehydration are water, sodium (Na), potassium (K), anions [usually chloride (Cl) and the alkali precursor lactate or citrate], and D-glucose (referred to as dextrose, abbreviated D).

### ORAL REHYDRATION

Oral rehydration is preferred in a child with mild to moderate dehydration who is able to drink fluids. A variety of commercially available solutions are designed specifically for children with gastroenteritis (e.g., Pedialyte, Infalyte); the Oral Rehydration Solution (ORS) developed by the World Health Organization (WHO) and United Nations International Children's Emergency Fund (UNICEF) is distributed and used widely in Third World countries. The composition of common oral fluids is given in Table 34-1. It is immediately apparent that many are not appropriate for use as oral rehydration solutions because of their high sugar content (which may aggravate diarrhea), high K (may cause hyperkalemia in a child with prerenal failure), or low Na content (ineffective rehydration).

### INTRAVENOUS REHYDRATION

Intravenous rehydration is used in children who are unable to take oral rehydration. The components of basic intravenous fluids are listed in Table 34-2. Normal saline (NS) is an isotonic solution that is used in acute resuscitation when the goal is acute volume expansion and restoration of vital signs. NS is available with 5 g/100 mL dextrose (D5NS). It should not be used for rapid infusion, as it may lead to hyperglycemia, glucosuria, and hence urine losses from osmotic diuresis. Half-normal saline (0.5NS) is a hypotonic solution and can lead to hemolysis if it is infused intravenously; therefore, D5 is added to yield D5½NS.

Table 34-1 **Composition of Common Oral Fluids**

|  | Sodium, mEq/L | Potassium, mEq/L | Sugar, g/100 mL | Alkali Source |
|---|---|---|---|---|
| Water | 0 | 0 | 0 | None |
| Kool-Aid | 1 | 1 | 10 | Citrate |
| Coca-Cola | 2 | 0 | 10.5 | Bicarbonate |
| Apple juice | 1 | 30 | 12 | Citrate |
| Orange juice | 1 | 55 | 12 | Citrate |
| Gatorade | 22 | 2.5 | 4.5 | Citrate |
| Pedialyte | 45 | 20 | 2.5 | Citrate |
| Oral Rehydration Solution | 75 | 20 | 1.35 | Citrate |

"Quarter"-normal saline (.02NS) is also hypotonic, and so D5 is added to yield D5¼NS. Lactated Ringer (LR) contains acetate as one of its anions, which acts as a source of alkali; hence, LR is considered a buffered solution. Rarely used in pediatrics, it is popular in surgical services.

Na is the ingredient necessary for volume expansion: It would be impossible to reverse shock with D5, and it would require twice the volume of D5½NS compared with NS. K is added depending on serum K and not until urine flow is documented. Glucose usually is added to intravenous (IV) fluids as D5 for two reasons: to buffer hypotonic solutions (that may lead to acute hemolysis) and to prevent short-term starvation and catabolism.

Table 34-2 **Components of Basic Parenteral Fluids**

|  | Na⁺ mEq/L | Cl, mEq/L | K, mEq/L | Lactate, mEq/L | Osmolarity, mOsm/L |
|---|---|---|---|---|---|
| Normal saline (NS) | 154 | 154 | 0 | 0 | 308 |
| Half-normal saline (0.5 NS) | 77 | 77 | 0 | 0 | 154 |
| "Quarter"-normal saline (0.2 NS)* | 30 | 30 | 0 | 0 | 60 |
| Lactated Ringer | 130 | 109 | 4 | 28 | 271 |

*The term "quarter" normal saline is technically inaccurate but commonly used for convenience. The solution is actually one-fifth normal saline.

## THE EUVOLEMIC CHILD

Calculation of fluid requirements in health (maintenance) and disease (deficits and ongoing losses) relies on a clear understanding of normal fluid and electrolyte physiology.

### NORMAL BODY COMPOSITION

Total body water in infants and children makes up a larger proportion of body weight than it does in adults. Water and electrolytes in the body are distributed into extracellular fluid (ECF) and intracellular fluid (ICF); ECF constitutes more of the body weight in infants than in adults (Table 34-3).

The composition of ECF is reflected in serum measurements. The main anion is Na (140 mEq/L), with minor contributions from K (3.5 to 5 mEq/L), calcium, and magnesium. The main cations are Cl (100 mEq/L) and bicarbonate (25 mEq/L), with minor contributions from phosphates and proteins. Acute weight loss is usually fluid loss, primarily from the ECF.

The major cation in ICF is K (150 mEq/L), with a minor contribution from Na (5 mEq/L) and others; the major anions are phosphates and proteins.

### NORMAL WATER AND ELECTROLYTE HOMEOSTASIS

#### WATER HOMEOSTASIS

Water is required for dissipation of heat and for solute excretion. Water is added to the body orally (drinks and foods), and endogenous water is generated from the oxidation of fat, carbohydrate, and protein. Water is lost through the urine (50 to 65 percent), insensible losses from the skin and lungs (30 to 40 percent), and a minor contribution from stools. In calculating fluid maintenance in pediatrics, it is assumed that the kidneys excrete the daily solute load in isotonic urine; that is, the kidneys do not concentrate or

Table 34-3 **Body Composition and Compartments: Changes during Growth**

| Age | TBW, % | ECF, % | ICF, % | Blood Volume, mL/kg |
|---|---|---|---|---|
| Premature | 80 | 45 | 35 | 80 |
| Full term | 75 | 40 | 35 | 70 |
| 1–12 months | 65 | 30 | 35 | 65 |
| 1–12 years | 60 | 20 | 40 | 60 |
| Adult male | 55 | 25 | 30 | 60 |
| Adult female | 50 | 20 | 30 | 60 |

TBW = total body water; ICF = intracellular fluid; ECF = extracellular fluid.

dilute the urine. In reality, antidiuretic hormone (ADH) regulates the amount of water excreted in the urine, and the urine concentration normally varies between 50 and 1200 mOsmol/kg.

## SODIUM HOMEOSTASIS

Body losses are always hypotonic. Urine Na is variable: It depends on Na intake and urine flow rate and is fine-tuned in the distal nephron by aldosterone; it averages 65 mEq/L. Fluids lost through the lungs have Na 15 mEq/L, stools 5 mEq/L, and skin < 40 mEq/L.

## POTASSIUM HOMEOSTASIS

Potassium is taken orally in variable amounts. Destruction of cells (hemolysis or rhabdomyolysis) generates significant amounts of K. Potassium losses in the urine depend on the glomerular filtration rate, the urine flow rate, the presence of aldosterone, and the anion content of urine. There is an insignificant amount of K in the stools that may increase with severe diarrhea.

K handling is dependent on renal and adrenal function. It can be affected by medications, including angiotensin-converting enzyme (ACE) inhibitors, diuretics, and sympathomimetics. Most K in the body is intracellular. The entry of K into cells is regulated by membrane pumps; it also is facilitated by insulin (alongside glucose), aldosterone, and sympathomimetics. The transfer of K across cell membranes can be affected acutely by the acid-base status (serum K increases in acidosis and decreases in alkalosis, being exchanged for protons).

Serum K imperfectly reflects total body K. However, as a rule, low K reflects low body K, whereas high serum K may accompany dehydration or decreased renal perfusion.

## ACID-BASE HOMEOSTASIS

The kidneys reabsorb all the bicarbonate filtered (proximal tubule) and excrete the daily acid production of 2 mEq/kg (distal tubule). There are no alkali requirements.

Acidosis in a dehydrated child may be due to loss of alkali (small intestinal fluid), renal hypoperfusion (decreased renal acid excretion), or starvation and tissue hypoperfusion (lactic acid production).

## MAINTENANCE REQUIREMENTS

Maintenance fluids commonly are calculated using the Holliday-Segar method, which assumes that 1 mL of water is needed for 1 calorie metabolized.

Caloric (and hence water) requirements are proportional to body weight in a stepwise fashion:

0–10 kg: 100 cal/kg
11–20 kg: additional 50 cal/kg for each kg over 10 kg
Over 20 kg: additional 20 cal/kg for each kilogram over 20 kg

Daily water requirements thus are calculated per day (or, in a shortcut method, directly per hour) as follows:

1–10 kg: 100 mL/kg per day (rounded to 4 mL/kg/h)
11–20 kg: 1000 mL + 50 mL/kg per day (additional 2 mL/kg/h)
> 20 kg: 1500 mL + 20 mL/kg per day (additional 1 mL/kg/h)

Example: The water requirement of a 6-kg baby is 6 kg × 100 mL/kg/day = 600mL/day (or 6 kg × 4 mL/kg/h = 24 mL/h). The water requirement of a 21-kg child is 1500 mL + 20 mL = 1520 mL/day (or 40 + 20 + 1 = 61 mL/h). There is a slight (but acceptable) variance in the results obtained by the two methods.

These estimates are for an otherwise healthy child. Fever increases the daily water requirement by 12 percent for each degree Centigrade (7 percent for each degree Fahrenheit). Activity increases the daily water requirement by 25 to 50 percent, and hypometabolic states (e.g., coma) decrease it by 20 to 25 percent. Sweat losses are additional.

The Na requirement in children is 3 mEq/kg per day. However, it is safe to give larger amounts since the kidneys can readily excrete Na loads as high as 10 mEq/kg per day, and very hypotonic solutions may cause hyponatremia as a result of a low glomerular filtration rate (GFR) in younger children. Further, since many hospital conditions (e.g., nausea, pneumonia, meningitis, or anesthesia) can induce ADH release and impair water excretion, many pediatricians consider it unsafe to use D5¼NS in children and use D5½NS instead.

The potassium requirement in children is 2 mEq/kg per day. However, if one has doubts, it is safer to give less than more; K, in the presence of compromised renal function, may lead to hyperkalemia and the risk of arrhythmias. The dictum is "no pee (urine output), no K."

Example: Write fluid orders for a 6-kg child placed NPO (nothing by mouth) in anticipation of elective surgery.

Maintenance fluid requirement: 6 kg × 100mL/kg/day = 600 mL/day
Na requirement: 3 mEq/kg/day × 6 kg = 18 mEq/day
K requirement: 2 mEq/kg/day × 6 kg = 12 mEq/day

In terms of solution choice, this would be provided by a solution containing Na 30 mEq/L and K 20 mEq/L. The closest commercially available solution is D5¼NS + 20 mEq/L K; practically, many pediatricians would prefer D5½NS + 20mEq/L K to avoid the risk of hyponatremia. The intravenous (IV) fluid rate will be 600 mL/day ÷ 24 h = 25 mL/h (shortcut method, 6 kg × 4 mL/kg/h = 24 mL/h).

## THE DEHYDRATED CHILD

### PATHOPHYSIOLOGY

Gastroenteritis in infants and children is usually viral and less commonly bacterial. Diarrhea increases both the volume of water lost through the stools and its electrolyte content. Na concentration in normal stools is negligible (5 mEq/L), but it increases with the severity of the diarrhea to reach 100 mEq/L in severe secretory diarrhea (e.g., cholera); still, the stools are always hypotonic. Vomiting alone usually leads to alkalosis (loss of HCl in gastric fluid), and diarrhea leads to acidosis through loss of bicarbonate-rich small intestinal fluid. Both vomiting and diarrhea lead to K losses.

### HISTORY

The history aims at defining the fluid deficit as well as possible electrolyte disturbances. The parent should be asked about the child's weight before illness to make it possible to calculate weight loss and the severity (percent) of dehydration. If a previous weight is not available, the severity of dehydration can be estimated from the physical examination.

The losses should be described (How many times did the child vomit? Can the volume be estimated? How many times did the child pass a stool? Can the volume be estimated?). In the hospital, diapers can be weighed to calculate output more precisely. Intake is noted carefully, including the volume of fluid taken orally and its composition (e.g., a child who took large amounts of tea or water may be hyponatremic). In addition to enteral intake and losses, the history should include fever, sweating, and mental status changes. Careful inquiry is made about the frequency and volume of urine output; this is often difficult to ascertain in a child with profuse diarrhea.

### PHYSICAL EXAMINATION

A full set of vital signs should be obtained. Special attention is paid to the fontanel (flat versus sunken), mucous membranes (moist versus dry), peripheral perfusion and pulses, skin turgor, and mental state. The magnitude of dehydration is best determined by recent weight loss. If that information is not available, the degree of dehydration is based on the clinical picture. The presence of tears when the child cries or urine in the diaper should be noted. Clinical assessment of the severity of dehydration is described in Table 34-4.

### LABORATORY EVALUATION

Laboratory evaluation may include a basic chemistry profile. Blood urea nitrogen (BUN) may be elevated, with an increased BUN/creatinine ratio; if dehydration is affecting renal perfusion, creatinine may be elevated as well. A child with isolated vomiting may have alkalosis because of the loss of

Table 34-4 **Clinical Assessment of Dehydration**

| Dehydration | Mild | Moderate | Severe |
|---|---|---|---|
| Percent body weight | < 5 | 5–10 | 10–15 |
| Skin turgor | Normal | Tenting | None |
| Skin color | Normal | Pale | Mottled |
| Fontanel | Flat | Soft | Sunken |
| Eyes | Normal | Deep | Sunken |
| Mucosa/lips | Moist | Dry | Parched |
| Central nervous system | Consolable | Irritable | Lethargic |
| Pulses | Normal | Fast | Thready |
| Capillary refill | Normal | 2–3 s | > 3 s |
| Urine output | Normal | Decreased | Anuric |

gastric HCl; however, most children with gastroenteritis are acidotic to some degree as a result of bicarbonate loss in the diarrheal fluid, decreased renal perfusion, and generation of lactic acid. Serum K is variable, depending on the magnitude of the deficit, renal perfusion, and transcellular shifts (e.g., acidosis). Urinalysis may reveal a high specific gravity and/or ketones.

## HYPERNATREMIC DEHYDRATION: NA > 150 MEQ/L

Hypernatremia is the "natural history" of unattended dehydration, since insensible losses and body fluids are always hypotonic; rarely, hypernatremia is due to intake of high solute (e.g., administration of improperly prepared oral hydration solution or excessively salted chicken soup). It usually is seen in very small infants (e.g., a newborn who is breast-feeding poorly) or in an illness with both severe vomiting and diarrhea.

In the presence of hypernatremia (and high plasma osmolality), fluid leaves the ICF. The advantage is that intravascular volume and vital signs are relatively preserved in hypernatremic dehydration compared with other forms of dehydration. The disadvantage is that cell shrinkage can lead to a physical reduction in the size of the brain, with attendant rupture of veins bridging to the cranial vault and hence intracranial hemorrhage. Intracranial hemorrhage should be suspected in a child with hypernatremia who has significant mental status changes that do not improve with management.

Hypernatremia can lead to transient insulin resistance and hence hyperglycemia; this hyperglycemia, coupled with ketoacidosis in a severely dehydrated child, may mimic diabetic ketoacidosis but resolves with proper hydration. Hypernatremic dehydration, especially if recurrent, raises the concern of diabetes insipidus.

## NORMONATREMIC DEHYDRATION (NA 130–150 MEQ/L)

Normonatremic dehydration is the most common type of dehydration. It usually is due to increased losses with an intake that closely replaces the proportion of water and electrolytes in the losses (e.g., Pedialyte, Gatorade).

## HYPONATREMIC DEHYDRATION (NA < 130 MEQ/L)

Hyponatremic dehydration occurs when gastrointestinal losses are replaced by solute-free fluids such as fruit juices, water, or sodas. Medical conditions such as adrenal insufficiency or cystic fibrosis may aggravate hyponatremia during dehydration. Hyponatremia, if severe, can lead to mental status changes, including disorientation, lethargy, and seizures. With hyponatremic dehydration, water shifts from ECF to ICF; hence, cardiovascular instability is greater than might be expected for the degree of dehydration.

### MANAGEMENT

In calculating the fluid and electrolyte needs of a child with dehydration, the deficits and maintenance needs are calculated separately and added. Additional calculations are the free-water requirement in hypernatremia and the extra Na requirement in hyponatremia. Ongoing losses are added if massive or if the disease is unusually prolonged.

The addition of potassium to IV fluids is contingent on an established urine output. An important point is that K extravasation into soft tissues at a high concentration can lead to soft tissue necrosis. Potassium at 20 mEq/L is safely given through a peripheral IV, and 40 mEq/L can be given if necessary. Higher concentrations (rarely needed) require a central line.

The child should be reevaluated periodically, with particular attention to signs and symptoms of dehydration or fluid overload. Intake and output should be charted carefully and reviewed. Any child on IV fluids should be weighed on a periodic basis.

### SHOCK

Shock, if present, should be treated immediately, with the aim of restoring vital signs and perfusion of vital organs. Shock is treated with a bolus of 20 mL/kg of NS given over 30 to 60 min and repeated if needed. Plasma expanders (e.g., fresh-frozen plasma, dextran, and 5% human albumin) rarely are needed in a previously healthy child. Vital signs, clinical status, and urine output should be monitored carefully; fluid overload may occur in a child with heart problems or established renal failure. Once fluid resuscitation is complete, it must be assumed that the patient still has severe dehydration, and deficits of water and electrolytes must be replaced accordingly.

## DEFICIT THERAPY

The estimate of water and solute deficits is based on documented weight loss (if available) or on a clinical assessment of the percentage of dehydration. It is assumed that all weight loss is due to loss of water and electrolytes, mostly from the ECF (60 percent) and the rest from the ICF (40 percent). For ease of remembering, it is assumed that ECF has only Na 140 mEq/L, and ICF only K 140 mEq/L. Remember, however, that hyperkalemia may occur easily in a dehydrated child and lead to dangerous arrhythmias; it is often best *not* to add K to IV fluids until urine output is well established and a low serum K is documented.

## HYPERNATREMIC DEHYDRATION

Hypernatremic dehydration requires more gradual and careful replacement of deficits. Rapid fluid replacement is dangerous, as cells adapt to a hyperosmolar state by generating "idiogenic" osmoles. Rapid infusion of hypotonic fluid would lead to a fluid shift intracellularly and hence to an increase in cell volume (including brain edema with consequent seizures or mental state changes). In practice, hypernatremia should be corrected at a rate of 0.5 to 1 mEq Na per hour, that is, over 48 to 72 h.

Example: A 6-kg baby comes in with 10 percent dehydration and a serum Na of 160 mEq/L.

Calculate the baby's water deficit: With 10 percent dehydration, the baby's water deficit is 600 mL with 60 percent from ECF (360 mL) and 40 percent from ICF (240 mL).

Calculate the baby's electrolyte deficits: Na deficit = 360 mL × 140 mEq/L = 50 mEq; K deficit = 240 mL × 140 mEq/L = 34 mEq.

Calculate the baby's maintenance fluid and electrolytes: Water 600 mL, Na 18 mEq, K 12 mEq.

Calculate the baby's total needs: Water 1200 mL, Na 68 mEq, K 46 mEq; the closest commercially available solution is D5½NS + 40 mEq/L K.

Calculate the rate of administration: 1200 mL/24 h = 50 mL/h, maintained over 48 h. Note that this rate is equal to twice maintenance. Be sure to monitor the Na closely.

## ISONATREMIC DEHYDRATION

Example: A 10-kg child presents with 10 percent isonatremic dehydration.

Calculate the child's deficits: Water deficit = 1000 mL of water, 60 percent (600 mL) from ECF and 40 percent (400 mL) from ICF. Na deficit is the Na contained in 600 mL of ECF (600 mL × 140 mEq/L = 84 mEq). K deficit is the K in 400 mL ICF (400 mL × 140 mEq/L = 56 mEq).

Calculate the child's maintenance: Water = 10 kg × 100 mL/kg/day = 1000 mL, Na = 3 mEq/kg/day × 10 kg = 30 mEq, K = 2 mEq/kg/day × 10 kg = 20 mEq.

Calculate the child's total needs: Water 2000 mL, Na 114 mEq, K 76 mEq. The closest commercially available solution is D5¾NS + 40mEq/L K. Three-quarter NS contains 115 mEq/L of both Na and Cl. Since the Na is normal in this patient, D5½NS with 40 mEq/L K also may be a reasonable choice.

Calculate the rate: 2000 mL/day or 83 mL/h (again, twice maintenance). It is traditional in isonatremic dehydration to give one-half of the water volume (in this case, 1000 mL) in the first 8 h and the other half (1000 mL) over the next 16 h; thus, the rate would be 1000 mL/8 h = 125 mL/h initially for 8 h and then 1000 mL/16 h = 63 mL/h for 16 h.

## HYPONATREMIC DEHYDRATION

Hyponatremia usually is due to intake of free water in excess of needed electrolytes; thus, there is a relative Na deficit over and above the deficits estimated in the usual fashion (i.e., 60/40 from ECF/ICF). This "extra" deficit can be calculated by knowing that 0.6 mEq/kg body weight raises serum Na by 1 mEq/L.

Example: A 6-kg baby comes with 10 percent dehydration and serum Na 120 mEq/L.

Calculate the baby's water deficit: With 10 percent dehydration, the baby's water deficit is 600 mL with 60 percent from ECF (360 mL) and 40 percent from ICF (240 mL).

Calculate the baby's electrolyte deficits: Na deficit is the Na of ECF (50 mEq); K deficit is the K of ICF (34 mEq).

Calculate the baby's "extra" Na deficit: Normal Na (140 mEq/L) – patient's Na (120 mEq/L) = 20 mEq/L. The amount of Na required to increase serum Na by 1 mEq/L = patient's weight (6 kg) × 0.6 mEq/kg = 3.6 mEq/L. Therefore, the amount of Na needed to increase the baby's serum Na by 20 is 20 mEq Na × 3.6 mEq/L = 72 mEq/L.

Calculate the baby's maintenance needs: Water 600 mL, Na 18 mEq, K 12 mEq.

Calculate the baby's total needs: Water 1200 mL, Na 140 mEq, K 46 mEq. This would be provided by a solution with Na 116 mEq/L and K 38 mEq/L; the closest commercially available solution is D5¾NS + 40mEq/L K.

Calculate the baby's fluid rate: 1200ml/24 h or 50 mL/h (i.e., twice maintenance).

Caveat: Rapid correction of hyponatremia in adults can lead to devastating neurologic deficits ("osmotic demyelination" or central pontine myelinolysis). Although this is rare in children, hyponatremia (like hypernatremia) should not be corrected with a change in serum sodium higher than 0.5 to 1 mEq/L per hour.

## SYMPTOMATIC HYPONATREMIA

Hyponatremia may present with seizures, typically if serum Na is < 120 mEq/L. In this situation, the initial goal of therapy is to raise the serum Na just enough to stop the seizures, usually to 120 mEq/L.

Example: A 6-kg baby comes in with seizures and serum Na 115 mEq/L. Calculate how much Na would (probably) stop the seizures.

Recall that 0.6 mEq Na/kg increases serum Na by 1 mEq/L. This baby would need 18 mEq Na to increase his or her Na by 5 mEq/L. Since this would have to be given rapidly, one might decide to use 3% NaCl ("hot salt"); hot salt has 0.5 mEq Na/mL, and so this baby needs 36 mL. This can be given safely over 1 h, with the infusion switched to the baby's calculated needs as soon as the seizure clinically abates.

## ACIDOSIS

Alkali replacement rarely is needed, as correction of hypoperfusion often leads to the resolution of acidosis. Administration of alkali also can result in "paradoxical" central nervous system acidosis, which may aggravate mental status changes. Correction may be considered in a child with severe acidosis (pH <7.15) with ongoing profuse diarrhea.

## ONGOING LOSSES

Most gastroenteritis is self-limited, and children are able to take fluids orally within 24 to 48 h. However, in cases in which ongoing losses are massive, their volume and composition can be added to IV fluids. The volume can be measured by weighing diapers in the case of infants; electrolyte content is estimated, or a fluid sample is sent to the laboratory for more accurate measurement.

## BIBLIOGRAPHY

Awazu M, Devarajan P, Stewart CL, et al. Maintenance therapy and treatment of dehydration and overhydration. In Ichikawa I, ed., *Pediatric Textbook of Fluids and Electolytes*. Baltimore: Williams & Wilkins, 1990: 417–428.

Centers for Disease Control and Prevention. http://cdc.gov.

UNICEF. http://unicef.org.

# NEUROLOGY

## Joseph Gigante

● LEARNING OJECTIVES

1. Recognize the signs and symptoms of cerebral palsy.
2. Be familiar with the multidisciplinary team approach to the management of children with cerebral palsy.
3. List the characteristics of the major neurocutaneous disorders.

## CEREBRAL PALSY

### INTRODUCTION

Cerebral palsy can be defined as a broad range of static, nonprogressive motor disabilities that present from birth to early childhood. Cerebral palsy occurs as a result of central nervous system (CNS) insults of congenital, hypoxic, ischemic, or traumatic origin. Motor involvement is always present, but additional neurologic, sensory, and mental deficits may occur as well. The clinical manifestations vary, depending on the nature and extent of the original injury. Characteristically, they are chronic throughout life and involve abnormalities in physical growth and mobility as well as intellectual, social, and emotional development. The incidence of cerebral palsy is approximately 2 in 3000 live births. The increasing number of extremely low-birthweight infants who survive the neonatal period may contribute to a rising incidence of cerebral palsy.

## PATHOPHYSIOLOGY

Numerous conditions can injure the developing brain and lead to cerebral palsy. The clinical presentation varies markedly, depending on the location, extent, and character of the CNS system insult. Functional deficits depend on the nature and severity of the injury and can range from slight coordination difficulties to complete quadriplegia with sensorimotor and cognitive involvement. Voluntary and involuntary motor performance, posture, and tone normally are coordinated by communication between the cerebral cortex, thalamus, basal ganglia, brainstem (medulla, pons, midbrain), cerebellum, and spinal cord with ascending and descending sensorimotor pathways. This complex network lends itself to injury at many different levels. The causes of cerebral palsy are numerous and can occur during the prenatal (e.g., congenital brain malformation, maternal bleeding, intrauterine infection), perinatal (e.g., ischemia, asphyxia, chorioamnionitis), or postnatal (e.g., prematurity/low birthweight, head trauma, CNS infections) period. Although there are many etiologies for cerebral palsy, many children with cerebral palsy have no identifiable cause. Cerebral palsy is classified according to the extremities involved (monoplegia—one limb involved; hemiplegia—one side of body involved; diplegia—lower limbs more affected than the upper limbs; quadriplegia—all extremities affected) and the characteristics of the neurologic dysfunction (spastic—60 percent of cases, marked by an increase in muscle tone; dyskinetic—20 percent of cases, marked by several movement disorders, such as dystonia or athetosis; ataxic—1 percent, marked by incoordination of movement and lack of balance; mixed—remainder of cases).

## HISTORY

Children with cerebral palsy may not have any apparent problems during the first few months of life. The clinical picture is progressive, although the CNS injury is not. An infant's motor skills during the first few months are primarily on a reflex basis, with little cortical involvement with movements. As the brain matures (myelinization of tracts), changes in the clinical picture occur that can range from mild to severe. The most common complaint by parents is concern about delayed development, and so a developmental history is important in patients with suspected cerebral palsy, with special attention to gross motor milestones. Affected children display a number of abnormal motor characteristics. The child may appear to be stiff (hypertonia), although during the first few months of life the infant may have decreased tone (hypotonia). Parents may notice fisting, strong hand preference before 12 months of age, movement of one limb less than the others (because of paresis), or excessive arching of the back.

As was noted earlier, a thorough prenatal, perinatal, and postnatal history should be obtained in an attempt to determine a cause for the cerebral palsy. The family history may reveal other relatives with cerebral palsy. Excessive lethargy and irritability, a high-pitched cry, and oral hypersensitivity are behaviors that may be present.

## PHYSICAL EXAMINATION

A number of findings may be noted on the neurologic and neuromuscular examination. Hyperreflexia with sustained ankle clonus is commonly present. Muscle tone usually is increased, but these infants initially may present with hypotonia. There may be decreased range of motion at a joint, especially the ankles or hips. Resistance to movement during range of motion may be indicative of spasticity. Abnormal movements such as athetosis, chorea, or dystonia may be evident. Persistence of primitive reflexes beyond 6 months of age (when they usually disappear) is another hallmark of cerebral palsy. Some of these primitive reflexes include the Moro reflex, asymmetric tonic neck reflex, and palmar grasp.

## LABORATORY AND RADIOGRAPHIC EVALUATION

An exclusive test for the detection of cerebral palsy does not exist. Therefore, the diagnosis is based on a thorough history, physical examination, and comprehensive neurologic assessment, as well as the exclusion of other diagnoses. Early on it may be difficult to distinguish cerebral palsy from a progressive neurologic disorder, and so tests to screen for a metabolic disorder and imaging of the brain may be indicated.

## MANAGEMENT

Successful management involves a multidisciplinary team of specialists, with services coordinated with an early intervention program in the school system. A variety of therapies, including physical, occupational, and speech-language therapy, address problems related to abnormal tone and positioning, fine and gross motor development, self-help/independence, and oral motor concerns (feeding and communication). Assistive devices such as splints can be used to control abnormal joint posture and prevent contractures. Some patients may need special seating or mobility aids (e.g., walkers or wheelchairs). A number of surgeries may be necessary, including orthopedic surgery (e.g., tendon lengthening and tendon transfers, surgery for scoliosis), neurosurgery (e.g., selective dorsal rhisotomy), or placement of a gastrostomy tube for patients with significant gastroesophageal reflux and aspiration. Medications such as diazepam and baclofen may be given to reduce muscle tone. Many patients with cerebral palsy have a seizure disorder, and so these patients are treated with anticonvulsants. Constipation is a common problem that is treated with stool softeners. More than half of affected children have mental retardation, and these children require special education. Parental and family education and support are vitally important.

Families need help with behavior management issues with the affected child in addition to counseling for social and emotional issues.

## NEUROCUTANEOUS DISORDERS

Neurocutaneous disorders (phakomatoses) are diseases that have in common lesions of the skin and brain. This occurs because the skin, teeth, hair, and nails have the same embryonic origin from neuroectoderm as the brain. Most of these diseases are inherited, and so a complete family history is important. The major neurocutaneous disorders are neurofibromatosis, tuberous sclerosis, Sturge-Weber disease, and ataxia-telangiectasia.

*Neurofibromatosis type 1 (NF-1)* is an autosomal dominant disease, and it is estimated that 1 in 3000 people have this disease. The diagnosis of NF-1 requires two or more of the following features:

1. Café au lait spots are present in over 90 percent of these patients. There typically are six or more of these macules over 5 mm in greatest diameter in prepubertal patients and over 15 mm in postpubertal patients. The margin of the spots may be smooth or irregular. The number of spots may increase after puberty.
2. Two or more Lisch nodules, which are pigmented hamartomas of the iris.
3. Two or more neurofibromas of any type or one plexiform neurofibroma.
4. Freckling in the axillary or inguinal region.
5. Optic glioma.
6. A distinctive osseous lesion such as sphenoid dysplasia or pseudoarthrosis.
7. A first-degree relative with NF-1.

*Neurofibromatosis type 2 (NF-2)* is diagnosed by the presence of bilateral acoustic neuromas or a first-degree relative with NF-2 and either a unilateral eighth cranial nerve mass or two of the following: neurofibroma, meningioma, glioma, schwannoma, and posterior subcapsular cataracts.

*Tuberous sclerosis* is an autosomal dominant disease that is characterized by the triad of skin lesions, mental retardation, and seizures. A variety of skin abnormalities are seen in patients with tuberous sclerosis, including *adenoma sebaceum*, which are angiokeratomas (angiofibromas) surrounding the sweat glands. They begin to appear at 2 to 5 years of age. They predominate in the malar regions of the face and appear as pink or red macules. *Shagreen patches* are uneven, thickened, elevated rough plaques of skin that have a predilection for the lumbar and gluteal regions. *Ash leaf spots* are flat, hypopigmented spots that are visible under a Wood's lamp. *Café au lait* spots also may be present. Seizures occur early in life and may be difficult to control. Mental retardation that is slowly progressive is seen. Periventricular tumors can occur, leading to hydrocephalus. Cysts and malignant tumors can develop in the heart, pancreas, peritoneal cavity, or kidneys. Renal hamartomas can result in hypertension and abdominal masses.

*Sturge-Weber syndrome* is thought to be a sporadic disease. It is characterized by facial hemangiomas (port-wine stain), meningeal hemangiomas, seizures, and mental retardation. A facial port-wine stain (capillary hemangioma) occurs unilaterally in the distribution of the trigeminal nerve. Meningeal hemangiomas involve the ipsilateral side of the brain. Calcium deposition becomes detectable in the gyri of the brain underlying the angioma, giving the classic radiologic picture of "tram track" or "railroad track" calcifications. Glaucoma can be seen in these patients if the vascular nevus involves the eye; thus, routine ophthalmologic evaluations are necessary in these patients.

*Ataxia-telangiectasia* is an autosomal recessive disorder that affects the skin, cerebellum, and immune system. Ataxia usually develops in the first 5 years of life, and other causes of ataxia should be ruled out. Telangiectasias, which occur most commonly in the conjunctiva and ears, typically occur in the second 5 years of life. Frequent infections, especially lung infections, occur secondary to immunologic dysfunction. Malignancies, especially lymphoma and leukemia, are seen in affected patients and are a leading cause of death, in addition to infections.

## BIBLIOGRAPHY

DeBella K, Szudek J, Friedman JM. Use of the National Institutes of Health criteria for diagnosis of neurofibromatosis 1 in children. *Pediatrics* 105:608–614, 2000.

Kuban KCK, Leviton A. Cerebral palsy. *N Engl J Med* 330:188–195, 1994.

# ORTHOPEDICS

## M. Robin English

● LEARNING OBJECTIVES

1. Know the presenting signs and symptoms for each of the diseases of the spine, hip, knee, leg, and elbow.

2. Understand the underlying etiology and/or pathophysiology for diseases of the spine, hip, knee, leg, and elbow.

3. Know the appropriate initial workup and management for diseases of the spine, hip, knee, leg, and elbow.

4. Describe the differences between fractures and sprains in children.

## INTRODUCTION

The pediatrician is often the first person to encounter orthopedic problems in childhood. The adolescent population frequently is affected by these diseases because adolescence is a time of rapid growth spurts. It is important to be able to identify orthopedic diseases and know when to refer to a pediatric orthopedic surgeon, because a few of these diseases require immediate surgical intervention. Traumatic problems such as fractures and sprains present acutely and usually with a concise history of an injury or fall. Other diseases, such as a slipped capital femoral epiphysis and Legg-Calvé-Perthes disease, may present with a longer history of pain or limp. The physical examination of children with orthopedic complaints should include the patient's general appearance and observation of posture and gait. The examination also should include visualization of the involved area without clothing, looking for symmetry or obvious skin lesions. If a particular limb or joint is affected, that area should be palpated gently to assess for masses, tenderness, or warmth, and range of motion should be tested as well. A thorough neurologic examination that focuses on muscle strength also is indicated.

One situation in which a complete orthopedic examination is indicated is the sports preparticipation physical examination. This almost always is performed by a primary health-care provider rather than an orthopedic surgeon. This evaluation includes a careful history of the athlete's past medical history, a family history of cardiovascular disease or syncope, and a history of medication use. A past history of injuries is critical, especially those involving paired organs. The examination should include a pupillary examination, a thorough heart and lung examination, and an abdominal examination. The musculoskeletal examination is important as well. All joints, including the neck and hip, should be evaluated for range of motion and swelling. All muscle groups should be tested for active and passive muscle strength.

Plain radiographs are often the diagnostic test of choice for orthopedic diseases. It is always helpful to get bilateral films, even if the complaint is unilateral. This allows for comparison to the "normal" side and can make identification of subtle changes possible.

Some orthopedic problems may occur in any area of the body, whereas others occur in specific bones or joints. This chapter is arranged by body area and discusses a few common orthopedic diseases in pediatrics. The typical history, physical examination (with specific maneuvers), diagnosis, and management are discussed for each entity.

## CONDITIONS AFFECTING ANY JOINT OR BONE

### FRACTURE

Fractures in children and adolescents are somewhat different from those seen in adults. When one compares injuries in children with similar injuries in adults, children are more likely to sustain a fracture than a tendon tear because the surrounding ligaments and tendons are stronger than the growing bone underneath, whereas adults have tears of the ligaments and tendons more often than they have fractures. Another feature of pediatric fractures pertains to the immaturity of the bone in that the affected bone may bow instead of break. Buckle fractures are caused by compression of the bone and are seen commonly in the distal radius. Greenstick fractures are those in which one side of the bone breaks while the other side bends. Growth plate, or physeal, fractures are common fractures in children. They can be difficult to see on radiographs and can be classified according to the Salter-Harris scheme (Table 36-1).

The history of the fracture is extremely important, especially in young preverbal children who may not be able to provide their own history. Infants

*Table 36-1*  **Salter-Harris Classification Scheme**

| Classification | Description |
| --- | --- |
| I | Fracture through physis |
| II | Fracture through physis and metaphysis |
| III | Fracture through physis and epiphysis |
| IV | Fracture through epiphysis, across physis, through metaphysis |
| V | Crush injury of physis |

and toddlers with fractures often present with refusal to move the affected limb, which is known as pseudoparalysis. The history should focus on the mechanism of the injury and whether it is consistent with the findings on physical examination. Child abuse perpetrators often provide a vague history of a fall or another event to explain an injury. A history that is inconsistent with the child's developmental age or one that changes from one examiner to another is suspicious for child abuse as well. Physical examination findings suggestive of a fracture include overlying bruising and point tenderness. If child abuse is suspected, a complete examination, including a skin and retinal examination, is warranted.

Anteroposterior and lateral plain radiographs of the affected area often show the fracture, but some fractures can be difficult to appreciate. Most fractures in pediatrics are closed fractures and can be managed by casting. Orthopedic consultation and/or follow-up are recommended.

## SPRAIN

A sprain is an injury to a ligament or joint capsule. The history may reveal a twisting mechanism or a direct, forceful blow. The physical examination usually reveals swelling and pain at the site of injury. If severe pain or bruising is present, radiographs may be indicated to rule out a fracture. Sprains are graded by the severity and degree of ligament tearing, and management is determined accordingly. Most sprains can be managed with rest, elevation, compression, and nonsteroidal anti-inflammatory drugs for severe pain.

## TENDINITIS

Tendinitis usually occurs as a result of excessive or repetitive use and therefore is seen commonly in adolescent athletes. The examination generally shows tenderness over the affected tendon. Management includes rest and nonsteroidal anti-inflammatory medications for pain.

# THE PEDIATRIC SPINE

## *SCOLIOSIS*

Scoliosis is defined as a lateral curvature of the spine greater than 10 degrees. The population most often associated with scoliosis is adolescent females, but other children may have scoliosis as well. The most common cause of scoliosis is idiopathic, which can occur in infants, older children, and adolescents. Scoliosis also can occur secondary to other causes, such as leg-length discrepancy. Congenital scoliosis is a result of abnormal vertebral development such as hemivertebrae or bar (failure to form spaces between vertebrae). Neuromuscular scoliosis can occur with both upper and lower motor neuron diseases such as cerebral palsy. Trauma and spinal cord tumors also can cause scoliosis.

The history should elicit the time course of the scoliosis if the parent or child has noticed it before. An important point to ask about is the presence of back pain or stiffness. Idiopathic scoliosis rarely causes back pain, and so pain should alert the examiner to the possibility of a tumor or infection. In adolescents, it is important to ask about pubertal changes, because puberty is a time of rapid growth, and curves can progress quickly with growth spurts. If puberty is complete, the curve is less likely to progress significantly. The history also should include a complete review of systems, including constitutional symptoms such as weight loss and fever, and the child's level of activity.

The physical examination should involve visualization of the child's posture and gait. The back should be examined without clothing for evidence of a curve and for symmetry of the scapulae and hips. Asymmetric skin folds can be a clue that scoliosis is present. Asymmetric hips may indicate leg-length discrepancy. The Adams test should be performed in all children. This involves having the child stand with the legs together and flex forward at the hips with the arms stretched out in front and the palms together. The presence of a hump on one side (which is caused by rib convexity) is very suspicious for a curvature with vertebral rotation. The degree of the curve can be measured with a scoliometer. The remainder of the examination should include a close inspection for lesions over the spine and other skin lesions and a complete neurologic examination.

When the physical examination is consistent with scoliosis, an anteroposterior and lateral radiograph of the entire spine is indicated, and curvature can be measured by using the Cobb angle. Most cases of idiopathic scoliosis are curved to the right in the thoracic area. If a different curve is present, the examiner should strongly consider another cause for the scoliosis.

Curves less than 20 degrees usually can be monitored and followed with subsequent radiographs. More severe curves should be referred to an orthopedic surgeon for evaluation. The child's pubertal stage is one determinant of whether bracing should be performed. Prepubertal children are more likely to undergo bracing because of the risk of progression with the adolescent growth spurt. Bracing prevents future curvature, but it does not correct existing curves. If an underlying cause for the scoliosis is found, further evaluation and/or treatment are indicated.

## THE PEDIATRIC HIP

### DEVELOPMENTAL DYSPLASIA OF THE HIP

Developmental dysplasia of the hip (DDH) is an abnormal relationship of the femoral head within the acetabulum and includes subluxation, frank dislocation, and instability. Early detection is important in determining the outcome, and so evaluation for DDH begins in the newborn nursery. Many cases of DDH are not evident at birth, and so periodic examination of the hips is indicated until the child is 12 to 18 months of age and is walking well.

Risk factors for DDH are female gender, family history of DDH, and breech presentation. Affected infants are often firstborns. Other musculoskeletal abnormalities, such as congenital torticollis and clubfoot, also may be present.

The examination of newborns and infants should include visual inspection of the hips. Asymmetric skin folds or unequal thigh lengths may be clues to the presence of dislocation. Range of motion also should be assessed. Up to 3 months of age, the Ortolani and Barlow maneuvers should be performed with the infant lying supine without a diaper to look for both subluxation and dislocation. The Ortolani maneuver is done by placing the thumb on the medial aspect of the knee and the middle finger over the greater trochanter while the hip is flexed. Simultaneously, the hip is abducted and gently pressed toward the examination table, with the middle finger placing gentle pressure anteriorly. This maneuver will reduce a dislocated femoral head, which will be felt as a "clunk." The Barlow maneuver is done with the hands in the same position. Pressure is applied posteriorly toward the examination table while the hip is flexed and abducted. A "clunk" will be felt as the previously reduced femoral hip is dislocated posteriorly. These maneuvers are less reliable and more difficult to do in children over age 3 to 4 months. At that age, a Galeazzi maneuver should be performed at all visits until the child is walking. This involves having the child lie supine with the knees flexed and the feet on the examination table. Asymmetry of the knees may indicate a posterior dislocation. Limitation of motion at the hip also may be a sign of hip dysplasia in older infants.

Orthopedic consultation should be obtained if the Barlow or Ortolani maneuver is positive at birth. If there is doubt about the examination, a repeat examination at age 2 weeks is indicated. If the diagnosis is still suspected after the 2-week examination, an ultrasound of the hips should be obtained. After 3 to 4 months of age, plain radiographs are more reliable in detecting dysplasia. Treatment consists of maintaining the hip in a flexed, abducted, and externally rotated position; this is done by placing the child in a Pavlik harness. Triple diapering is ineffective and delays more appropriate treatment.

## LEGG-CALVÉ-PERTHES DISEASE

Legg-Calvé-Perthes (also known as Perthes) disease is caused by idiopathic avascular necrosis of the femoral head. It affects boys age 4 to 8 years most commonly, and it usually occurs unilaterally. The history usually reveals a limp of several weeks' duration, and the parents may be unable to identify the exact time of onset. These children may complain of pain in the hip, thigh, or knee. The physical examination typically reveals limited internal rotation and abduction of the hip. An antalgic gait usually is seen, and these children are otherwise well-appearing.

Plain radiographs of the hips are the diagnostic method of choice and reveal flattening and sclerosis of the femoral head on the affected side. Orthopedic consultation is required, although young children with mild involvement may be only observed. The therapy is aimed at preventing further femoral head deformity and improving range of motion. Bracing, casting, and surgical containment are all possible treatments. The age at presentation and the degree of involvement are important determinants of the therapeutic approach.

## SLIPPED CAPITAL FEMORAL EPIPHYSIS

Slipped capital femoral epiphysis (SCFE) is seen most commonly in the adolescent population. The femoral head becomes displaced, or "slips" on the femoral neck. The exact etiology is unknown but may be related to endocrinologic disorders or excessive forces caused by obesity. Slips may be acute or chronic and are usually unilateral. The history from a patient with an acute displacement may include sudden severe hip pain. Children with chronic slips usually complain of limp and vague, gradual hip pain, which may be referred to the knee. Affected adolescents are almost always obese. If a child who is nonobese and is younger than adolescent age presents with SCFE, an endocrinologic evaluation should be considered. The examination typically reveals limitation of hip flexion, abduction, and internal rotation, which may be more severe in an acute displacement.

If SCFE is suspected, anteroposterior and frog-leg radiographs of the hips bilaterally are indicated. Both views are necessary, because anteroposterior views may not reveal the displacement as well as frog-leg views do. If the diagnosis is confirmed, orthopedic consultation is indicated urgently. Surgical treatment involves the placement of a screw to stabilize the femoral head on the femoral neck. If this procedure is delayed, avascular necrosis of the hip can occur.

## THE PEDIATRIC KNEE AND LEG

### OSGOOD-SCHLATTER DISEASE

Osgood-Schlatter disease (OSD) is a common cause of knee pain in the adolescent population. It results from avulsion of the patellar tendon from its insertion point on the tibial tubercle and is seen most commonly in athletes. It may be due to increased use of the quadriceps muscle, which puts tension on the patellar tendon.

The exact time of onset of the pain may be difficult to elicit, and adolescents may present with pain for several weeks. The pain is usually worse with exercise and is relieved with rest. Affected adolescents also may complain of knee swelling. The examination shows localized pain and swelling over the tibial tubercle. Range of motion is usually normal. A hip examination is indicated because of the possibility of referred pain.

Radiographs are not always indicated to make the diagnosis if the history and examination are consistent with OSD, but they can be helpful to rule out other diseases. Radiographs may show abnormal ossification at the tubercle or occasionally an avulsion fracture. The mainstay of treatment is rest, although adolescents with mild OSD may continue to be active in sports. Knee pads and ice may be helpful. Long-term complications are unusual, but some adolescents have a persistent "bump" on the knee into adulthood.

### TIBIAL TORSION

Internal tibial torsion is a common cause of in-toeing that affects children age 12 to 18 months. It is thought to be due to intrauterine molding, but it is recognized only after a child begins to walk. The child's gait typically shows in-toeing that is fixed from one step to another, and the physical examination reveals that the lateral malleolus is anterior to the medial malleolus (normally the lateral is posterior to the medial in the plane of the body). No radiologic studies are required. Tibial torsion typically resolves as the child improves his or her walking balance and therefore usually requires no treatment.

### KNEE BOWING

Most children under age 3 years have a somewhat bowed appearance to the legs, which is normal. More severe bowing can be physiologic; it results from intrauterine molding and resolves without treatment. Severe bowing also can be caused by rickets or Blount disease, which is an abnormality of the medial proximal growth plate of the tibia. Plain radiographs of the legs bilaterally should be obtained in children with severe bowing, but most cases resolve.

## THE PEDIATRIC ELBOW

### NURSEMAID'S ELBOW

Nursemaid's elbow, or subluxation of the radial head, is a common injury in children under 5 years of age. It occurs when the arm is pulled up by the caregiver either to prevent a fall or to lift the child. A pop may be felt by the caregiver, but the lack of this history does not rule out the diagnosis. Children present with the arm held in flexion and pronation against the body. Tenderness over the radial head may be seen. The external appearance of the arm is normal. If bruising is seen or tenderness is palpated over another part of the arm, a fracture or another injury should be suspected.

If the history and physical examination are consistent with nursemaid's elbow, a maneuver to reduce the dislocation may be attempted. This is done by placing pressure on the radial head with the thumb while simultaneously flexing and supinating the arm. A palpable pop may be felt under the thumb with this maneuver; another indication that the dislocation has been reduced is increased movement and use of the arm, which usually occur within minutes to hours. After successful reduction, further treatment usually is not required, but the child may experience pain at the elbow for a few days. The parents should be cautioned not to lift the child by one arm to avoid recurrence. If any doubt about the mechanism of injury exists or if the physical examination is not typical, plain radiographs of the elbow should be obtained. In nursemaid's elbow, the radiographs are typically normal. Orthopedic consultation usually is not required unless a fracture is seen on radiographs.

## CONCLUSION

Pediatric orthopedic problems are important for the pediatrician to recognize so that timely evaluation and treatment can be initiated. The pediatric skeleton is unique; therefore, many diseases are seen only in this growing population. The history and physical examination, along with plain radiographs, are usually sufficient to make a diagnosis. Orthopedic consultation is required immediately for some diseases; others can be treated successfully or observed by the primary care provider.

## BIBLIOGRAPHY

Eiff MP, Hatch RL. Boning up on common pediatric fractures. *Contemp Pediatr* 20:30–59, 2003.

Goldberg MJ. Early detection of developmental hip dysplasia: Synopsis of the AAP clinical practice guideline. *Pediatr Rev* 22:131–134, 2001.

Kautz SM, Skaggs DL. Getting an angle on spinal deformities. *Contemp Pediatr* 15:111–128, 1998.

Krowchuk DP. The preparticipation athletic examination: A closer look. *Pediatr Ann* 26:37–47, 1997.

Richards BS. Slipped capital femoral epiphysis. *Pediatr Rev* 17:69–70, 1996.

Waanders NA, Hellerstein E, Ballock RT. Nursemaid's elbow: Pulling out the diagnosis. *Contemp Pediatr* 17:87–96, 2000.

Wall EJ. Osgood-Schlatter disease: Practical treatment for a self-limiting condition. *Physician Sports Med* 26:29–34, 1998.

# PEDIATRIC PULMONARY SYSTEM

*Gregory Plemmons*

## LEARNING OBJECTIVES

1. Know the classification system for asthma severity.
2. Describe the initial management of an acute asthma exacerbation.
3. List some of the causes of wheezing.
4. State the presenting signs and symptoms of bronchiolitis.
5. List the various causes of pneumonia based on age.
6. Describe the etiology and pathophysiology of cystic fibrosis.

## INTRODUCTION

The respiratory system has unique importance among children. Unlike most other organ systems, the airways and lungs of the developing fetus are largely undeveloped and unused before birth. With the first cry, air exchange begins. Still, almost 95 percent of the alveoli, or air sacs, develop after birth, making infants and small children uniquely susceptible to lung injury, whether from infection or from premature birth. Indeed, unlike the case in adults, the most common cause of cardiac failure in children is respiratory failure. Disorders of the respiratory system remain the most common cause of morbidity and hospitalization in children, whether from asthma, bronchiolitis, or pneumonia or from other disorders. An understanding of lung development and the presentation of illness in children is crucial in the art and practice of pediatrics.

## HISTORY

Pulmonary disorders may present with a variety of colorful descriptions. Parents may report cough, wheezing, noisy breathing, or even "rattling in the chest." Older children may complain of dyspnea, shortness of breath, or, rarely, chest pain. Fortunately, most pulmonary disorders rarely remain silent.

*Cough.* The pediatric cough is often more of a nuisance and source of worry to parents than to the child. Parents sometimes describe coughs as "wet" (suggesting mucus or sputum production) or "dry" (suggesting airway irritation). The pediatric cough rarely can be described as productive or nonproductive, since most children are unable to produce sputum on command before school age.

*Wheezing.* Parents may report wheezing, which truly may represent bronchoconstriction, but often the term *wheezing* is used nonspecifically to describe any noisy breathing, whether caused by stridor, true bronchoconstriction, or upper airway congestion.

*Stridor.* Stridor may be inspiratory, expiratory, or both and generally implies noisy breathing associated with upper rather than lower airway obstruction.

*Shortness of breath (dyspnea) and chest pain.* Young infants or children rarely are able to report a sensation of dyspnea, inability to move air, or chest pain, unlike teenagers and adults, who are able to communicate these symptoms.

### PHYSICAL EXAMINATION

The approach to examining an anxious child may be daunting because a careful cardiopulmonary examination requires a quiet child. However, a pediatric examiner can ascertain much simply by observing the child's breathing from across the examination room after requesting that a parent lift up a shirt or undress the patient. One of the first priorities in evaluating sick children is to determine if a child is in respiratory distress and obtain a rapid but systematic assessment. Is the child comfortable or ill-appearing? Is the child running around the examination room, chatting or babbling, or inactive and unable to vocalize? Are any indicators of respiratory distress (grunting, flaring, retractions) present? Is there any noise in the examination room? In extreme disruptions of breathing, true wheezing or stridor may be heard from across the examination room.

A careful observer may be able to determine the respiratory rate from a few feet away by monitoring chest wall movement. Tachypnea is a fairly sensitive finding for detecting pneumonia in children; the World Health Organization (WHO) concluded in 1990 that tachypnea is the most useful and objective sign for identifying pneumonia in children, especially if radiography is not readily available. For a more detailed description of the physical examination of the chest, see Chap. 3.

## RADIOGRAPHIC EVALUATION

*Chest radiography* is a mainstay in the evaluation of pulmonary disease. Anteroposterior (AP) views are generally adequate in a young infant. Lateral views may be obtained in an older child to evaluate the retrocardiac area and potential lower and middle lobe infiltrates, which may be masked by the cardiac silhouette on AP views.

*Computed tomography (CT) of the chest* offers additional anatomic information and is particularly useful in the evaluation of abnormalities (e.g., lung abscesses, masses, pleural effusions, congenital abnormalities) for which surgical intervention may be required.

*Barium swallow (upper gastrointestinal series)* is one of the best modalities to evaluate swallowing function and aspiration in infants and children and also may aid in the detection of anatomic abnormalities.

*Technetium scan* or *milk scan* is somewhat similar to the upper gastrointestinal (GI) series but may offer additional information on the risk of aspiration.

## OTHER EVALUATIONS

*Pulse oximetry,* sometimes called the "fifth vital sign," offers a quick assessment of oxygenation status by utilizing hemoglobin absorption of specific light wavelength.

*Bronchoscopy* may be both diagnostic and therapeutic. Direct visualization of pulmonary structures allows the collection of tissue or other material for further evaluation and also may be used to retrieve foreign bodies or relieve plugging if needed.

*Arterial blood gases (ABGs)* offer information on oxygenation and acid-base status and are obtained most often in the critical care or emergency setting. Rising $P_{CO_2}$ may be indicative of impending respiratory failure.

*Pulmonary function tests (PFTs)* are primarily helpful in differentiating between restrictive (e.g., muscular dystrophy) and obstructive (asthma) lung disease.

## DISEASES AND CONDITIONS

### ASTHMA

Asthma is the leading cause of pediatric hospitalization in the United States, and its prevalence among children under 18 years of age has doubled over the last two decades. Significant disparities continue to exist between populations: African-American children have higher rates of prevalence, hospitalization, and death compared with Caucasian children. Once thought to be primarily bronchoconstrictive and reversible in nature, asthma increasingly is viewed as a chronic disease that may lead to decreased long-term lung function if treated improperly.

## DIAGNOSIS

The diagnosis of asthma remains largely clinical. Most patients present with a history of cough, wheezing, or both. A history of other atopic disease (eczema, allergic rhinitis) or a family history of asthma is also suggestive. Radiographic findings may include increased bronchial wall markings, airway hyperinflation, and atelectasis, but these findings may be indistinguishable from those in patients with bronchiolitis. Chest radiographs also may be normal in children with asthma. Pulmonary function tests and spirometry may offer additional data on reversible airway obstruction but are difficult to perform in infants and preschool children. Often a clinical response to bronchodilator therapy is used to support a diagnosis of asthma.

Much more is understood now about the inflammatory component of asthma. The National Asthma Education and Prevention Program (NAEPP), under the guidance of the National Institutes of Health (NIH), has convened three expert panels and published two sets of evidence-based guidelines, offering practitioners improved classification of disease severity and recommendations for therapy (Table 37-1).

## MANAGEMENT

Although new therapies continue to be developed, educating the family about the disease and encouraging avoidance of triggers are crucial to preventing exacerbations. Known triggers in children include exercise, weather changes, cold air, allergens (dust, cockroach antigens, animal dander, pollen), air pollution, tobacco smoke exposure, gastroesophageal reflux, viral respiratory infections, and even emotional status.

Most asthma medications are delivered largely by inhalation, using a metered-dose inhaler (MDI) or a nebulizer, reducing the risk of systemic absorption and potential side effects. Still, only approximately 10 percent of most medications are delivered directly to the lungs, even with proper technique; use of a spacer can double this rate. MDIs have been used over the last 50 years but require coordination and some skill. Consideration of the age and development of the child may favor a nebulizer over the use of MDIs, although MDIs used with a spacer and face mask have been shown to be effective in the delivery of medication even in young children if administered properly.

### Short-Acting $\beta_2$ Agonists (Bronchodilators)

Before the widespread use of albuterol, epinephrine was used to treat the acute bronchoconstrictive phase of asthma. Albuterol is more $\beta_2$-specific and is

*Table 37-1* **Classification of Asthma Severity\***

## Clinical Features Before Treatment

| | Symptoms† | Nighttime Symptoms | Lung Function |
|---|---|---|---|
| STEP 1<br>Mild<br>Intermittent | • ≤ 2 times a week<br><br>• Asymptomatic<br><br><br><br>• Exacerbations<br>brief (from a<br>few hours to a<br>few days);<br>intensity may vary | ≤ 2 times a month | • $FEV_1$ or PEF<br>≥ 80% predicted<br>• PEF variability<br>< 20%<br>Normal PEF<br>between<br>exacerbations |
| STEP 2<br>Mild<br>Persistent | • > 2 times a week<br>but < 1 time<br>a day<br>• Exacerbations<br>may affect<br>activity | > 2 times a month | • $FEV_1$ or PEF ≥<br>80% predicted<br>• PEF variability<br>20–30% |
| STEP 3<br>Moderate<br>Persistent | • Daily<br>• Daily use of<br>inhaled short-<br>acting $\beta_2$-agonist<br>• Exacerbations<br>affect activity<br>• Exacerbations<br>≥ 2 times a<br>week; may last<br>days | > 1 time a week | • $FEV_1$ or PEF =<br>60–80% predicted<br>• PEF variability<br>> 30% |
| STEP 4<br><br>Severe<br><br>Persistent | • Continual<br><br>• Limited physical<br>activity<br>• Frequent<br>exacerbations | Frequent | • $FEV_1$ or PEF ≤<br>60% predicted<br>• PEF variability<br>> 30% |

\*The presence of one of the features of severity is sufficient to place a patient in that category. An individual should be assigned to the most severe grade in which any feature occurs. The characteristics noted in this table are general and may overlap because asthma is highly variable. Furthermore, an individual's classification may change over time.

†Patients at any level of severity can have mild, moderate, or severe exacerbations. Some patients with intermittent asthma experience severe and life-threatening exacerbations separated by long periods of normal lung function and no symptoms.

$FEV_1$ = forced expiratory volume in 1 second; PEF = peak expiratory flow.

currently the most widely used bronchodilator. Side effects include tachycardia, hyperactivity, and, with repeated short-term use, occasional hypokalemia.

### Inhaled Corticosteroids

With increasing recognition of the inflammatory component of asthma and the delayed response, inhaled corticosteroids are a mainstay of prevention. Side effects include the possible risk of growth suppression in children. The most widely used inhaled corticosteroids in children currently are fluticasone and budesonide. Newer corticosteroids have first-pass metabolism in the liver with reduced systemic effects, and long-term risk of growth suppression appears to be minimal in all but those receiving high doses.

### Long-Acting $\beta_2$ Agonists

Salmeterol was the first long-acting $\beta_2$ agonist, having been introduced in 1994. It remains a useful adjunct to other therapies in moderately to severely persistent asthmatic patients and often is used in combination with inhaled corticosteroid products.

### Leukotriene Inhibitors

Leukotriene inhibitors were introduced in the mid-1990s and have been shown to reduce airway inflammation as well. Zafirlukast (Accolate), zileuton, and montelukast (Singulair) are taken orally; only montelukast is approved for children under 12 years of age.

### Other Medications

Cromolyn sodium (Intal) is an inhaled medication and a mast cell stabilizer and has an excellent safety profile. Historically used as a preventer, it has been superseded largely by inhaled corticosteroids in part because of their increased efficacy and rates of compliance, since cromolyn must be administered at least three to four times per day. Anticholinergics such as ipratropium (Atrovent) have been shown to be useful in the acute (bronchoconstrictive) phase and may be used in the emergency room or critical care setting in the case of status asthmaticus. The use of methylxanthines such as theophylline has declined because of their limited efficacy, the need to monitor blood levels, and their side-effect profile.

In managing patients with asthma in an outpatient setting, it is crucial to ensure that family members know how to administer medications properly and are aware of the importance of preventive medications in preventing exacerbations. Practitioners frequently "step up" or "step down" therapy on the basis of the patient's response to medication and symptomatology.

*Status asthmaticus* is a medical emergency; it refers to a condition in which the patient is unresponsive to bronchodilator therapy. Albuterol frequently is given continuously, and systemic doses of corticosteroids may be given as well as supplemental oxygen. Additional interventions may include the administration of ipratropium, terbutaline, and intravenous magnesium sulfate, all of which may produce bronchodilation. Status asthmaticus generally requires admission and monitoring in an emergency or critical care setting and is a leading cause of pediatric hospitalization.

## BRONCHIOLITIS

### PATHOPHYSIOLOGY

Bronchiolitis is an infectious lower respiratory tract illness that is almost always viral in origin. It is characterized by small airway inflammation and obstruction and may be virtually indistinguishable from an asthma exacerbation. Bronchiolitis is one of the leading causes of hospitalization among children under 2 years of age.

Several viruses have been identified as bronchiolitis pathogens. Respiratory syncytial virus (RSV) is the leading cause of infection and is ubiquitous; by 3 years of age, virtually 100 percent of children have become infected. Other viruses include parainfluenza virus, influenza virus, adenovirus, rhinovirus, and metapneumovirus.

### HISTORY AND PHYSICAL EXAMINATION

Infants and young children may first develop a prodrome of rhinorrhea and slight cough, followed by tachypnea, expiratory wheezing, crackles, rhonchi, fever, and poor oral intake. Moderate to severe cases may present with lethargy, occasional apnea, hypoxemia, and respiratory distress.

### LABORATORY AND RADIOGRAPHIC EVALUATION

Rapid detection tests for RSV and influenza are available, but the diagnosis of bronchiolitis remains a largely clinical one. Radiographic findings may be identical to those found in asthma (hyperinflation, atelectasis), show consolidation, or even be normal.

### PREVENTION

As with all viral infections, frequent hand washing is recommended. RSV, for instance, may be viable on countertops for several hours. Universal respiratory precautions and isolation are used frequently for hospitalized children who are infected. Immunoprophylaxis also is offered currently in the United States for those infants and children at greatest risk for disease severity (premature infants, infants with significant lung disease, and children with cyanotic heart disease). Palivizumab is a humanized monoclonal mouse antibody that may be given to these groups monthly as an intramuscular injection and provides some passive immunity. The cost remains substantial, however, and reduction of hospitalization (40 to 60 percent) has remained modest at best. Research continues on RSV vaccines.

## MANAGEMENT

Treatment even at the turn of the twenty-first century remains largely supportive. For hospitalized children, adequate hydration and oxygenation generally are provided. Because there is significant overlap between bronchiolitis and asthma and because bronchiolitis may be the initial presentation for many children who go on to develop asthma, medications such as bronchodilators (albuterol, epinephrine) and corticosteroids historically were used to treat children with bronchiolitis as well, with variable responses. Benefits from inhaled bronchodilators or oral or inhaled corticosteroids in most evidence-based reviews remain questionable. Ribavirin, a synthetic nucleoside analog that inhibits viral replication, appears to offer little additional benefit, even in severely affected children.

## REACTIVE AIRWAY DISEASE: THE CONUNDRUM

Students may be confused between asthma and bronchiolitis and may have heard the term *reactive airway disease*. Research has failed to unravel the following scenario: Does bronchiolitis cause asthma to develop in some children, or do presymptomatic children with asthma have a propensity to infection? The answer remains unclear. Only about a third of children under age 3 years who are diagnosed with bronchiolitis go on to develop clinical signs of asthma. Members of this subgroup may respond to bronchodilator therapy, and often the term *reactive airway disease (RAD)* has been used to describe any child under 3 years of age who wheezes. It is useful to remember that there are occasionally other causes of wheezing as well, hence the caveat "all that wheezes isn't asthma."

## OTHER CAUSES OF WHEEZING

*Gastrointestinal reflux disease (GERD)* may produce microaspiration and bronchospasm in young children and infants. *Foreign body aspiration* may produce wheezing, usually monophonic and frequently unilateral, depending on the site of obstruction. *Cystic fibrosis (CF)* is an inherited metabolic disorder that may produce wheezing and significant bronchoconstriction. *Croup* (laryngotracheobronchitis) and anatomic obstructions of the airway (e.g., *vascular ring, tracheoesophageal fistula*) may present with wheezing in addition to stridor.

### PNEUMONIA

Community-acquired pneumonia is an acute infectious lower respiratory tract infection that is characterized by an inflammatory response in the alveolar spaces. Classic symptoms at presentation include fever, cough, tachypnea, varying degrees of respiratory distress, and, less commonly, vomiting, abdominal pain, or chest pain. Findings on auscultation (crackles, rhonchi, and rales) as well as respiratory distress, although fairly specific, are not very sensitive. As was mentioned earlier, the respiratory rate is a fairly sensitive marker for detecting disease, especially when chest radiography is not readily available.

There is no acceptable gold standard for the diagnosis of pneumonia. Lung fluid rarely is obtainable, and sputum or nasopharyngeal cultures may reflect colonization rather than true infection. Further, a variety of organisms have been proved to cause pneumonia in children. Chest radiography occasionally may help distinguish between bacterial and viral causes, since consolidation often is associated more with bacterial causes, but viral pathogens occasionally may produce consolidation and bacterial pathogens often may produce interstitial patterns more commonly associated with viral processes. Further, common atypical pathogens such as *Mycoplasma pneumoniae* may mimic both radiographic patterns. Still, clinicians frequently rely on physical examination and chest radiography to determine the best course of therapy and often base empirical treatment on the child's age and risk factors rather than on radiographic findings (Table 37-2).

In children with chronic medical conditions, clinicians also must consider other pathogens. For instance, children who are neurologically impaired are at increased risk for aspiration pneumonia, and anaerobic pathogens normally found in mouth flora may cause disease. Children with immunodeficiency may be at increased risk for infection with unusual organisms, such as fungal or mycobacterial pathogens. Children with cystic fibrosis are susceptible to recurrent infections with *Staphylococcus aureus* and *Pseudomonas* species.

There is strong evidence that antibiotics are beneficial in the treatment of bacterial pneumonia; there has been a 97 percent decrease in the rate of mor-

*Table 37-2* **Etiology of Pediatric Pneumonia by Age**

|  | Neonates | 6 Months– 4 Years | 4 Years and Up |
|---|---|---|---|
| *Streptococcus agalactiae* (group B streptococcus) | +++ |  |  |
| *Streptococcus pneumoniae* | + | + | + |
| *Mycoplasma pneumoniae* |  | + | +++ |
| *Chlamydia pneumoniae* |  | + | +++ |
| Viral | + | +++ | + |
| Respiratory syncytial virus, influenza, adenovirus, rhinovirus, metapneumovirus |  |  |  |

tality from pneumonia over the last century. Ideally, the etiology of a specific agent should guide therapy, but the rapid ability to differentiate between viral and bacterial disease is still outside the realm of office-based practitioners.

As with many other common pediatric infectious diseases, two questions face the clinician in treatment decisions: what is the likelihood of bacterial disease? and, if it is likely, what is the best antibiotic choice empirically? Not surprisingly, evidence-based guidelines are lacking and controversial. Some experts feel that excluding bacterial infection is impossible and that all these children should receive antibiotic therapy. For infants and preschool children, coverage for *Streptococcus pneumoniae* usually is recommended; for older children, coverage for atypical bacteria such as *M. pneumoniae* is considered. In addition to antibiotics, a hospitalized child may require intravenous fluids for dehydration and oxygen therapy. Some pyogenic bacterial pathogens may produce substantial complications. *Staphylococcus aureus* may produce lung abscesses, and *Strep. pneumoniae* occasionally may produce substantial pleural effusions that may require surgical drainage.

## CROUP (LARYNGOTRACHEOBRONCHITIS)

Croup is a syndrome that is fairly specific to children. It is characterized by a barking cough, hoarseness, stridor, and, in severe instances, respiratory distress, and the most common forms are infectious. Croup incidence peaks in the second year of life, and because of its viral etiology, croup often occurs biannually, most often in the spring and fall. It is caused primarily by parainfluenza viruses; less common causes include RSV, influenza virus, and adenovirus. The airway of a toddler seems peculiarly sensitive to infections with these viruses, as the same viruses may manifest with less severe presentations in an older adolescent and an adult, such as cold symptoms and laryngitis. Croup is often much more dramatic. Typically beginning with a prodrome of rhinorrhea, cough, congestion, and fever, croup is followed by a characteristic bark or seal-like cough, hoarseness, and, in severe instances, stridor and respiratory distress.

The diagnosis remains largely clinical. Confirmatory studies include neck radiographs to exclude other important causes of acute stridor such as epiglottitis or bacterial tracheitis. However, the "steeple sign," which often is described on a frontal view of the neck, is not pathognomonic for croup and is not always present. Although viral cultures may provide interesting epidemiologic data, they currently play no role in the initial diagnosis and acute management of croup.

### MANAGEMENT

#### Humidified Air
Despite its long-standing use, there is no strong evidence that humidified air is beneficial for patients with croup. Humidified air as a treatment for stri-

dor was introduced in the 1800s, when diphtheria was a common cause of upper airway obstruction. In addition to steaming showers and vaporizers, countless pediatricians have recommended taking children outside into the cool night air for relief (indeed, this 3:00 a.m. tradition seems almost a ritual of parenthood), but again, there is only anecdotal evidence for the efficacy of cool air or humidity. No controlled trials have been published to date.

### Nebulized Epinephrine

Nebulized epinephrine produces immediate, although short-term, relief of moderate to severe airway obstruction in children with croup. Since its introduction in the late 1960s, mortality and morbidity rates associated with croup have declined steadily, and the need for emergency tracheostomy has been virtually eliminated. A racemic mixture of D- and L-isomers has been used traditionally in the United States. Initially thought to have fewer cardiac effects, racemic epinephrine now appears to have no substantial benefit or side-effect profile compared with L-epinephrine, which is used throughout the United Kingdom and Australia. Historically, patients who received racemic epinephrine were admitted to the hospital or observed for several hours because of concern that epinephrine increased the severity of symptoms after its effects waned (sometimes called the *rebound phenomenon*). However, this has not been substantiated. Epinephrine appears to mask clinical deterioration rather than contribute to it. With the advent of corticosteroids, it may be safe to discharge patients from the hospital or outpatient setting after a period of observation if there is no evidence of worsening status.

### Corticosteroids

For patients with moderate to severe symptoms from croup, there is strong evidence that corticosteroids are effective. Corticosteroids were first shown to benefit children hospitalized for croup both by improving clinical symptoms and by reducing the need for intubation. They now clearly play a role in the outpatient setting as well for moderate to severe cases of croup. Several randomized clinical trials have demonstrated that corticosteroids produce faster clinical improvement, reduce the need for other interventions (such as epinephrine), reduce the amount of time spent in the emergency department, and reduce the need for hospitalization. Corticosteroids may be given orally, intramuscularly, or via inhalation. Oral administration appears to be as efficacious as the intramuscular route and is less painful.

## CYSTIC FIBROSIS

### PATHOPHYSIOLOGY

Although this genetic disorder can involve many organ systems, the respiratory system is the most commonly affected and contributes overall to the increased morbidity and mortality in patients with CF; currently, the median age of survival is 30 years. A defect in a single gene on chromosome 7 that encodes a cyclic adenosine monophosphate (cAMP)-regulated chloride channel [the cystic fibrosis transmembrane conductance regulator (CFTR)] produces an inability to transport chloride ions, leading to decreased fluid secretion and obstruction of organs such as the lungs and pancreas. Other subtle defects in organ systems are being recognized at the molecular level as well, but the historic diagnostic triad of elevated sweat chloride concentration, pancreatic insufficiency, and chronic pulmonary disease stands as a hallmark of this disease.

## HISTORY AND PHYSICAL EXAMINATION

The presentation may vary, often with findings specific to the age of the child. Neonates and infants often present with GI problems such as meconium ileus, jaundice, and, rarely, hypochloremic alkalosis caused by salt loss. Beyond infancy, failure to thrive is a very common presentation and is usually the result of pancreatic insufficiency. Respiratory symptoms are also common. Pneumonia, especially recurrent, in any child with the diagnosis of failure to thrive should prompt an evaluation for CF.

## LABORATORY AND RADIOGRAPHIC EVALUATION

Occasionally, the diagnosis may be suspected by family history, since inheritance is autosomal recessive and an estimated 5 percent of Americans currently carry at least one allele for the disease. CF is more common in Caucasians. Several states have instituted newborn screening programs. The most common genetic mutation, $\Delta 508$, currently accounts for about 70 percent of all reported mutations. Because the genotype does not always correlate with the degree of clinical disease, the sweat test remains a gold standard in the diagnosis of CF. Most commonly, a small electric current is applied to the skin to induce sweat, which is analyzed for chloride content. A sweat chloride concentration greater than 60 mEq/L in the presence of clinical findings is diagnostic.

## MANAGEMENT

Because the lungs of most children with CF soon fill with viscous secretions as they mature and other subtle defects at the epithelial level may contribute to impaired clearance as well, airways soon become colonized with bacteria that are difficult to eradicate. *Staphylococcus aureus* and *Haemophilus influenzae* predominate in infancy and early childhood. By adolescence, most children become colonized with *Pseudomonas* species, which often are tenaciously mucoid and, unfortunately, frequently are drug-resistant by adolescence. Pulmonary exacerbations often are heralded by increased cough and sputum production, dyspnea, poor appetite, weight loss, fatigue, changes in PFTs, radiographic or examination findings, or, rarely, hemoptysis. Any or all of these changes may indicate exacerbation and the need for treatment or hospitalization.

## NUTRITION

Many children with CF demonstrate significant malabsorption and also eventually develop increased metabolic needs as a result of pulmonary insufficiency, and so maximizing nutrition for these patients is a cornerstone of therapy. Most of these children are placed on supplemental pancreatic enzymes as well as supplements of fat-soluble vitamins (vitamins A, D, E, and K) at the time of diagnosis. As pulmonary disease progresses, the increased metabolic needs of these individuals often require caloric supplementation and, rarely, gastrostomy placement.

## ANTIBIOTICS

Antibiotics frequently are used to treat pulmonary exacerbations, and the choice often is based on sputum cultures or, in young children, throat swabs. Since it is impossible to eradicate organisms in these individuals, the goals for therapy are to suppress the organisms to levels at which lung function can be preserved and airway scarring can be avoided. Frequently the pharmacokinetics of individuals with CF are different, requiring higher doses. Antibiotics may be given orally, via nebulization, and, in moderate exacerbations, intravenously.

## OTHER THERAPIES FOR LUNG DISEASE

Because mucus is often thick and tenacious, chest physiotherapies (ranging from clapping and postural drainage to newer mechanized devices such as the flutter vest) frequently are employed in both hospital and outpatient settings. Recombinant human deoxyribonuclease, given as an inhalation, also appears to help mucus clearance. Since airway inflammation and occasional bronchospasm are common, many of the medications used in asthma therapy (bronchodilators and corticosteroids) often are used in CF patients as well. For many adult patients, lung transplants are currently the only viable option for end-stage disease. Although much has been understood about CF at the genetic and molecular levels over the last 20 years, genetic interventions unfortunately have not been as forthcoming.

Infrequently, some patients with advanced pulmonary disease may develop bronchiectasis (distention and weakening of bronchi and bronchioles) and subsequent dilation of bronchial arteries, which may produce hemoptysis (life-threatening in rare instances). Spontaneous pneumothorax also may occur. Patients with CF are also at increased risk of allergic bronchopulmonary aspergillosis, a hypersensitivity reaction to *Aspergillus* species.

## HYALINE MEMBRANE DISEASE, BRONCHOPULMONARY DYSPLASIA, AND CHRONIC LUNG DISEASE

As was mentioned in the introduction to this chapter, infants, especially premature infants, are particularly susceptible to lung injury for several reasons. First, surfactant is not produced in utero in sufficient quantities until the last trimester. By lowering surface tension, it tremendously improves oxygenation. Infants born before 34 to 35 weeks may lack surfactant and develop *hyaline membrane disease (HMD)*, which may require intubation and mechanical ventilation to provide oxygenation. Artificial surfactant often is used routinely in the neonatal intensive care unit (NICU) setting and has improved the survival of premature infants greatly. Even with surfactant therapy, however, the lungs of the smallest and most premature infants are susceptible to injury from mechanical ventilation, barotrauma, and even oxygen (from toxic free-radical formation). *Bronchopulmonary dysplasia (BPD)* often is used to describe the condition in these infants and is loosely defined as oxygen dependence after birth in the face of radiographic changes. The term *chronic lung disease (CLD)* often is used to describe this condition, particularly in infants who may or may not have been premature but have other significant perinatal complications (e.g., meconium aspiration, diaphragmatic hernia) that required mechanical ventilation in the postnatal period.

Oxygen supplementation may be needed several months to years after birth to maximize growth. These infants are at risk for pulmonary edema as well. Mild fluid restriction and diuretics such as furosemide often are used to reduce lung edema. The side effects of diuretics may include electrolyte disturbances, bone loss, and nephrocalcinosis. The caloric needs of an infant with significant BPD can be astounding. Many infants may require 180 to 190 kcal/kg per day, almost double the daily requirement of healthy term infants, and so infant formula frequently is modified to provide additional calories. As was mentioned earlier, infants with BPD and CLD are at increased risk of significant bronchiolitis.

## BIBLIOGRAPHY

Chavasse R et al. Short acting beta agonists for recurrent wheeze in children under two years of age. *Cochrane Database Syst Rev* 1, 2005.

Dowell SF, Kupronis BA, Zell ER, et al. Mortality from pneumonia in children in the United States, 1939 through 1996. *N Engl J Med* 342(19):1399–1407, 2000.

National Institutes of Health. *Guidelines for the Diagnosis and Management of Asthma.* Publication 97-4051, July 1997.

Patel H, Platt R, et al. Glucocorticoids for acute viral bronchiolitis in infants and young children. *Cochrane Database Syst Rev* 1, 2005.

# PEDIATRIC

# RHEUMATOLOGY

*Michael A. Barone*

## ● LEARNING OBJECTIVES

1.  Describe a general approach to children with suspected rheumatic disease.
2.  List the disorders that exhibit clinical overlap with rheumatologic disease.
3.  List the differences between systemic-onset arthritis, polyarticular arthritis, and pauciarticular arthritis.
4.  List the criteria for the classification of systemic lupus erythematosus.
5.  State the criteria for the diagnosis of Kawasaki syndrome.
6.  List the presenting signs and symptoms of reactive arthritis, rheumatic fever, and Lyme disease.

## GENERAL CONSIDERATIONS

Individually, pediatric rheumatic diseases are not common. Taken as a group, however, these illnesses represent a notable aspect of any pediatrician's practice. Their complexity and clinical overlap with so many other diseases (particularly infectious diseases) mandate awareness and diagnostic skill on the part of the practitioner.

At their core, the diseases in the realm of pediatric rheumatology are related to immune dysregulation. Instead of directing its defenses at offending organisms or antigens, the immune system attacks target organs, leading to acute and chronic inflammation with resulting signs and symptoms. Although the etiologies of these diseases are unknown, certain environmental and genetic risk factors have been elucidated. Furthermore, specifics of the nature of the inflammation response in each disease are changing treatment modalities from the use of nonspecific immunomodulatory agents [steroids, intravenous immunoglobulin (IVIG)] to the use of specific agents such as antibodies (Ab) against inflammatory cytokines [e.g., Ab versus tumor necrosis factor $\alpha$ (TNF-$\alpha$)].

## THE APPROACH TO A CHILD WITH SUSPECTED RHEUMATIC DISEASE

The diagnosis of a child with rheumatic disease is especially challenging because of the time needed for signs and symptoms to develop. Certain diagnostic criteria may not be met for months or in some cases years. During this time, repeated evaluations are performed, with the most important components being the interval history and noting any changes in the physical examination findings. In this process, one must be aware of the clinical overlap that rheumatic diseases may have with infectious diseases, malignancies, and orthopedic disorders (Table 38-1). For example, high fevers are characteristic of systemic-onset juvenile rheumatoid arthritis but also may be seen in a child with leukemia.

As many pediatric rheumatic diseases include joint involvement, a history of arthralgia and arthritis should be investigated. Specific characteristics, including the number of joints involved, migration of pain, and the time of day when symptoms are worse (e.g., morning stiffness in juvenile rheumatoid arthritis), are important historic features. Associated symptoms such as weight loss, recent history of pharyngitis (e.g., acute rheumatic fever), and recent diarrhea (reactive arthritis) also should be elicited. Although fatigue is often a nonspecific symptom, it may be reflective of the anemia of chronic disease. Furthermore, the specific presence of muscle weakness may serve as an important clue for disorders such as dermatomyositis.

The family history should be reviewed for rheumatic diseases and other autoimmune diseases, such as inflammatory bowel disease or autoimmune hypothyroidism. Finally, the current functional level of the patient and the specifics of any disability are worth assessing. Has the child been performing poorly at school or have there been multiple school absences? Are the child's symptoms present only in certain environments, such as school (e.g., school refusal)?

At any one time, the physical examination may be diagnostic of specific illness or may be normal. This again is due to the latency in the development of physical findings. As each body system may be involved, a thorough physical examination is essential. A reduced weight for height should be noted if present. Growth parameters should be put in the context of any recent changes in height and weight velocity. Vital signs may reveal tachycardia (anemia) or fever. Abnormal features may be seen on the eye exami-

*Table 38-1* **Childhood Disorders That Exhibit Clinical Overlap with Rheumatologic Disease**

*Arthritis Caused by Infectious Diseases or Trauma*
  Pyogenic (septic) arthritis (e.g., staphylococci, group A streptococci)
  Lyme disease
  Gonococcal arthritis (adolescent)
  Viral arthritis (e.g., parvovirus)
  Traumatic injury with or without hemarthrosis
  Transient synovitis ("toxic synovitis")
*Other Infectious Diseases*
  Osteomyelitis
  Bacterial endocarditis
  Adenovirus infections
  Brucellosis
  Epstein-Barr virus infections
  Leptospirosis
*Malignancies*
  Leukemia
  Osteosarcoma
  Ewing sarcoma
  Neuroblastoma
*Orthopedic Disorders*
  Slipped capital femoral epiphysis
  Legg-Calvé-Perthes disease
  Chondromalacia
  Blount disease
  Growing pains
*Psychogenic Disorders*

nation [juvenile rheumatoid arthritis (JRA)] or in the oral cavity [mouth ulcers in systemic lupus erythematosus (SLE)]. The cardiorespiratory examination may reveal a friction rub (pericarditis in SLE or JRA) or evidence of pleural effusion. Abdominal examination may reveal hepatosplenomegaly (systemic-onset JRA). Careful examination of the extremities may demonstrate arthritis or muscle weakness. A complete dermatologic examination may reveal specific signs such as malar rash (SLE) or periorbital violaceous edema suggestive of dermatomyositis.

Laboratory evaluation can be considered in terms of both specific and nonspecific tests. General nonspecific markers of inflammation include the erythrocyte sedimentation rate (ESR) and C-reactive protein (CRP). Their profiles differ in that the ESR generally takes a few days to increase in any infectious or inflammatory condition and stays elevated for a longer duration. The CRP rises and falls more quickly in response to an infectious or inflammatory stimulus. Other general tests, such as chemistry profiles and the complete blood count, may serve to evaluate target organ damage and assess for evidence of chronic disease. Certain tests, such as creatine phosphokinase, should be done if there is suspicion for dermatomyositis. Urinalysis can be useful in evaluating for concomitant nephritis (SLE).

More specific tests to evaluate for rheumatic disease exist but should not be used as screening tests in the absence of a reasonably supportive history and/or examination, in which case their interpretation can be difficult. Although also nonspecific for rheumatic versus infectious diseases, the antinuclear antibody (ANA) may be useful if it is of sufficiently high titer ($\geq$ 1:80). Although it may seem logical that children with JRA would have a positive rheumatoid factor (RF), this is not the case, with only 10 to 15 percent of those children being RF-positive. Rheumatoid factor also may be positive in children with SLE, but the majority of those patients are negative. The list below summarizes other autoantibodies that have enhanced specificity for certain diseases.

| Autoantibody | Disorder |
| --- | --- |
| Anti-SSA (Ro)/SSB (La) | SLE, Sjögren syndrome |
| Anti-Smith | SLE |
| Anti-double-stranded DNA | SLE |
| Antiribonucleoprotein (RNP) | Mixed connective tissue diseases |

## RHEUMATIC DISEASES OF CHILDHOOD

The remainder of this chapter focuses on three pediatric rheumatic diseases of significance. Although many such disorders exist, knowledge of juvenile rheumatoid arthritis, systemic lupus erythematosus, and dermatomyositis is essential for a pediatrician. Also included are the classic vasculitis syndromes of Henoch-Schönlein purpura (HSP) and Kawasaki syndrome (KS). HSP and KS are disorders that may be classified differently; for example, there is growing evidence that Kawasaki syndrome may be related in part to viral infection. However, their clinical overlap with other rheumatic diseases makes their discussion here relevant. Finally, a description of acute rheumatic fever, reactive arthritides, and Lyme disease (a disorder with a known infectious etiology) is included.

## JUVENILE RHEUMATOID ARTHRITIS

Juvenile rheumatoid arthritis is a group of disorders with three primary patterns of onset: pauciarticular JRA, polyarticular JRA, and systemic-onset

JRA. When these types are taken together, JRA is the most common pediatric rheumatic disease.

## EPIDEMIOLOGY

Although studies vary, the estimated incidence of JRA is 10 to 15 cases per 100,000 children per year. Prevalence figures are also difficult to assess but are generally estimated at 80 to 100 cases per 100,000 children. By convention, JRA is defined as arthritis before age 16. The peak age of onset is between 1 and 3 years of age. Overall, affected girls outnumber affected boys by 2 to 1. Each subtype of JRA has a slightly different peak age and gender, as discussed below.

## PATHOPHYSIOLOGY

There is no single known cause of JRA. As with many autoimmune diseases, the pathogenesis of JRA is thought to be related to a specific trigger in a genetically susceptible host. Infections, particularly viral, have been implicated as possible triggers, although none have been specifically determined. The immune dysregulation in JRA is mediated at the level of T cells, and responses of autoimmunity toward the synovium can be demonstrated. Activation of T cells leads to other components of the immune system becoming involved, such as B cells and the complement cascade. Cytokine release causes migration of inflammatory cells, leading to direct tissue damage.

Certain human leukocyte antigen (HLA) types have an association with JRA, including DR8 (pauciarticular), DR4 (systemic-onset and polyarticular with positive rheumatoid factor), and DP3 (polyarticular with negative rheumatoid factor).

## CLINICAL MANIFESTATIONS

From a clinical perspective, JRA is diagnosed as an illness lasting 6 weeks or longer (beginning before age 16 years) that is characterized by arthritis that includes obvious effusion or swelling of the joints or two of the following: joint tenderness with motion, decreased range of joint motion, and increased joint warmth. Individual clinical and laboratory characteristics of the different types of JRA onset are summarized in Table 38-2.

Pauciarticular (oligoarticular) JRA accounts for 40 percent of all cases of JRA. Four or fewer joints are involved, and systemic signs and symptoms such as fever, fatigue, and organomegaly are rare. Large joints typically are involved, and many patients can present with single-joint involvement (monarthritis). Insidious eye disease (uveitis) may be present in a significant number of female patients, necessitating eye examinations every 3 to 6 months. This is particularly true for children with a positive ANA. Patients with eye disease tend to have a favorable prognosis for arthritis even in the

Table 38-2  **Subtypes of Juvenile Rheumatoid Arthritis**

|  | **Pauciarticular** | **Polyarticular** | **Systemic Onset** |
|---|---|---|---|
| Percent of cases | 40% | 50% | 10% |
| Subtypes | Early onset (EO) | Rheumatoid factor–postive (RF+) | |
| | Late onset (LO) | Rheumatoid factor–negative (RF-) | |
| Age of onset | (EO): 1–5 years | Age 1–3 and adolescence (RF-) | No age peak |
| | (LO): ≥ 7 | Adolescence (RF+) | |
| Gender predominance | (EO): Female (LO): Male | Female (RF+ and RF-) | Females = males |
| Number of joints involved | 4 or fewer | 5 or more | Generally 5 or more |
| Types of joints | (EO): Large joints | Large and small joints | Large and small joints |
| Eye disease (uveitis) | (EO): 20–30% | 5% | Rare |
| Notes | (LO): HLA B27+ | Systemic features may be seen; RF+ adolescent girls much like adult rheumatoid arthritis | Patterned high spiking fevers Salmon rash |

setting of severe uveitis. Some patients with pauciarticular JRA (those with positive RF) may go on to develop progressive polyarthritis.

Polyarticular JRA is defined as arthritis in five or more joints. Some patients exhibit arthritis in 20 or more joints. Elbows, ankles, wrists, and knees may be involved as well as the interphalangeal joints in the hands. Uveitis is less common than it is in pauciarticular disease, but these patients may have systemic symptoms such as those seen in systemic-onset JRA. Older patients with positive RF can resemble adults with rheumatoid arthritis.

Systemic-onset JRA has no gender predilection and can manifest as systemic symptoms without the presence of arthritis for many months. It is therefore difficult to diagnose. Systemic involvement is characterized by high spiking fevers [> 39°C (102.2°F)] in a once- or twice-per-day pattern. There may be hypothermia after the fever resolves. Rash often accompanies the fever and appears as transient salmon-colored macules. In addition to multijoint arthritis, other manifestations of JRA include serositis (pericarditis, pleuritis), lymphadenopathy, and organomegaly. Originally described by George Still, this form of JRA often is referred to as *Still's disease.*

### LABORATORY EVALUATION

In JRA, the medical history relating to disease onset, types of joints involved, and presence or absence of systemic symptoms plays a large role in one's expectation of the utility of the laboratory evaluation. Inflammatory markers such as CRP and ESR typically are elevated, but normal values do not exclude the diagnosis. Although ANA and RF tests do not have a universal profile across the subtypes of JRA, some characteristics are worth noting. Fewer than 10 percent of patients with systemic-onset JRA will be ANA-positive, whereas as many as 60 percent of patients with pauciarticular disease will be. Virtually all these patients are RF-negative except for older patients with polyarticular disease. In the interpretation of RF and ANA tests, one must keep in mind that illnesses such as infection with Epstein-Barr virus also may cause positive test results. Synovial fluid analysis can show a great range of results in JRA. Median fluid total white blood cell (WBC) counts are 10,000 WBC/mm$^3$, with a range of polymorphonuclear neutrophils of 20 to 90 percent. Synovial fluid glucose levels also may be low.

### MANAGEMENT

Many children with JRA need only nonsteroidal anti-inflammatory medications for symptom relief and return to functionality. Some patients need additional or alternative medications. Although glucocorticoids are generally effective as powerful immunomodulating agents, their long-term use is associated with many side effects. Currently, less toxic and more specific anti-inflammatory medications are offered in a stepwise therapeutic approach. Methotrexate and sulfasalazine are used as second-line therapy, with more powerful (and toxic) immunosuppressants such as azathioprine and cyclophosphamide being reserved for children with severe disease. Other therapies include periodic infusions of IVIG, etanercept (TNF-α fusion protein), and infliximab (monoclonal antibody to TNF-α). Evaluation and treatment by a qualified physical therapist should be done in children with moderate to severe involvement. Experienced ophthalmologists should treat chronic uveitis. Topical steroids with or without mydriatics can be used.

## SYSTEMIC LUPUS ERYTHEMATOSUS

Systemic lupus erythematosus is a complex multisystem autoimmune disorder characterized by the production of autoantibodies and immune complex formation. SLE should be distinguished from neonatal lupus erythematosus, a disorder of newborns in which the transplacental passage of maternal antibody leads to the characteristic findings.

## EPIDEMIOLOGY

SLE is the second most common rheumatic disease in childhood. A female predominance is present in both prepubertal patients (4 to 1) and postpubertal patients (8 to 1). African Americans and Asians are affected with SLE more often than whites are. Prevalence rates of SLE vary, but approximately 100 patients per 100,000 childhood population have SLE. The incidence is less than 1 patient per 100,000 childhood population per year.

## PATHOPHYSIOLOGY

As with most autoimmune disorders, the exact cause of SLE is not known, although it is felt to be related to certain stimuli in a genetically susceptible host. Medications and hormonal changes have been implicated. Infections also have been thought to contribute to the pathogenesis of SLE. Epstein-Barr virus (EBV) has come under scrutiny because of evidence that EBV infection is more common in SLE patients than in controls. Certain human leukocyte antigen types (HLA DR2 and HLA DR3) are seen more commonly in patients with SLE. It is therefore not surprising that the disorder is more common in first-degree relatives of those already affected with SLE.

As was stated above, the hallmarks of SLE are the production of autoantibodies and the circulation and deposition of immune complexes. Through complement fixation and recruitment of inflammatory cells, the immune complexes lead to tissue damage at various body sites. Other manifestations of the dysregulation of the immune system include B-cell abnormalities. Patients with SLE have polyclonal B-cell activation, increased number of B cells, and hypergammaglobulinemia. T-cell abnormalities exist as well, with a notable feature being an impaired ability of T cells to suppress B-cell production of antibody. Sustained high levels of immunoglobulin can contribute to antibody-mediated autoimmune phenomena such as hemolytic anemia and thrombocytopenia. Patients with SLE also are known to have abnormal apoptosis (programmed cell death) in some proinflammatory cells.

## CLINICAL MANIFESTATIONS

Despite some useful laboratory tests, SLE remains a clinical diagnosis. Although originally used to identify patients for research studies, the information in Table 38-3 often is used as a set of diagnostic criteria, with patients said to have SLE if they manifest 4 of the 11 components. The three most common presenting features are arthritis, renal involvement, and skin involvement. In addition to target organ and tissue involvement, systemic symptoms such as weight loss, fatigue, and fever are common.

*Table 38-3* **Criteria for Diagnosis of Systemic Lupus Erythematosus\***

| Criterion | Definition |
| --- | --- |
| 1. Malar rash | Fixed erythema, flat or raised, over the malar eminences, tending to spare the nasolabial folds |
| 2. Discoid rash | Erythematous raised patches with adherent keratotic scaling and follicular plugging; atrophic scarring may occur in older lesions |
| 3. Photosensitivity | Skin rash as a result of unusual reaction to sunlight, by patient history, or by physician observation |
| 4. Oral ulcers | Oral or nasopharyngeal ulceration, usually painless, observed by physician |
| 5. Arthritis | Nonerosive arthritis involving two or more peripheral joints, characterized by tenderness, swelling, or effusion |
| 6. Serositis | Pleuritis—convincing history of pleuritic pain or rubbing heard by a physician or evidence of pleural effusion *or* Pericarditis—documented by electrocardiography or rub or evidence of pericardial effusion |
| 7. Renal disorder | Persistent proteinuria greater than 0.5 g/d or greater than 3+ if quantification not performed *or* Cellular casts—may be red cell, hemoglobin, granular, tubular, or mixed |
| 8. Neurologic disorder | Seizures—in the absence of offending drugs or known metabolic derangements, e.g., uremia, ketoacidosis, or electrolyte imbalance *or* Psychosis—in the absence of offending drugs or known metabolic derangements, e.g., uremia, ketoacidosis, or electrolyte imbalance |
| 9. Hematologic disorder | Hemolytic anemia—with reticulocytosis *or* Leukopenia—less than 4000/mm$^3$ total on two or more occasions *or* Lymphopenia—less than 1500/mm$^3$ on two or more occasions *or* Thrombocytopenia—less than 100,000/mm$^3$ in the absence of offending drugs |

*(continued)*

*Table 38-3* **Criteria for Diagnosis of Systemic Lupus Erythematosus\* (continued)**

| Criterion | Definition |
| --- | --- |
| 10. Immunologic disorder | Anti-DNA: antibody to native DNA in abnormal titer *or* Anti-Sm: presence of antibody to Sm nuclear antigen *or* Positive finding of antiphospholipid antibodies based on (1) an abnormal serum level of IgG or IgM anticardiolipin antibodies, (2) a positive test result for lupus anticoagulant using a standard method, or (3) a false-positive serologic test for syphilis known to be positive for at least 6 months and confirmed by *Treponema pallidum* immobilization or fluorescent treponemal antibody absorption test |
| 11. Antinuclear antibody | An abnormal titer of antinuclear antibody by immunofluorescence or an equivalent assay at any point in time and in the absence of drugs known to be associated with "drug-induced lupus" syndrome |

*The proposed classification is based on 11 criteria. For the purpose of identifying patients in clinical studies, a person shall be said to have systemic lupus erythematosus if any 4 or more of the 11 criteria are present, serially or simultaneously, during any interval of observation.

Source: Tan EM, Cohen AS, Fries JF, et al. The 1982 revised criteria for the classification of systemic lupus erythematosus. *Arthritis Rheum* 25:1271–1277, 1982; Hochberg MC. Updating the American College of Rheumatology revised criteria for the classification of systemic lupus erythematosus [letter]. *Arthritis Rheum* 40:1725, 1997.

Approximately 60 to 75 percent of these patients demonstrate some manifestation of lupus nephritis. Renal disease may be subclinical, but the clinical manifestations include proteinuria, hematuria, hypertension, and renal failure. The World Health Organization (WHO) offers a classification scheme for lupus nephritis that ranges from class I (normal) to class VI (glomerular sclerosis).

Disease of the central nervous system (CNS) occurs in approximately 25 percent of patients with SLE. Manifestations include depression, cognitive impairment, seizures, and peripheral neuropathy. Headache often is seen in SLE patients and must be approached carefully. Most headaches respond to typical analgesics, but when severe, headaches may be a marker for CNS infection or cerebral vein thrombosis.

Dermatologic involvement in SLE is common. The malar rash (butterfly rash) of SLE can be seen in more than 50 percent of affected children. Other lesions of vasculitis (e.g., petechiae) are common. Approximately 30 to 40 percent of children with SLE develop alopecia or photosensitivity. Overall, skin involvement in SLE is present in approximately 80 percent of patients.

Polyarthritis with arthralgia is present in 80 to 90 percent of patients with SLE. Joint involvement is generally migratory, and the symptoms last 24 to 48 h. SLE also can cause myositis.

Blood disorders are seen commonly in SLE. They range from depression of cell lines (e.g., thrombocytopenia, leukopenia, lymphopenia), to anemia of chronic disease, to hemolytic anemias. The antiphospholipid syndrome (APLS) refers to the presence of antibodies to phospholipids that include anticardiolipin and the lupus anticoagulant. Patients with APLS have an increased tendency for venous thrombosis but also may present with arterial occlusion or fetal loss in adolescent females.

Cardiopulmonary involvement generally manifests as inflammation of serosal surfaces such as pericarditis and pleuritis. Pulmonary hemorrhage and myocarditis may be seen in SLE.

## LABORATORY EVALUATION

Nonspecific markers of inflammation such as ESR and CRP typically are elevated. Complement levels (C3, C4) are low because of activation of complement by immune complexes. Evidence of chronic disease (anemia) or other cytopenias (thrombocytopenia, leukopenia) may be noted. A urinalysis should be performed to evaluate for proteinuria, hematuria, and urinary sediment. Spinal fluid analysis and neuroimaging [magnetic resonance imaging (MRI) with angiography] should be considered in patients with new or deteriorating CNS symptoms.

The autoantibody profile in SLE is characterized by both sensitive and specific laboratory markers. Virtually all SLE patients have a positive ANA; this finding, however, is not specific for SLE, as a positive ANA also can be seen in JRA, scleroderma, and mixed connective tissue disease. Anti-double-stranded-DNA antibodies have much greater specificity, and their levels correlate with disease activity, particularly nephritis. Anti-Smith antibodies also are highly specific for SLE but are less prevalent in patients (lower sensitivity). Although neither specific nor sensitive, antibodies to other nuclear antigens, such as anti-Ro/SS-A and anti-La/SS-B, also may be found in SLE.

## MANAGEMENT

Therapy for SLE is directed at maximizing function and limiting potential complications such as end-organ damage. Experienced rheumatologists can match the intensity of the treatment to the severity of the patient's disease. Nonsteroidal anti-inflammatory agents, hydroxychloroquine, and corticosteroids are used for mild disease manifesting as systemic symptoms, dermatologic disease, and arthritis. As severity increases, glucocorticoids (at higher doses) and other immunosuppressive agents (e.g., methotrexate, cyclophosphamide) become the mainstays of treatment. Virtually all patients with renal involvement require glucocorticoids or more intense therapy. In the most severe cases, therapies such as IVIG and plasmapheresis can be used, but data in pediatric patients are very limited.

Whether the infections are due to intrinsic disease activity or immunosuppressive therapy, patients with SLE are at risk for secondary infections with common and opportunistic organisms. They therefore should be monitored closely for any infectious complications and treated aggressively. Thrombosis in patients with APLS is treated with anticoagulant therapy. With current standards of care, the prognosis for survival is 90 percent 5 years after diagnosis.

## JUVENILE DERMATOMYOSITIS

As the name implies, dermatomyositis is a rheumatic disorder with muscle and skin involvement. It often includes constitutional symptoms such as fever, weight loss, and fatigue.

### EPIDEMIOLOGY

The incidence of juvenile dermatomyositis (JDM) is approximately 0.5 cases per 100,000 childhood population per year. Females are twice as likely to be affected as males. JDM is rare before the age of 5 years, and the average age of onset is 7 years. There is no significant racial predilection.

### PATHOPHYSIOLOGY

JDM is a vasculitis without a known cause. The immune dysregulation consists of, among many abnormalities, lymphocytes that can cause a direct cytotoxic effect on muscles. In addition, immune-complex formation and complement activation play a role.

Many infectious agents have been implicated in JDM, but evidence is inconclusive. Enteroviruses, *Toxoplasma gondii,* and respiratory viruses such as Coxsackie virus and influenza virus have been investigated.

### CLINICAL MANIFESTATIONS

Systemic symptoms such as fever and fatigue generally present with findings of rash and proximal muscle weakness. Severe muscle involvement may cause inability to walk and inability to sit because of weak back and neck muscles. Virtually all these children demonstrate a rash, with the majority showing at least one of the characteristic patterns of the following: (1) heliotrope rash, (2) Gottron papules, and (3) periungual capillary changes. The heliotrope rash refers to a violet discoloration of the upper eyelids. Gottron papules are scaly erythematous lesions on the dorsum of the hand over the metacarpophalangeal joints and the proximal interphalangeal joints. Periungual skin can become erythematous, and abnormal capillary "loops" may be seen.

Other physical findings in JDM include calcinosis (deposition of calcium into muscle and other soft tissue) and cardiac involvement (myopathy, conduction abnormalities).

## LABORATORY EVALUATION

Tests such as a complete blood count (CBC) and inflammatory markers (ESR, CRP) are useful. Anemia of chronic disease may be present, and inflammatory markers usually are elevated. As a rule, muscle enzyme levels (lactate dehydrogenase, creatine phosphokinase, aldolase, and aspartate aminotransferase) are elevated. Further investigation of myositis can be done with electromyography, MRI, or muscle biopsy. Many of these children have a positive ANA, and very few have a positive rheumatoid factor.

## MANAGEMENT

A multidisciplinary approach to therapy includes medications, physical therapy (joint range of motion), and occupational therapy (daily activities, assistance with swallowing if necessary). The pharmacologic treatment of choice is glucocorticoids, although for severe disease, other immunosuppressants, such as methotrexate, azathioprine, and cyclosporine, have been used. The antimalarial hydroxychloroquine also has shown effectiveness in juvenile dermatomyositis.

# VASCULITIS SYNDROMES

## KAWASAKI SYNDROME

Kawasaki syndrome is a vasculitis disorder of childhood that is characterized by prolonged fever of 38.9°C (102°F) for 5 or more days and at least four of the following five features (the illness should not be explained by another identifiable cause):

1. Nonexudative bulbar conjunctivitis with limbic sparing
2. Polymorphous rash (generally not vesicular)
3. Mucous membrane changes, including pharyngitis, changes to the tongue, and red, fissured dry lips
4. Acral changes: erythema to palms and soles, edema of hands and feet (particularly the dorsal surfaces)
5. Cervical lymph node: unilateral ≥ 1.5 cm node without suppuration

### EPIDEMIOLOGY

The first cases of Kawasaki syndrome may have been described in the late 1800s through autopsies of children who had died of a febrile illness and hemopericardium (secondary to coronary rupture). The disease as it currently is known originally was described as the "mucocutaneous lymph node syndrome" by Dr. Kawasaki in 1967. Today astute observation by clinicians leads to a current incidence of approximately 3000 to 4000 cases per year in the United States. Seventy-five percent of these children are less than age 5 years, and the peak incidence occurs between 3 and 11 months of age. KS may be seen in children less than age 6 months and adolescents, but in these age groups fewer diagnostic criteria may be apparent. Among all ethnic groups, Asians have the highest incidence.

## PATHOPHYSIOLOGY

The cause of KS is unknown. Many viruses (parvovirus, EBV) and bacteria (*Staphylococcus aureus, Streptococcus pyogenes*) have been implicated. Infectious agents have been considered carefully because in many ways KS behaves like an infectious disease. It is more common in the late winter in the United States, and it affects certain age groups. Recently, a newly described coronavirus was shown to be linked epidemiologically to KS.

Patients with KS demonstrate an inflammatory cascade with T-lymphocyte stimulation. One theory of the pathogenesis is based on the action of superantigens, examples of which are the streptococcal pyrogenic exotoxins A/B and staphylococcal toxic shock syndrome toxin-I (TSST-I). Superantigens cause abnormal interaction of the beta chain of the T-cell receptor and the major histocompatibility complex (MHC) class II molecule on the antigen-presenting cell. This leads to T-cell activation with resultant autoimmunity phenomena. The vasculitis that ensues may involve any of the medium-size arteries, but the coronary arteries are at particular risk. As the vessel wall is damaged, aneurysms may form, leading to possible thrombus formation in the coronary arteries.

## CLINICAL MANIFESTATIONS

The main physical features are included in the diagnostic criteria discussed above. Other findings that are not part of the case definition may be seen in KS. At the time of diagnosis, a desquamating rash may be seen in the perineum or in intertriginous areas such as the anterior neck fold. Right upper quadrant pain may be seen as a result of hydrops of the gallbladder. Males may show swelling in the tip of the penis, and arthritis may occur with a slight predominance in girls. Most children with KS are irritable. If a lumbar puncture is performed, aseptic meningitis may be seen. The classic desquamation in the periungual areas (around the nails) rarely is seen at diagnosis as it tends to appear 10 to 20 days after the onset of illness. Most children, if the disorder is properly recognized, are treated before this time.

Kawasaki syndrome is the most common cause of acquired heart disease in the United States. Cardiac involvement can consist of myocarditis and pericarditis in the acute phase. Coronary artery aneurysms are the most feared complication, with a 25 percent likelihood in untreated patients and a 2 to 3 percent likelihood in properly treated patients.

The differential diagnosis of KS consists of infectious illnesses such as those due to parvovirus, adenoviruses, enteroviruses, and measles; hypersensitivity reactions; and toxin-mediated staphylococcal and streptococcal diseases such as toxic shock syndrome, scarlet fever, and scalded skin syndrome.

## LABORATORY EVALUATION

Kawasaki syndrome is a clinical diagnosis, and no single test is diagnostic. Inflammatory markers (CRP, ESR) typically are elevated. The CBC may show an increased WBC count with a left shift and a pattern of toxic vacuolization in the white blood cells. Although the platelet count is usually normal at diagnosis, it rises during the convalescent phase of the illness; this marker often serves to confirm the diagnosis. Liver function tests [aspartate aminotransferase (AST), alanine aminotransferase (ALT), gamma-glutamyl aminotransferase (GGT)] may be elevated. Some patients exhibit hypoalbuminemia, as can be seen in other vasculitis syndromes. The spinal fluid may reveal a sterile pleocytosis, and the urinalysis often reveals pyuria with a negative bacterial culture (sterile pyuria).

Possible aneurysms of the coronary arteries should be examined by echocardiography at the time of diagnosis and 6 to 8 weeks after onset. Some physicians also recommend an echocardiogram after the acute phase of the illness at approximately 2 weeks after onset.

## MANAGEMENT

In 1988, the American Academy of Pediatrics endorsed a regimen of high-dose IVIG (2 g/kg) and aspirin to treat Kawasaki syndrome. This standard of care remains in effect today, with the IVIG generally given as a single dose and aspirin being given at a high dose (80 to 100 mg/kg) during the early portion of the acute phase and then at a low dose (3 to 5 mg/kg per day) throughout the convalescent phase of the illness. Aspirin then is discontinued, assuming no coronary aneurysms. Children with coronary artery involvement should be managed by an experienced pediatric cardiologist. These children generally remain on aspirin therapy and may be candidates for vascular remodeling agents such as abciximab. Patients on long-term aspirin should be vaccinated against influenza. Any child who has received IVIG should have live virus vaccines [e.g., measles-mumps-rubella (MMR), Varivax) delayed for 11 months as vaccines are less immunogenic during this period because of treatment.

## HENOCH-SCHÖNLEIN PURPURA

Henoch-Schönlein purpura is a common vasculitis syndrome in children that is characterized by purpuric skin lesions without thrombocytopenia, abdominal pain with possible gastrointestinal (GI) bleeding, arthralgia, and nephritis.

## Epidemiology

HSP may follow an upper respiratory tract infection, although in the age groups affected (children ages 3 to 10 years), an antecedent upper respiratory infection (URI) seems so common that this finding is rather nonspecific. Boys are affected twice as much as girls, and the incidence is approximately 10 per 100,000 childhood population per year. This is felt to be an underestimate, however, since many children are evaluated and treated by a primary care physician and thus never get reported.

## Pathophysiology

HSP also is known as *anaphylactoid purpura*. It is a leukocytoclastic vasculitis with immunoglobulin A (IgA)-predominant immune-complex deposition in vessels, most notably the postcapillary venules. This immune complex deposition can occur in the skin and glomeruli. The cause of HSP is not known, although as with Kawasaki syndrome, many infectious agents have been implicated. Although organisms such as parvovirus, *Mycoplasma pneumoniae*, and *Campylobacter jejuni* have been suggested, the organism that has come under the greatest scrutiny is group A β-hemolytic streptococcus (*Strep. pyogenes*). Studies have shown that up to 30 percent of these patients have evidence of an antecedent or current streptococcal infection at the time when HSP is apparent. Other possible causes of HSP may be drug hypersensitivity, food allergy, and reaction to insect stings.

## Clinical Manifestations

Among the features mentioned above, the rash of "palpable purpura" is the most common. Involvement is generally below the waist. Some children may show swelling of hands, feet, and periorbital regions. Edema to dependent areas such as the scrotum may occur.

Approximately half of children with HSP have clinical GI involvement. Vasculitis of the intestinal vessels can cause abdominal pain, microscopic stool blood loss, or frank GI bleeding as manifested by hematemesis or hemochezia. Intussusception may occur. In HSP, intussusception demonstrates the uncharacteristic features, often involving only the small bowel (ileoileal) and showing a different age distribution (older children) than does typical intussusception.

Nephropathy occurs in approximately one-third of children with HSP, with involvement ranging from mild nephritis (hematuria, proteinuria) to acute renal failure. As renal disease may not be apparent until weeks to months after the onset of HSP, it is important to screen patients with urinalyses throughout the follow-up period.

Joint involvement is seen in 50 to 75 percent of patients with HSP. Typical involvement is arthralgia of the knees and ankles with tender periarticular swelling. Joint erythema and effusions are unusual. Most symptoms resolve within a week.

## LABORATORY EVALUATION

HSP is a clinical diagnosis, but some laboratory tests can be helpful, including urinalysis and tests for occult blood in the stool. If a child exhibits hematuria and proteinuria, demonstration of normal complement levels (C3, C4) can differentiate nephritis of HSP from the more common poststreptococcal glomerulonephritis, which classically manifests with low serum complement.

The CBC is not diagnostic but may show anemia caused by GI blood loss. A mildly elevated WBC count can be seen, and the platelet count is usually normal. Inflammatory markers such as CRP and ESR can be mildly elevated or normal. Elevated serum IgA and immunoglobulin M (IgM) are seen in approximately 50 percent of these patients.

## MANAGEMENT

Children with HSP need not be admitted to the hospital if the supportive measures of pain control, hydration, and nutrition can be done at home. Pain control with analgesics or anti-inflammatory medications such as acetaminophen and ibuprofen is generally effective. Children may require hospitalization if further supportive care is necessary or if abdominal complications such as severe GI bleeding and intussusception are present. Many physicians administer steroids (prednisone 2 mg/kg per day) to children with severe abdominal pain or GI hemorrhage. Children with significant renal involvement should be referred to a pediatric nephrologist.

## INFECTIONS AND INFLAMMATORY DISEASES

### RHEUMATIC FEVER

Rheumatic fever occurs 2 to 3 weeks after an episode of tonsillopharyngitis caused by group A β-hemolytic *Strep. pyogenes* (GABHS).

## EPIDEMIOLOGY

The current incidence of rheumatic fever is approximately 1 to 2 per 100,000 childhood population per year. In the early twentieth century, incidence rates were 50 to 100 times higher. The incidence dropped even before the introduction of antibiotics, suggesting that poverty and crowding were risk factors that contributed to the population burden of this disease. Outbreaks may occur if particular "rheumatogenic" serotypes of GABHS emerge. The most recent outbreak in the United States occurred in the late 1980s.

Similar to the clinical syndrome of streptococcal pharyngitis, the peak age of onset of rheumatic fever is ages 5 to 15 years, with rheumatic fever being a rare finding in children age 4 or younger. Rheumatic heart disease is the most common worldwide cause of acquired heart disease.

## PATHOPHYSIOLOGY

The actual mechanism by which GABHS leads to a multisystem inflammatory disease is not known. The most accepted theory focuses on immunologic cross-reactivity between certain GABHS antigens and human tissue occurring in a genetically susceptible host. During infection with GABHS, antibodies to streptococcal M proteins may attack host brain, joint, and myocardial tissue. Substances elaborated by certain strains of GABHS, specifically superantigens such as streptococcal pyrogenic exotoxins A and B, also may play a role in rheumatic fever through T-cell activation.

The resultant process is a vasculitis of the small vessels. Inflammatory infiltrates can occur in synovial tissue as well as in the endocardium and myocardium, leading to degeneration of collagen.

## CLINICAL MANIFESTATIONS

The original clinical criteria for rheumatic fever were published in the 1940s by Dr. T. Duckett Jones and were revised in 1992 (Table 38-4). With some exceptions, to make the diagnosis of rheumatic fever, a patient should have evidence of an antecedent infection with GABHS and fulfill two major criteria or one major criterion and two minor criteria. Exceptions may include patients with isolated chorea or rheumatic carditis.

*Table 38-4* **Revised Jones Criteria for Rheumatic Fever, 1992**

| Major Criteria | Minor Criteria |
|---|---|
| Carditis | Clinical |
| Polyarthritis | Fever |
| Erythema marginatum | Arthralgia |
| Arthritis | Laboratory |
| Subcutaneous nodules | Elevated erythrocyte sedimentation rate, C-reactive protein |
| | Prolonged PR interval |
| Supporting evidence of group A β-hemolytic *Streptococcus pyogenes* infection: | |
| • Elevated or increasing streptococcal antibody titer | |
| • Positive throat culture or rapid streptococcal antigen test | |

Source: Special Writing Group of the Committee on Rheumatic Fever, Endocarditis, and Kawasaki Disease of the Council on Cardiovascular Disease in the Young of the American Heart Association. Guidelines for the diagnosis of rheumatic fever: Jones criteria updated 1992. *JAMA* 268:2069–2073, 1992.

The arthritis of rheumatic fever manifests in 60 to 70 percent of patients. Large joints are mainly involved in a migratory pattern. The physical examination reveals a swollen erythematous joint with evidence of effusion. Pain is a predominant symptom and can be so excruciating that children may complain about even the light touch of a bedsheet.

Rheumatic carditis may be absent or subclinical or may present as severe pancarditis. Cardiac involvement is present in 50 to 60 percent of children with rheumatic fever and is a more specific finding than is arthritis. The endocardium and myocardium are most affected, although pericarditis also may occur. The resulting signs and symptoms include cardiomegaly, conduction abnormalities, murmurs of valvular insufficiency (predominantly affecting the mitral and aortic valves), and congestive heart failure.

Sydenham chorea, also known as St. Vitus dance, occurs in approximately 15 percent of children with rheumatic fever. Although frank chorea is characterized by involuntary, uncoordinated movements, other features include emotional lability and cognitive deficits. Classic physical findings include a characteristic "bag of worms" movement of a protruded tongue and the milkmaid's grip, an irregular contraction of the patient's hand when the patient is asked to grip the examiner's fingers.

Erythema marginatum and subcutaneous nodules are the least common findings. Erythema marginatum presents as an erythematous serpiginous rash on the trunk and extremities. Subcutaneous nodules are mobile 1- to 2-cm lesions found along the extensor surfaces of tendons near joints. Their presence correlates with the presence of rheumatic heart disease.

## LABORATORY EVALUATION

Patients should clinically fulfill the revised Jones criteria. A preceding GABHS infection may be evaluated by throat culture or rapid streptococcal antigen at the time of evaluation or the measurement of streptococcal antibody titers, specifically antistreptolysin O (ASO) or anti-DNase B. The majority of patients (80 to 90 percent) have high titers to one or both of these antibodies. A fourfold rise in antibody titer adds further credibility to a preceding GABHS infection. Inflammatory markers such as ESR and CRP usually are elevated and are considered part of the minor criteria. Electrocardiography may reveal first-degree atrioventricular (AV) block (PR prolongation), and echocardiography should be used to evaluate for myocarditis, pericarditis, and valvular disease.

## MANAGEMENT

The arthritis of rheumatic fever responds well to aspirin therapy. The dramatic response to treatment with salicylates often is felt to strengthen the conviction in the clinical diagnosis. Aspirin also can be used to treat mild carditis, assuming no cardiac failure. For those with severe carditis, glucocorticoids are administered over a period of 2 to 4 weeks with tapering doses at the end of therapy. For children with debilitating chorea, anticonvulsants such as phenobarbital or sedative medications such as haloperidol can be used.

All patients with rheumatic fever should receive therapy for streptococcal pharyngitis even if the throat culture is negative at the time of presentation. Secondary prevention to prevent recurrences of rheumatic fever is accomplished with long-term antibiotic prophylaxis. For those with carditis, intramuscular penicillin therapy is given every 3 to 4 weeks into adulthood. Certain compliant patients may use daily oral antibiotic therapy. Primary prevention of rheumatic fever is accomplished by the prompt diagnosis and treatment of GABHS pharyngitis.

## REACTIVE ARTHRITIS

Although the arthritis of rheumatic fever is technically a reactive arthritis, two other forms are notable. The first is arthritis that is precipitated by infection of either the genitourinary or the gastrointestinal tract. In this case, most patients are HLA B27–positive. Offending organisms are typically *Salmonella, Shigella, Campylobacter, Yersinia*, and *Chlamydia*. The second reactive arthritis occurs after group A streptococcal infection in children who do not meet the clinical criteria for rheumatic fever.

### EPIDEMIOLOGY

Reactive arthritis may be seen in approximately 2 percent of individuals with infection of the GI tract caused by one of the offending organisms. Rates as high as 10 percent have been suspected in *Yersinia* infections. Reactive arthritis caused by *Chlamydia* infections is more common in adolescents in light of the incidence of infection in that age group. The incidence of post-streptococcal reactive arthritis (PSRA) is approximately 1 patient per 100,000 children per year, but this may reflect underreporting.

### PATHOPHYSIOLOGY

Arthritis syndromes after GI or genitourinary (GU) infection correlate strongly with HLA B27–positive tests. This is not true for PSRA. The role of HLA B27 in the actual pathogenesis of arthritis is unclear, but the arthritis possibly is due to similarities between microbial antigens and host antigens causing an autoimmune phenomenon in these genetically predisposed individuals. PSRA has a shorter latency than does rheumatic fever, but the pathogenesis is felt to be similar (see "Rheumatic Fever," above).

### CLINICAL MANIFESTATIONS

For reactive arthritis caused by GI or GU disease, symptoms of the inciting infection may have occurred 1 to 4 weeks before the development of arthritis. Patients with bacterial gastroenteritis may report syndromes specific to the particular offending organism. For example, a history of bloody stools and abdominal pain could suggest *Salmonella* or *Shigella* infection. Reactive arthritis generally affects the large joints of the lower extremities but may involve the spine after infection with certain organisms (e.g., *Yersinia*). The duration of joint involvement is typically weeks to months. Infection of the urethra or cervix with *Chlamydia trachomatis* may cause abnormal penile or vaginal discharge, dysuria, or pelvic inflammatory disease in females. Infection also can be asymptomatic. When coupled with conjunctivitis, the reactive arthritis after *Chlamydia* infection may be referred to as Reiter syndrome. This also can be seen after dysenteric diarrhea, particularly with *Campylobacter* infections.

PSRA is seen 7 to 10 days after a GABHS infection, more rapidly than the typical appearance of rheumatic fever. As a result, many patients demonstrate evidence of acute pharyngitis. Large joints (knees, ankles) of the lower extremities usually are involved, and in contrast to rheumatic fever, the arthritis is nonmigratory and may last much longer. The mean duration is 8 to 10 weeks. Although these children are not felt to meet the criteria for rheumatic fever at the time of diagnosis, approximately 5 percent develop cardiac involvement.

## LABORATORY EVALUATION

As with many of the disorders described in this chapter, mild anemia and elevations of ESR and CRP can be seen. Occasionally, arthrocentesis with examination and culture of synovial fluid is needed to rule out acute joint infection, for example, to rule out septic arthritis with *Salmonella*. Although attempts should be made to culture the offending organisms, stool cultures for enteric organisms and throat cultures for GABHS may be negative. In this case, a history suggestive of a particular symptom complex (e.g., dysentery) or measurement of antibody levels such as ASO can be helpful to document recent past infection. In the case of *Chlamydia*, rapid diagnostic tests such as gene probe or polymerase chain reaction on urine specimens may be performed.

Because of the small but significant percentage of children with PSRA who have subclinical cardiac involvement, there should be a low threshold for electrocardiography (ECG) and echocardiography evaluations.

## MANAGEMENT

In evaluating a child with reactive arthritis, consideration must be given to treating the inciting infection. GABHS infections and *Chlamydia* infections should be treated with appropriate regimens. Treatment of GI infections should be done only in certain patients with acute infectious symptoms (e.g., *Shigella*). Longer-term antibiotics are not thought to improve the course of reactive arthritis.

SECTION IV / SELECTED TOPICS

Pharmacotherapy for reactive arthritis generally consists of nonsteroidal anti-inflammatory drugs (NSAIDs) or glucocorticoids. Steroids may be given systemically or as intraarticular injections. For patients with severe, relapsing symptoms, sulfasalazine may be used. Unlike children with rheumatic fever, children with PSRA do not have a dramatic response to aspirin therapy, and typically NSAIDs are used. Although most children with reactive arthritis do not demonstrate a relapsing course, those who do should be evaluated by a physical therapist during the course of medical therapy. For children with PSRA and no evidence of carditis, the American Heart Association recommends 1 year of antibiotic prophylaxis, using regimens similar to those used for rheumatic fever. If, during that time, the child develops signs of carditis, the diagnosis should be reclassified as rheumatic fever and the child should remain on secondary antibiotic prophylaxis until age 21.

## LYME DISEASE

Lyme disease is a tick-borne infectious disease that can cause a multisystem acute and chronic inflammatory disorder. A great deal is known about the microbiologic etiologic agent, *Borrelia burgdorferi*, and its common vectors, *Ixodes scapularis* and *I. pacificus*. The discovery of these agents is part of the fascinating history of Lyme disease, which began with a group of concerned mothers in Old Lyme, Connecticut, in the mid-1970s. An unusual cluster of juvenile rheumatoid arthritis cases was brought to the attention of state health officials. Surveillance over the ensuing summer revealed even more cases and a geographic disparity, with more cases on the east side of the Connecticut River. A case definition then was developed for Lyme arthritis. Eventually, a tick was recovered from a child affected with Lyme arthritis. The tick, *I. scapularis* (commonly known as the deer tick), was known to be more common on the river's east side.

With a possible vector known, the search began for an infectious cause. It ultimately was discovered that serum from those with Lyme arthritis reacted with a bacteria isolated from the gut of this tick. In recognition of the work of the entomologist Dr. Willy Burgdorfer, this spirochete was named *Borrelia burgdorferi*. The two-year life cycle of the *Ixodes* tick was elucidated further. Humans were determined to be incidental hosts for the second and third of three necessary blood meals in the maturity cycle of the tick. The primary hosts are the white-footed moose and the white-tailed deer. During a blood meal, the *Borrelia* in the tick midgut is transmitted to humans if the tick is attached for 48 h. This can result in asymptomatic infection or a clinical syndrome denoted by three phases: early localized disease, early disseminated disease, and late disease.

### EPIDEMIOLOGY

Lyme disease is seasonal, with peaks in spring, summer, and early fall in accordance with the tick life cycle and the more limited use of protective clothing (e.g., long pants) in the population in which the disease is seen. Although some areas of the United States have no clinical Lyme disease, other areas, such as the eastern seaboard from Maryland to New Hampshire and parts of Wisconsin, are hyperendemic. With *I. pacificus* as a vector, a cluster of Lyme disease also exists in California, particularly northern California. In the United States the annual incidence estimates range from 100 to 1000 cases per 100,000 population, depending on the area reporting. Children age 5 to 9 are the highest-risk group. Lyme disease also is seen in Europe and Asia.

## PATHOPHYSIOLOGY

A local inflammatory reaction consisting of primarily lymphocytes and macrophages is responsible for the rash (erythema migrans) that appears at the site of tick attachment. In untreated patients, spirochetes then may enter a bloodborne phase that clinically correlates with the manifestations of early disseminated disease. Through this process, involvement of joints, the heart, and the central nervous system can occur. The degree to which the organism itself or the host response (cytokines) contributes to inflammation is not fully known. Even after eradication of organisms, however, some patients may go on to develop a more chronic, reactive arthritis. HLA DR2 and HLA DR3 seem to correlate with this.

## CLINICAL MANIFESTATIONS

Many patients are asymptomatic. Those with symptoms are thought to progress through three stages but may present at any stage of the illness.

*Early localized disease* is the characteristic rash of erythema migrans (EM) 1 or 2 weeks after the tick bite. This rash generally is found in the axillae or groin, which are typical sites for tick attachment. At diagnosis, only 20 to 30 percent of patients can recall a tick bite, although it is felt that among those with clinical Lyme disease, 80 to 90 percent will develop EM. The rash begins as a small macule and expands circumferentially. Most lesions show homogenous erythema, although a minority can show central clearing. Patients may complain of pruritus or systemic symptoms such as fever and malaise, but the majority are asymptomatic.

*Early disseminated disease* is due to hematogenous spread of spirochetes. The onset is typically 7 days to a few months after the tick bite. Systemic symptoms such as fever, headache, malaise, and myalgias are common. Cutaneous, cardiac, and neurologic involvement can occur. Multiple EM lesions can be seen in approximately 25 percent of patients. This finding is not due to multiple tick bites but rather to the spirochetemia. Cardiac involvement is unusual in children but may consist of conduction abnormalities (AV block) with resultant syncope and myocarditis. In children, neurologic involvement in early disseminated disease is more common than carditis. Aseptic meningitis or meningoencephalitis may be seen. Children can present with severe headache, occasionally fever, and meningismus. Palsy of the seventh cranial nerve, although less common in children than in adults, is a classic finding. Patients with facial nerve palsy may not demonstrate other signs of CNS involvement such as nuchal rigidity and encephalopathy.

The latency between the tick bite and the appearance of *late Lyme disease* is thought to be months to years in untreated patients. Arthritis is the typical manifestation, usually in the large joints. Swelling and erythema can be marked, but joints are often less painful than the examination would suggest. Joint involvement lasts 1 to 2 weeks. If untreated, the arthritis may become migratory and episodes may demonstrate longer duration. Neurologic involvement may also occur in late Lyme disease; this often is referred to as tertiary neuroborreliosis. This syndrome of indolent encephalopathy, cognitive defects, and cranial and peripheral neuropathies is rare in children.

## LABORATORY EVALUATION

The ESR and CRP may be elevated in patients with early disseminated or late disease. Fluid analysis of an arthritic joint can reveal a wide range of cell counts from 1000 to over 50,000 $WBC/mm^3$. A cerebrospinal fluid (CSF) pleocytosis can be seen in those with neurologic involvement of early disseminated disease, with the cell count ranging from approximately 20 to 300 $WBC/mm^{3.}$

Specific tests for Lyme disease are primarily antibody-based. Since their interpretation can be difficult, it is crucial to use a reliable laboratory. It is also best to use these tests to investigate further a reasonable clinical suspicion of Lyme disease that is based on a supportive history and physical examination. Diagnosing Lyme disease on the basis of serologic evidence alone can cause a clinician to miss other relevant diagnoses.

Early localized Lyme disease is a clinical diagnosis that is based on the EM rash. Antibodies to *B. burgdorferi* may not be present yet in patients with EM, as IgM may not peak until 4 to 6 weeks after infection. Patients with later stages of Lyme disease virtually all have detectable antibody. Enzyme-linked immunosorbent assay (ELISA) is the first line of testing for Lyme antibody. Because of false positives, confirmatory testing needs to be done with the Western blot technique, which has the ability to differentiate IgM and IgG. False-positive ELISA testing may be seen in viral illnesses (e.g., EBV), connective tissue disorders (e.g., SLE), and syphilis. Western blot analysis generally is considered a true positive if 2 of 4 IgM bands are positive and 5 of 10 IgG bands are positive. Antibodies to *B. burgdorferi* also may be elaborated in the CSF. The results of these studies should be interpreted by a reputable reference laboratory. Other techniques, such as polymerase chain reaction (PCR), may be useful for synovial fluid. Detection of *B. burgdorferi* antigen in urine is available, but the use of this test is not recommended.

## MANAGEMENT

Treatment for Lyme disease varies with the stage of the illness. For treatment to be effective, a strong clinical and/or laboratory diagnosis should exist. If the incorrect illness is diagnosed, it seems logical that treatment will fail. Consideration also should be given to the possibility of coinfection with other tick-borne diseases, such as ehrlichiosis.

For early localized disease, amoxicillin (25 to 50 mg/kg/24 h divided into two doses) can be used in children less than 8 years old. For children age 8 years and older, doxycycline 100 mg in two divided doses is preferred. The duration of therapy is 14 to 21 days.

Treatment of some forms of early disseminated and late Lyme disease may be performed with oral antibiotic regimens. Children with multiple EM lesions as part of early disseminated disease can be treated with amoxicillin or doxycycline (doses given above) for 21 days.

Children with new-onset arthritis can be treated with amoxicillin or doxycycline (doses given above) for 28 days.

Treatment of children with CNS disease is more complex. Among patients who present with facial palsy, studies show that oral doxycycline is effective. Some patients with isolated facial palsy, however, may have a CSF pleocytosis despite a lack of the symptoms of meningitis. Therefore, the decision to perform a lumbar puncture on these children can present a dilemma. Some experts recommend that all children with a seventh nerve palsy undergo lumbar puncture. If a CSF pleocytosis exists, they are treated with parenteral antibiotics for CNS disease (see below). Other physicians feel that if a patient has no clinical signs of CNS disease beyond the facial nerve palsy, a lumbar puncture is not indicated and oral antibiotics should be used. In light of the higher likelihood of a CSF pleocytosis in Lyme-related facial palsy in children versus adults, this author prefers CSF analysis in all children who present with isolated facial palsy.

If CNS disease is present, as manifested by clinical signs and symptoms or by CSF pleocytosis, penicillin or a third-generation cephalosporin (ceftriaxone, cefotaxime) should be administered intravenously for 14 to 28 days. Lyme carditis is treated with similar regimens of parenteral antibiotics. Patients with refractory or recurrent arthritis (beyond 2 months from the original treatment) should be treated with one additional course of the parenteral antibiotics listed above for 14 to 28 days. All these regimens generally require long-term intravenous (IV) line placement [peripherally inserted central catheter (PICC) line or central line].

Efforts should be focused on the prevention of Lyme disease. Effective practices include wearing protective attire to prevent ticks from attaching to the lower legs (long pants), walking in the center of paths away from low-lying plants or grasses, and the use of insect repellent. For children, low concentrations of DEET (N,N-diethyl-m-toluamide) or a permethrin are effective.

Children should be inspected for ticks after outdoor play, with particular attention to the groin, axillae, and belt line. If a tick is attached, it should be removed with tweezers by grasping the tick as close to the skin as possible and using gentle force to remove as much of the tick as possible. Antibiotic prophylaxis to prevent Lyme disease hardly ever is indicated after a tick bite, even in a highly endemic area. There is currently no available vaccine against Lyme disease.

## BIBLIOGRAPHY

American Academy of Pediatrics. Lyme disease. In Pickering LK, ed., *Red Book: 2003 Report of the Committee on Infectious Diseases,* 26th ed. Elk Grove Village, IL: American Academy of Pediatrics, 2003: 407–411.

Athreya BH. A general approach to management of children with rheumatic diseases. In Cassidy JT, Petty RE, eds., *Textbook of Pediatric Rheumatology,* 4th ed. Philadelphia: Saunders, 2001: 189–213.

Jarvis JN. Juvenile rheumatoid arthritis: A guide for pediatricians. *Pediatr Ann* 31:437, 2002.

Passo MH. General approach to rheumatologic disease in children and adolescents. In Rudolph CD, Rudolph AM, Hostetter MK, et al, eds., *Rudolph's Pediatrics,* 21st ed. New York: McGraw-Hill, 2003: 829–832.

Petty RE, Cassidy JT. Kawasaki disease. In Cassidy JT, Petty RE, eds., *Textbook of Pediatric Rheumatology,* 4th ed. Philadelphia: Saunders, 2001: 580–594.

Petty RE, Cassidy JT. Systemic lupus erythematosus. In Cassidy JT, Petty RE, eds., *Textbook of Pediatric Rheumatology,* 4th ed. Philadelphia: Saunders, 2001: 396–449.

Silverman ED. Pediatric systemic lupus erythematosus. In Rudolph CD, Rudolph AM, Hostetter MK, et al, eds., *Rudolph's Pediatrics,* 21st ed. New York: McGraw-Hill, 2003: 847–851.

# TRAUMA AND EMERGENCY
# MEDICINE

### *Lynn M. Manfred*

## LEARNING OBJECTIVES

1. Evaluate and initiate treatment of common acute medical illnesses in pediatric patients.
2. Recognize the common toxidromes and initiate management of suspected poisonings and ingestions in pediatric patients.
3. Know how to initiate management and then summon help in caring for a critically ill child.

## INITIAL EVALUATION

### ABCDs

The initial approach to all patients should be the same: Is the patient sick or not sick? Is the patient stable or not stable? One commonly used way to address these questions is the ABCD method:

- *Airway* is assessed first. Is it open? Most often the child has positioned herself or himself with an open airway. If this is not the case, position the neck in an extended position for children and in a "sniff" position for infants. The sniff position is achieved by placing a towel under the shoulders of an infant, which allows the neck to be extended but not enough to close off the airway. Keep the neck stabilized while protecting the airway.
- *Breathing* then can be assessed. Look at the chest wall to see if it is moving. Listen to the chest on both sides in the axillary line to hear that air is

moving. Is there enough air moving? Is the patient breathing too fast? Are the breath sounds similar between the two sides? Is the pulse oximetry reading >93 percent? If breathing is not adequate, reposition the neck and recheck it. If it is still inadequate, add oxygen and initiate assistance with breathing. Assistance with breathing may consist of bag-to-mouth ventilation. If the patient is not conscious or has a large oxygen requirement, intubation and mechanical ventilation should be initiated. Reassess as soon as one of these is in place and periodically while the child is in the emergency department.

- *Circulation* is assessed next. Feel for a central pulse. In adults a carotid pulse is good, but in young children this can be difficult to assess. Therefore, in preschool children, check a femoral or brachial pulse. If this is adequate, check a more peripheral pulse, such as a radial or posterior tibial pulse. If these pulses are found, check a blood pressure. If you cannot feel pulses or get a blood pressure that is appropriate for age, order intravenous (IV) fluids that will stay in the intravascular space, such as normal saline and albumin. Blood should be ordered if the low blood pressure is from blood loss.
- *Disability* entails doing a brief neurologic evaluation. Check the pupils, assess if they are equal, and make sure they respond to light similarly. This will alert you early to narcotic poisoning or impending herniation of the brain into the small space occupied by the brainstem. When these tests are normal, you should check the patient's level of consciousness. For children, the AVPU method is used commonly:
  - A = alert
  - V = responds to verbal stimuli
  - P = responds to pain only
  - U = unresponsive

Many trauma specialists use the Glasgow Coma Scale to assess trauma in older children and adults. Younger children are not developmentally able to respond to some of these questions, making the scale less useful for preschoolers. The following step adds to the ABCDs:

- *Evaluate for injury and manage the environment* next. The patient is undressed and assessed both front and back for signs of trauma, fractures, wounds, bleeding, and other injuries. Carefully keep the neck and back stable until they have been evaluated for injuries and protected from further injury. Don't forget to cover the patient or place the patient on a warming bed once this survey is done. Patients can become hypothermic, especially infants who have a high ratio of surface area to body mass.

# SHOCK

Shock is a condition in which the necessary nutrients, including oxygen, do not reach the brain and other tissues of the body. Normal physiologic function is maintained by adequate delivery of nutrients to the tissues. The determinants of adequate delivery are oxygen delivery to the blood (oxygen saturation), oxygen-carrying capacity (hemoglobin), and cardiac output (stroke volume × heart rate). Stroke volume is controlled by preload or filling volume, myocardial contractility, and afterload.

In early shock, the body attempts to compensate by preserving blood flow to vital tissues and organs. Early or compensated shock is revealed by the physiologic response to low intravascular volume or functional hypovolemia. Tachycardia is usually the first physiologic change, but mild tachypnea, capillary refill delayed by 2 to 3 s, orthostatic changes in blood pressure and/or pulse, and mental status changes such as depressed mental state, irritability, or crankiness are often present.

Late or uncompensated shock is present when the body's circulation no longer can meet the metabolic demands of the body. The tissues then shift to the much less efficient anaerobic metabolism. Anaerobic metabolism cannot support the necessary functions of the body, and the cells begin to swell and die. Clinically, the tachycardia and tachypnea worsen and visible signs of shock appear, including a pale or dusky skin color, cool extremities, and prolonged capillary refill. All organs are subject to inadequate perfusion and ischemia to a varying degree.

Many common childhood illnesses can cause shock, including infections, dehydration, and trauma. Each one disrupts one or more of the mechanisms that support the delivery of oxygen and nutrients to the tissues. For example, bleeding secondary to trauma decreases the hemoglobin concentration and decreases the preload, which decreases the stroke volume and cardiac output. Compensatory vasoconstriction also increases the afterload, further decreasing cardiac output.

The underlying etiology of the shock should be evaluated and treated while one is supporting the ABCDs.

## TYPES OF SHOCK

### HYPOVOLEMIC SHOCK

The hallmark of hypovolemic shock, the most common cause of shock in children, is a decrease in the circulating blood volume. Worldwide, this often is caused by diarrhea and sometimes is complicated by vomiting. Other causes of hypovolemic shock include blood loss (from trauma or gastrointestinal bleeding,) low oncotic pressure (burns, low-protein states caused by nephrotic syndrome or low protein production), and osmotic diuresis.

## DISTRIBUTIVE SHOCK, OR "THIRD SPACING"

Vascular system vasodilation in response to inappropriate stimuli causes blood and fluid to pool in inappropriate areas. Anaphylaxis, sepsis, central nervous system (CNS) injury, and intoxication all can cause inappropriate vasodilation of one or more vascular beds. The resulting decrease in preload can cause a decrease in cardiac output.

## CARDIOGENIC SHOCK

Cardiogenic shock results when the myocardium is not able to pump out sufficient blood volume despite normal preload and afterload. Therefore, cardiac output cannot keep up with the demand, resulting in the symptoms of heart failure. Rales, an $S_3$ sound, hepatomegaly, and venous congestion all can be apparent. The etiologies include toxic myocardial damage, viral myocarditis, congenital cardiac diseases and their complications, metabolic disorders (hypoglycemia, hypoxia, hyperthyroidism), and deposition diseases such as hemochromatosis and Fabry disease.

## INCREASED AFTERLOAD

Obstruction from aortic valve disease, subaortic outlet obstruction, coarctation of the aorta, or severe vasoconstriction all can increase afterload to the point where the pumping action of the heart cannot overcome the pressure and supply the necessary peripheral blood flow.

## TREATMENT OF SHOCK

The ABCDs of emergency management constitute good initial management of shock. First the patient must be ventilated and optimally oxygenated. Table 39-1 describes the overview of the treatment process.

When a child presents in shock without obvious trauma or a history of heart disease, one should consider infectious causes: meningitis, sepsis, pneumonia, and pyelonephritis.

Children frequently present to the emergency room after a few hours to days of an acute illness when they have gotten much sicker. Some of them have a fever; others are hypothermic. Most are pale and tachycardic with some depression of sensorium. These children need urgent evaluation and treatment. The ABCDs are covered above, but as soon as they are accomplished, a search for the source of the illness must be done efficiently. Vital signs help identify a child who is hypoxic and probably has pneumonia. Flexion of the neck in a child over age 18 months uncovers the stiff neck of meningitis. Mottling and poor perfusion suggest septic shock. If the child is in moderate to severe shock, the administration of broad-spectrum antibiotics should be considered to treat presumed sepsis, in addition to fluids given to support blood pressure. As soon afterward as possible, cultures should be obtained. The organism and the site of infection determine the

*Table 39-1* **The Initial Management of Shock**

*Airway:* Be certain the airway is patent and monitor that it remains patent. Expect that the patient's airway muscles will have less tone and that the patient may need to be intubated to maintain the airway.

*Breathing:* Supply as much oxygen as possible to facilitate oxygen delivery to the tissues. Higher oxygen concentrations can be delivered to cells when 100% oxygen is delivered through an endotracheal tube compared with a mask.

*Assess metabolic state:* Check oxygenation, glucose, electrolytes, and blood counts.

*Circulation:* Establish venous access in a large central vessel with two large-bore needles if possible. Infuse isotonic fluids, normal saline 20–40 mL/kg initially. Blood should be given if there has been blood loss, or albumin can be given based on the clinical picture.

*Drug Therapy:* Give a positive inotropic agent such as dopamine, epinephrine, or isoproterenol to support tissue perfusion. Treat any metabolic abnormalities discovered in the laboratory work such as hypoglycemia, acidosis, and anemia.

*Empirically Treat:* Transfuse a bleeding patient, give antibiotics to a febrile or hypothermic patient, and consider whether any other treatment might be beneficial. Give oxygen, thiamine, glucose, and naloxone for an obtunded patient without a focus. The risk of each is small. Steroids for meningitis, insulin for severe hyperglycemia, $\beta_2$ agonists for status asthmaticus, and antidotes to toxins can all help improve outcomes of shock.

*Focus treatment* to address the specific disease process. Choose a specific antibiotic, a specific antidote, or treatment.

duration and type of therapy. Any child with depressed sensorium should have glucose and oxygen checked and corrected if they are low.

Dehydration is possible if a child has had severe and persistent vomiting or diarrhea. Rapid replacement of intravascular fluid by boluses of 10 to 20 mL/kg is necessary to perfuse vital organs and is diagnostic for dehydration.

## BURNS AND THERMAL INJURIES

### BURNS

Burns are common in children age 1 to 5 years and can be life-threatening. Young children have less subcutaneous tissue and are prone to greater injury after the same amount of heat exposure. As with other emergency evaluations, the ABCDs should be assessed and stabilized first. Then the degree of disability is established by rating the depth of the burn, the percentage of body surface area that is burned, and the location of the burn.

The depth of the burn is described as the degree of burn, with the lowest numbers being the least severe. First-degree burns are superficial, involving the epidermis, and do not blister and rarely scar, though they may have hyperpigmented areas as they heal. They are red, the skin is intact, and they hurt because the nerves are injured but not dead. Severe sunburn is an example of a first-degree burn. Second-degree burns are deeper, going into the dermis, and they often blister and also hurt. Superficial second-degree burns are often very painful, red, and swollen. They can heal in a couple of weeks with minimal scarring. Deeper second-degree burns may be less painful, but they have a wet or oozing surface and are in part pale. They probably will scar or require grafting to cover the burned areas. Third-degree burns are "full-thickness" burns of the dermal layers and subcutaneous tissue. They appear leathery on the skin surface and do not hurt because the entire nerve ending is destroyed. They take a long time to heal.

The percentage of body surface area involved is determined crudely by the rule of nines. For older children and adolescents, the head, one arm, the front of one leg, the back of one leg, the anterior trunk to the pelvis, and the posterior trunk each represent about 9 percent of the body surface area. For infants, 18 percent of the body surface area is on the head and the legs have less than 9 percent each. These are general estimates; more detailed charts are available in emergency medicine and surgery textbooks.

Burns to distal areas and specialized tissues often feature more ischemic injury, and so face, hand, foot, ear, and perineal burns all warrant hospitalization and special care. Circumferential burns also put distal areas at risk for ischemia as the injured area swells, and so these children often are admitted for frequent examinations and treatment of areas of poor blood flow.

Confounding variables in the treatment of burns are the type of burn (electrical and chemical burns are likely to cause much more severe injuries than is immediately apparent), lung injury resulting from smoke inhalation, eye injuries from flash fires or splash chemical burns, major trauma, and pre-existing medical problems all increase the level of care burn patients require.

## HYPOTHERMIA

Infants and the elderly are the most susceptible to hypothermia, or core temperatures of less than 35°C (95°F). Hypothermia is a common consideration when there is immersion in cold water or on extremely cold and windy days. However, hypothermia also must be considered when patients are underdressed or wet on breezy days when there is conductive and convective heat loss. Infants have less ability to vasoconstrict and maintain core body temperature. Medications and cardiorespiratory diseases make it harder to maintain core temperature and increase the risk of hypothermia.

Treatment consists of gradual warming by using external measures, warm humidified oxygen, and warm IV fluids.

## HEAT INJURIES

Heat injuries are most likely to happen when the weather suddenly becomes warmer and more humid. Heat injuries range from the relatively mild heat cramps (muscles cramping after vigorous exercise in high temperatures) to heat stroke, in which circulation collapses because of extreme temperature elevation and loss of the ability to dissipate heat. The extremes of age are most prone to the more severe forms of heat-related illnesses, and health-care providers must have a high index of suspicion during times of extremely hot temperatures and high humidity.

# SYNCOPE

Syncope is loss of consciousness resulting from a temporary lack of oxygen or glucose supply to the brain. The etiologies of syncope fall into the categories of cardiovascular and neurologic. The cardiovascular etiologies can be separated into cardiac and vascular. Syncope of cardiac origin includes structural lesions such as aortic stenosis, obstructive cardiomyopathy [e.g., idiopathic hypertrophic subaortic stenosis (IHSS)], pulmonary hypertension, and heart failure (hypothyroidism, infiltrative diseases, and muscle damage from infection or a toxin).

Cardiac arrhythmias also can cause syncope. Atrioventricular (AV) block, prolonged QT syndrome, and sick sinus syndrome all cause sudden death and should be sought actively. Supraventricular tachycardia (SVT) also can present as either palpitations or syncope.

Vascular syncope is the result of inappropriate vasodilation from hypovolemia, autonomic insufficiency, or metabolic abnormality such as hypoglycemia, hypoxia, or acidosis.

Neurologic causes of syncope are most commonly seizures, but syncope can result from the drop attacks of narcolepsy, atonic seizures, and poor cerebral perfusion caused by hyperventilation or breath-holding spells.

The two most common causes of syncope are innocent vasovagal episodes and breath-holding spells. Teenagers are most prone to vasovagal episodes, with 25 to 50 percent of teens having at least one episode. A triggering event such as pain or surprise, should be elicited. There should be no persistent pain, loss of consciousness should be brief, and the patient otherwise should be well. Young children are most likely to have breath-holding spells. The spell usually is provoked by sudden pain or anger. The child holds his or her breath until he or she passes out, and then the child resumes breathing and quickly "pinks up."

A thorough investigation must be made of any patient who has syncope during or after exercise or has syncope associated with chest pain, palpitations, or respiratory distress or has a family history of sudden death (prolonged QT). See Chap. 27 for a more detailed discussion of syncope.

## ACUTE ALLERGIC REACTIONS

### ANAPHYLAXIS

#### PATHOPHYSIOLOGY

Anaphylaxis is the end-organ result of the release of vasoactive compounds such as histamine from mast cells and basophils. This usually is triggered by immunoglobulin E (IgE), but "anaphylactoid" reactions can result from a physical or mechanical insult to mast cells and basophils that causes the release of the same histamine compounds and a similar though usually less severe reaction.

The most common causes of anaphylaxis are foods (peanuts, milk protein, shellfish, eggs), hymenoptera stings (bees, wasps, etc.), medications (antibiotics, immunotherapy, aspirin, and anti-inflammatories), and latex.

#### CLINICAL MANIFESTATIONS

The spectrum of anaphylaxis ranges from hives that can be treated locally to respiratory compromise or hypotension and cardiac arrest. Commonly there is involvement of the skin, including hives, flushing, pruritus, and angioedema, which causes the patient to seek care. Respiratory symptoms are frequently present and can include acute bronchospasm, laryngeal edema, and upper airway swelling. Vasodilation also can occur, causing hypotension and poor myocardial perfusion and resulting in myocardial damage and arrhythmias. Gastrointestinal involvement results in any combination of nausea, vomiting, diarrhea, and abdominal pain.

#### MANAGEMENT

Management of anaphylaxis varies depending on symptom severity and the organs involved. Hives and pruritus can be treated with an antihistamine such as diphenhydramine orally and with oral steroids if the area involved is extensive or if there is respiratory involvement. If there is respiratory or cardiovascular involvement, management entails securing the airway, administering oxygen, assuring adequate ventilation and circulation, and then treating the allergic cause with vasoconstrictors such as epinephrine, antihistamines of both the $H_1$ and $H_2$ types, and corticosteroids. Any patient who has had a reaction that involves the cardiac or respiratory system should have an Epi-Pen available for accidental reexposure to the triggering substance.

## STATUS ASTHMATICUS

Status asthmaticus is one of the most common allergic reasons for emergent evaluation. Often the patient has the chronic inflammatory condition of asthma and has received a triggering insult such as infection, exposure to allergens, exercise, or irritant exposure. Some patients have a slow progressive course, and others acutely decompensate. Treatment focuses on restoring normal respiratory function as quickly as possible. Initially, the mainstay of treatment is an inhaled $\beta_2$ agonist. Nebulized medication and medication inhaled with a mask and a spacer appear to be equally effective. Ipratropium added to the inhaled medications may decrease secretions and lower hospital admission rates. Supplemental oxygen is given and has been shown to be beneficial. Unless an underlying reason can be found for the exacerbation, steroids usually are given. Early administration of steroids may decrease the admission rate. If an underlying infection is found, it is treated.

Poor prognostic indicators for quick recovery are persistent tachypnea, hypoxia, retractions, tachycardia, mental status changes, poor air movement, and rising or normal $Pco_2$ as well as increased pulsus paradoxus.

# CENTRAL NERVOUS SYSTEM PROBLEMS

## MENTAL STATUS CHANGES

Changes in the level of consciousness are common causes for visits to the emergency room. The history is key here. Were the changes gradual or rapid in onset? Gradual changes over days suggest the slow development of a metabolic problem, drug use, or a tumor. Diabetes, hypercalcemia, and renal or liver failure all can cause depression of the central nervous system (CNS). Drug use often is associated with a change in behavior and withdrawal from social circles and family. Tumors may have accompanying headache, focal neurologic signs on examination, or change in personality over the preceding weeks.

Rapid-onset mental status changes (over a few hours) suggest acute ingestion, head injury, or CNS infection. The presence of a fever and changes in mental status mandate an investigation of the CNS for meningitis, encephalitis, and brain abscess. If there are any focal or localizing signs or a suggestion of increased intracranial pressure (ICP), the CNS should be imaged before lumbar puncture is done.

Closed head injuries can cause a number of changes in mental status. Immediate loss of consciousness or seizure at the time of the injury probably has no prognostic significance. Conversely, gradual changes over hours to days after the injury suggest the accumulation of blood or swelling of the brain that is progressing. Localizing findings are particularly worrisome. Vomiting, delayed seizures, and progressive crankiness all suggest the progression of the intracranial process and should be evaluated quickly. High fevers can cause temporary changes that can be ameliorated with antipyretics.

## LOSS OF CONSCIOUSNESS

Often loss of consciousness is a synonym for syncope. However, this could be the postictal phase of a seizure or could be due to the ingestion of a sedating substance. Common sedatives that are widely available include antihistamines, cough and cold preparations, narcotics, and psychiatric medications.

## SEIZURES

Seizures are a common reason for patients to present to the emergency room. Generalized tonic-clonic seizures are the most common. If fever is present, CNS infection must be excluded. Meningitis and encephalitis always entail some mental status changes, and the patient should have either a stiff neck (in children older than 18 months) or focal neurologic findings.

Febrile seizures are common. Children present with brief, nonfocal seizures, usually in the presence of a new fever. If the seizure is generalized, lasting less than 10 to 15 min, with a rapid return to normal mental status, it is most likely an innocent febrile seizure. These children usually are back to their normal behavior by the time they get to the emergency room. Atypical febrile seizures can last longer than 15 min or have a focal component. A complex febrile seizure has the highest likelihood of being recognized later as the first idiopathic seizure. However, this occurs in less than 12 percent of what initially are called febrile seizures.

A first seizure that is prolonged and has a postictal phase but has no localizing signs and no associated laboratory changes is probably innocent. Generally, if the neurologic exam is normal, the patient will not be treated for seizures as the risk-benefit ratio favors no treatment. Treatment is initiated when multiple seizures have occurred or if there is an abnormal neurologic examination. Imaging of the CNS is warranted when there are any focal abnormalities, changes in mental status, or developmental delay.

## ATAXIA

The many causes of ataxia can be separated by time course. Ataxia that presents in the emergency room is almost always acute. A subacute onset of ataxia and chronic progressive ataxia usually are caused by tumor (roughly two-thirds of pediatric brain tumors are infratentorial) or hydrocephalus or are metabolic in origin. They also can be distinguished by physical findings that are symmetric, such as weakness and sensory losses.

Acute ataxia has to be evaluated urgently (Fig. 39-1). Patients with fever and/or symptoms of increased ICP need a computed tomography (CT) scan and a lumbar puncture followed by treatment of the meningitis,

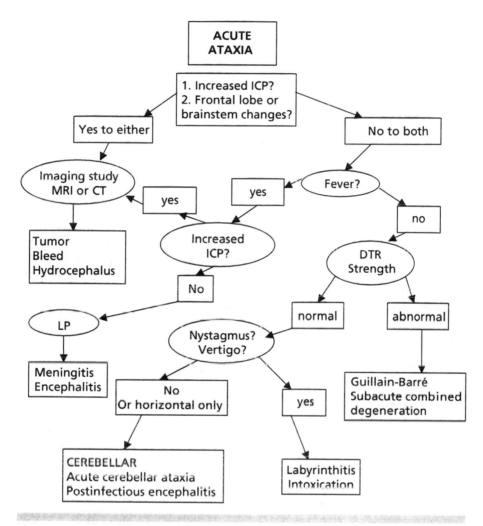

*Figure 39-1* **The Evaluation of Acute Ataxia**

encephalitis, or increased ICP. Neurologic evaluation of strength, deep tendon reflexes (DTR), and sensation as well as evaluation of the patient for
nystagmus will distinguish between a cerebellar process such as acute cerebellar ataxia or labyrinthitis and a peripheral process such as Guillain-Barré
syndrome.

## CHANGES IN MOTOR FUNCTION

When children present to the emergency room with changes in motor function, they need a thorough neurologic examination. The distribution of

motor weakness, involvement of DTR, sensory changes, and whether there is cranial nerve or cognitive involvement taken together will define whether it is a central neurologic problem (stroke, tumor, or brain abscess), cord lesion (transverse myelitis, spinal cord compression from trauma, lymphoma, sarcoma, or neuroblastoma), infection, peripheral neuropathy (acute polyneuritis, myasthenia gravis, or botulism), or motor function that is the issue. Once the location is determined, the appropriate evaluation can be ordered.

## SWOLLEN OR RED EYE

Children can present with swollen red eyelids with or without fever. The clinician must distinguish between swelling of the lid and proptosis (protrusion of the eye forward in the socket). Limitation of extraocular eye movements caused by one or two muscles is pathognomonic for a mass in the orbit. Most often this is pus, but it can be tumor. A CT scan of the orbit defines the mass. Infections usually are caused by *Staphylococcus* sp. or *Streptococcus* sp. now that most children are immunized against *Haemophilus influenzae* type B.

The swollen lid is usually allergic or a cellulitis. Allergic reactions can be quite asymmetric but are usually pruritic and often give a gritty sensation in the anterior eye. Other allergic symptoms should be present. Cellulitis of the eyelid usually results from a bite or trauma that introduces an infection.

Less commonly, children present with pain in the eye. Visual acuity should be evaluated, and a foreign body sought. If acuity is abnormal or the foreign body is not superficial, urgent ophthalmologic consultation is necessary.

## PSYCHIATRIC EMERGENCIES

### SUICIDE ATTEMPT OR IDEATION

Suicide attempts and ideation, or thoughts of suicide, must be taken seriously, especially in children and adolescents. Girls attempt suicide more often than boys do, but boys are much more likely to die from their attempts. Suicide and suicide attempts are often impulsive acts by a child or adolescent who has experienced personal stress or pressure; this makes it harder to predict which children are in imminent danger. More than three-quarters of all suicide attempts involve ingestions.

In the emergency room, rapid assessment of the history of the suicide attempt, the potential lethality, the child's mental status, and the strengths and supports in the child's life are key to deciding whether the child needs to be hospitalized.

An underlying medical cause for the suicide attempt should be sought as well as looking for underlying diseases that might create comorbidity. Psychiatric consultation is necessary for all attempts and for all severely depressed children.

## PANIC/ANXIETY

Adolescents occasionally present to the emergency room with acute anxiety reactions such as panic. These reactions often present as chest pain or difficulty taking a deep breath, but evaluation reveals no underlying lung or cardiac disease. Often there are family members with panic disorder. Once toxic and medical etiologies are excluded, a patient with anxiety may be treated acutely with benzodiazepines or beta blockers. Follow-up with psychiatric or primary care services is necessary.

## PSYCHOSIS

Adolescence is a common age of onset for psychosis. Psychosis is marked by changes in higher-order thinking such as cognition, perception, mood, and reality testing. Often there is a personal or family history of psychiatric disease, and the psychosis is of gradual onset once it is recognized. New-onset psychosis must be distinguished from manic-depressive illness, which also entails disordered thoughts, cognition, and perception. A history of depressive episodes, a quick onset of illness, and a recent decline in functional abilities all favor a bipolar diagnosis.

Acute psychosis with abnormal vital signs, changes in consciousness, or abnormal laboratory studies marks the type of psychosis that has an underlying medical etiology. Ingestions; metabolic disorders such as hypoglycemia, hypocalcemia, and vitamin $B_{12}$ deficiency; and renal or liver disease all can cause an acute change. The underlying medical disorder is treated, and then further evaluation is required.

## RESPIRATORY PROBLEMS

Acute respiratory problems are some of the most common causes of emergency room visits in children. Asthma is discussed above under "Allergic Conditions."

## APNEA, SUDDEN INFANT DEATH SYNDROME, AND APPARENT LIFE-THREATENING EVENTS

Sudden infant death syndrome (SIDS) is the death of a child in the first year of life when no apparent cause can be found after examining the child's history, establishing the location of the death, and doing a complete postmortem evaluation. The majority of SIDS deaths occur in the second to sixth month of life and in the winter. There is an increased risk in families that have had prior SIDS deaths, families with smokers in the house, and low-income families.

An apparent life-threatening event (ALTE) is a change in color and/or tone associated with gagging and choking, apnea, or upper airway obstruction that prevents air movement. Witnesses often are worried that the infant is dying. The etiologies of ALTEs are listed by organ system in Table 39-2. About half of the cases of ALTE can be classified into one of these categories.

Less than 10 percent of children with ALTEs have SIDS, and less than 10 percent of children who die of SIDS have had an ALTE. However, children with many of the diagnosed ALTEs are at risk for morbidity from their seizures or from reflux and aspiration.

Table 39-2 **Etiologies of Apparent Life-Threatening Events**

| Organ System | Specific Diagnoses |
| --- | --- |
| Respiratory | Respiratory syncytial virus and other respiratory viruses |
| | Sepsis or pneumonia |
| | Pertussis |
| | Chlamydia |
| | Tracheomalacia |
| | Upper airway obstruction |
| | Breath-holding spell |
| Nonaccidental trauma | Battered child |
| | Drug use or abuse |
| | Drug withdrawal |
| Cardiovascular | Congenital heart disease, especially with shunting or cyanosis |
| | Arrhythmia |
| | Cardiomyopathy |
| | Vasovagal response to pain or other stimuli |
| Neurologic | Seizure |
| | Apnea of infancy |
| | Central nervous system infection: meningitis or encephalitis |
| | Brain tumor |
| | Structural lesion: Arnold-Chiari malformation |
| | Central hypoventilation |
| | Increased intracranial pressure |
| | Sleep disorder breathing |
| Gastrointestinal | Gastroesophageal reflux |
| | Gastric distention |
| | Abnormal swallowing |

The key to the diagnosis of an ALTE as well as its underlying etiology is a careful history obtained from the caregiver. Eyes deviated in one direction or repetitive movements suggest seizures. An association with feeding and vomiting suggests reflux. Fever suggests an infectious etiology. Premature infants are at risk of CNS immaturity and the apnea of prematurity.

The "Back to Sleep" program of the America Academy of Pediatrics has promoted education about sleeping positions and tobacco exposure avoidance, both of which have known associations with apnea and SIDS.

## UPPER AIRWAY OBSTRUCTION AND INFECTION

Children and infants who present to the emergency room in respiratory distress or unable to swallow often have some sort of upper airway issue. If they are in respiratory distress, they usually are working hard to breathe and generating a noise called stridor. This inspiratory noise is diagnostic of airway obstruction above the thorax. In children less than 6 weeks old, the etiology of the stridor is usually tracheomalacia. The normally soft cartilaginous rings are too soft to keep the airway patent, and the stridor becomes more severe when the child is stressed by feeding, the supine position, or congestion from an upper respiratory tract infection or gastroesophageal reflux.

The most common etiologies of acquired stridor include the aspiration of foreign bodies, croup, and, rarely, epiglottitis. Infants and toddlers who explore their world by putting novel items in their mouths most commonly aspirate small objects. Toys, beads, buttons, coins, and foods that are not cut small enough are aspirated. Plastic and food items are not visible on x-ray, but metal objects are. Once one is certain that the object is in the airway, laryngoscopy or bronchoscopy can be used to retrieve objects that will not pass through the gastrointestinal tract.

Croup is a viral upper airway soft tissue infection that presents with a distinctive barky cough that usually starts in the evening and gets progressively worse. A soft tissue x-ray of the neck shows the steeple sign that demonstrates the subglottic edema. Cool air or warm mist often ameliorates milder cases that are without stridor at rest. Severe cases can obstruct the upper airway. Racemic epinephrine and other β agonists will shrink the edema in the upper airway and make breathing easier. These agents have a short half-life, and respiratory distress can recur when they wear off. Therefore, severe cases must be admitted or observed in the emergency room until they clearly are not going to recur. Moderate and severe cases can improve more quickly with the early administration of oral or intramuscular (IM) steroids.

Older children presenting with "croup," especially at atypical times of the year, could have spasmodic croup, angioedema, or a retropharyngeal foreign body.

Epiglottitis presents as the acute onset of severe respiratory distress and high fever and causes a young child to sit in the sniffing position to open the airway as much as possible. Epiglottitis is much less common than it was before children were vaccinated against *H. influenzae* and pneumococci. Nonetheless, it has not been eradicated and is a potentially lethal disease. A child with possible epiglottitis should not be forced to lie down or have any medical instrumentation of the mouth or airway until both equipment and personnel are available to perform an immediate tracheostomy if needed.

School-age children and older children can present with severe sore throat and difficulty swallowing that mark tonsillar and peritonsillar abscesses. Both present with unilateral pain and swelling that make swallowing even saliva difficult. The diagnosis is made by direct visualization, and treatment consists of drainage and antibiotics. Occasionally, intravenous fluids are necessary until the child can tolerate sufficient oral fluids.

Retropharyngeal abscess is an infection of the posterior pharynx nodes that progresses to cellulitis and abscess. The typical patient is a child less than 2 years old who has a high fever and increased respiratory noise and work and who presents with an extended neck, drooling, and an airy "hot potato" voice. Intravenous antibiotics are needed, and some true abscesses require surgical drainage if the airway is compromised or there is progression despite antibiotic treatment.

Ludwig angina is a cellulitis of the space below the floor of the mouth. Poor dentition or trauma to the floor of the mouth introduces oral flora into this space. It is often rapidly progressive as infection spreads from the mucosa of the mouth toward the hyoid bone and impinges on the airway. These children are at risk of sudden death from airway occlusion and need to be monitored closely.

## LOWER AIRWAY PROBLEMS

Asthma and foreign body aspiration were discussed above. Aspiration of foreign bodies into the lower respiratory tract often causes a ball-valve phenomenon with an expiration-inspiration cycle. This allows air in with inspiration and traps the air in expiration. This leads to the physical findings of localized inspiratory whistling. Comparing inspiratory and expiratory chest x-rays or right and left lateral decubitus films in children too young to cooperate with inspiratory and expiratory films may demonstrate the trapped air on the side of the foreign body.

Pneumonia can present with the abrupt onset of fever, chills, and increased work of breathing. Younger children are more likely to present with systemic symptoms and little or no cough or chest findings on physical examination. Therefore, a high index of suspicion of respiratory causes of fever must be maintained in patients with an increased respiratory rate, an increased heart rate, and/or a mild decrease in pulse oximetry. Children with lower lobe pneumonia may present with abdominal pain. The common bacterial causes of pneumonia are pneumococcus, streptococcus, and mycoplasma, though the latter rarely causes hypoxia.

Aspiration pneumonia presents similarly, but the etiologic agents are the oral flora. Most patients with aspiration pneumonia have underlying mental status changes, developmental delay, chronic respiratory illnesses, or gastroesophageal reflux. In addition to the pneumonia, they are likely to get bronchospasm and chemical pneumonitis.

Bronchiolitis is a clinical syndrome that usually is seen in infants who present with fever, coryza, and increased respiratory noise. Respiratory syncytial virus (RSV) and parainfluenza virus are common causes of bronchiolitis. Chronically ill children are particularly vulnerable to this disease; this is why premature infants with congenital heart disease and chronic respiratory disease are given anti-RSV immunoglobulin for the winter months for the first 18 months of life. Apnea and wheezing are common comorbidities. Wheezing associated with bronchiolitis usually is not responsive to inhaled bronchodilators.

## DROWNING AND NEAR DROWNING

Submersion injuries are the second most common accidental cause of death in children. Any collection of water, indoors or outdoors, can cause drowning. Submersion may cause acute and severe laryngospasm that prevents water and air from entering the lungs. Cardiovascular collapse and loss of consciousness soon follow. If this is not reversed in 4 to 6 min, severe CNS insult occurs that can be irreversible.

Alternatively, fluid may be aspirated into the lungs, increasing the alveolar-to-arteriolar gradient so that little oxygen can cross into the bloodstream. Hypoxia causes cardiac and CNS damage that is permanent if it is not reversed quickly.

Assessing a child who has been submerged requires observation and warming to close to room temperature. A child who fell through the ice may appear dead until warmed to 33 or 34°C (91.4 to 93.2°F). Alternatively, a child who was submerged in warm bath water may appear fine on arrival in the emergency room only to deteriorate as the damage done to the lungs causes progressive hypoxia. Associated injuries such as hyperextension neck injuries must be assessed as well.

## POISONINGS AND INGESTIONS

### INITIAL EVALUATION

The best treatment of poisonings and ingestions is prevention. Pediatricians spend much of their well-child visits discussing ways to prevent accidents and ingestions. Using cabinet and drawer locks and storing medications and cleaning supplies out of sight and/or out of reach help a parent prevent ingestions.

Once a child is discovered with a potentially toxic substance in his or her mouth, decontamination should be attempted. Wash absorbed toxins off skin surfaces, remove the child from the area where inhaled toxins are present, and clear the area of the substance. For oral ingestions, sweep the mouth for any solid that has been taken in but not swallowed.

Once they are in the emergency room, the initial evaluation of patients with toxic ingestions should be similar to that of trauma patients (Table 39-3): Check the ABCDs (see Table 39-1). The airway needs to be clear of all foreign matter, and the patient needs to be moving air independently. If the patient is not doing this, secure the airway and either bag or mechanically ventilate the patient. Check central and peripheral pulses as well as perfusion and then secure intravenous or intraosseous access before attempting treatment of the ingestion. Patients whose airway, breathing, and circulation are intact are considered for disability and decontamination. If the patient is sedated or comatose, evaluation of serum glucose and oxygenation should be done, and this should be treated if low. If these values are normal and the patient has a toxidrome consistent with narcotic intoxication, naloxone is given.

Patients who have ingested large amounts of toxic substances, especially those with anticholinergic effects that will delay gastric emptying, could receive gastric lavage. The toxic risks to the patient must be weighed against the risk of aspiration during the procedure. Patients who have ingested substances other than hydrocarbons, heavy metals, or digoxin often are given charcoal to bind the ingested substance in the gastrointestinal tract and carry it out in the stool. Charcoal has the added advantage of binding substances that have gotten into the bloodstream and are undergoing enterohepatic circulation. This lowers the blood level much faster. Binding the substance in the GI tract encourages secretion into the GI tract. Cathartics such as sorbitol may be added to the charcoal or given separately to hasten the movement through the gastrointestinal tract and theoretically decrease absorption. Sorbitol should be used with caution in young children because it may cause dehydration and electrolyte abnormalities.

The evaluation of toxic ingestions is similar to the evaluation of patients in general:

1. Consider the host. Toddlers "get into things" and in exploring them will eat or drink some. Therefore, they ingest what are usually smaller quantities of substances. Because of their small body size, even small amounts of medications and other highly toxic items can cause physiologic problems in children. In contrast, adolescents who ingest things often take larger amounts and are likely to hide the ingestion for longer periods than do toddlers.

*Table 39-3* **Physical Examination Clues to Toxic Ingestions (Toxidromes)**

| Clinical Clues | Possible Toxin |
|---|---|
| 1. Sedative poisoning | Narcotics |
| Pinpoint pupils | Codeine, morphine |
| Coma/central nervous | |
| system depression | Hydrocodone, oxycodone |
| Ataxia | Clonidine |
| Hypotension | Sedatives |
| Hyporeflexia | Barbiturates |
| Respiratory depression | Other hypnotics |
| | Benzodiazepines |
| 2. Sympathomimetic poisoning | Caffeine |
| Delirium and psychosis | Cocaine |
| Excitation/irritability | Amphetamine |
| Tremor/myoclonus | Dexamphetamine |
| Fever | Methamphetamine |
| Tachycardia | Theophylline |
| Hypertension | |
| Mydriasis | |
| Diaphoresis | |
| Seizures | |
| 3. Anticholinergic poisoning (the Mad Hatter from *Alice in Wonderland*) | |
| Mad as a hatter (delirium) | Tricyclic antidepressants |
| Dry as a bell | Antihistamines |
| Blind as a bat (mydriasis) | Carbamazepine |
| Red as a beet (flushed) | |
| Hot as Hades (fever) | |
| Tachycardia | |
| Arrhythmias | |
| Hypertension | |
| Seizures | |
| 4. Cholinergic poisoning (DUMBBELS) | |
| Diarrhea | Organophosphates |
| Urination | Muscarinic mushroom poisoning |
| Miosis and muscle weakness | |
| Bronchorrhea or bronchospasm | |
| Bradycardia or tachycardia | |
| Emesis | |
| Lacrimation | |
| Salivation and seizures | |
| Plus confusion, fasciculations | |

*(continued)*

*Table 39-3* **Physical Examination Clues to Toxic Ingestions (Toxidromes) (continued)**

| Clinical Clues | Possible Toxin |
| --- | --- |
| 5. Skin color | |
|    a. Cyanotic on oxygen | Methemoglobinemia |
|    b. Red | Antihistamines, alcohol, atropine, carbon monoxide, cyanide |
| 6. Hyperventilation and fever | Salicylates |
| 7. Extrapyramidal syndromes | Phenothiazine |
| | Metoclopramide |
|      Torticollis | Compazine |
|      Dystonic reactions | |
|      Trismus | |
|      Ataxia | |
|      Tongue movements | |
|      Oculogyric movements | |
|    Hypotension | |
|    Hypothermia | |
|    Tachycardia | |
|    Tachypnea | |
|    Tremor and seizures | |
|    Sedation or coma | |
| 8. Oral burns: caustic compounds | Lye |
| 9. Distinctive odors | |
|    a. Volatile hydrocarbons | |
|      i. Gasoline | Gasoline |
|      ii. Toluene | Toluene |
|      iii. Nail polish remover | Acetone, isopropyl alcohol, or phenol |
|      iv. Benzene | Benzene |
|    b. Mothballs | Naphthalene |
|    c. Wintergreen | Methyl salicylate |
|    d. Garlic | Organophosphates or heavy metals |
|    e. Almond | Cyanide |

2. Look to see that the patient's ABCDs are safe while you gather the history. Check the chart of clinical syndromes (Figure 39-3) to see what toxins are possible on the basis of the general examination of the patient.

3. Gather the history. What did the child ingest? About how much could the child have gotten? How long ago could the ingestion have occurred? What else is available in the house that the child also might have gotten into? What has happened since the ingestion? (Has the child vomited,

| Ingestion | Antidote |
|---|---|
| Acetaminophen | N-acetylcysteine (NAC) |
| Benzodiazepines (lorazepam, clonazepam, diazepam, etc.) | Flumazenil |
| Beta blockers | Glucagon |
| Calcium channel blockers (nifedipine, diltiazem, verapamil, nicardipine, etc.) | Calcium chloride or gluconate |
| Carbon monoxide | Oxygen, hyperbaric oxygen |
| Digoxin | Fab (digoxin-specific) antibodies |
| Ethylene glycol | Ethanol |
| Heavy metals (iron, lead, arsenic, mercury, etc.) | Chelating agents |
| Methanol | Ethanol |
| Narcotics | Naloxone (Narcan) |
| Nitrites | Methylene blue |
| Organophosphates | Atropine: muscarinic antagonist Pralidoxime: activates cholinesterase |
| Oral hypoglycemics | Glucagon or glucose |
| Phenothiazine | Diphenhydramine or benztropine |
| Warfarin | Vitamin K |

Figure 39-2 *Antidotes and Treatments for Common Ingestions*

had a seizure, passed out, etc.?) Has the child ingested things previously? Are there any underlying medical conditions?

4. Perform the physical examination, looking for some of the physical findings that are particular to certain toxidromes.
5. Laboratory evaluations may be used to measure specific levels or look for toxicities such as hypoglycemia in ethanol ingestions and metabolic acidosis in many kinds of ingestions (Figure 39-3). X-rays may reveal the presence of radiopaque substances such as iodine, iron, lead, or extended-release medications.
6. Assessment of the data. Is the patient ill or likely to become ill from this ingestion? If the answer to this question is yes, a management plan is in order. What other diagnostic studies are necessary? What antidotes and supportive measures should be used? What should be monitored for changes?

## EVALUATION AND MANAGEMENT OF COMMON POISONINGS

If the patient is ill or likely to become ill from the ingestion, one should consult POISINDEX or another commonly used and frequently updated toxi-

**M**ethanol and ethanol
**U**remia
**D**iabetic or other ketoacidosis
**P**araldehyde or **p**henformin
**I**ron
**L**actic acidosis
**E**thylene glycol
**S**alicylates
**I**soniazid
**T**oluene

*Figure 39-3* **Etiologies of High Anion Gap Acidosis (MUDPILES IT)**

cology reference or a toxicologist either locally or at the Rocky Mountain
Poison Control Center (1-800-222-1222). What are the common effects of this
substance? This will help the clinician determine what further evaluation
and monitoring need to be done (see Table 39-3).

## BIBLIOGRAPHY

Crain EF, Gershel JC. *Clinical Manual of Emergency Pediatrics*, 4th ed. New York:
    McGraw-Hill, 2003.
Fleisher GR, Ludwig S, eds. *Textbook of Pediatric Emergency Medicine*, 4th ed.
    Philadelphia: Lippincott Williams & Wilkins, 2000.

NOTE: Page numbers followed by *f* indicate figures; those followed by *t* indicate tables.

CPSIA information can be obtained at www.ICGtesting.com
Printed in the USA
LVOW07s1420290815

451888LV00010B/136/P